MW00468838

Nursing at Home

Nursing at Home

A Practical Guide to the Care of the Sick
and the Invalid in the Home
Plus Self-Help Instructions for the Patient

By Page Parker
and Lois N. Dietz, R.N., M.P.H.

Illustrations by G. P. Parker

With special thanks to Gloria Zellmer, Ph.D., R.D., for
reviewing the material on nutrition.

CROWN PUBLISHERS, INC., NEW YORK

Inquiries should be addressed to Crown Publishers, Inc., One Park Avenue, New York, N.Y. 10016
Printed in the United States of America
Published simultaneously in Canada by
General Publishing Company Limited

Library of Congress Cataloging in Publication Data

Parker, Page, 1913–
Nursing at home.

Includes index.
1. Home nursing. 2. Care of the sick.
I. Dietz, Lois N., joint author. II. Title.
[DNLM: 1. Home nursing. WY200 P242n]
RT61.P33 1979 649.8 79-11087
ISBN 0-517-52836-3

Contents

Preface vii
Acknowledgments viii

Part One: You—the Nurse

1 Just You Two Together 3
2 Be Yourself 4
3 Home Not the Hospital 6
4 You and the Doctor 8
5 When to Call the Doctor 11
6 When the Doctor Visits 15
7 The Visiting Nurse Program 18
8 Sickroom Equipment You'll Need 20
9 The Supplies You'll Need 55
10 The Medicinals Your Patient Needs 59
11 Germs, Viruses, and Bacteria 62
12 If It's Catching 66
13 Making the Bed 70
14 How to Move Your Patient Safely—for Both of You! 81
15 Bedsores and What to Do About Them 90
16 Handicap Aids 95
17 Foot Care 103
18 The Body/Back Rub 113
19 Temperature 117
20 Pulse 129
21 Respiration 132
22 Blood Pressure 135
23 Wash and Bath Times 142
24 The Sitz Bath 159
25 The Enema 161
26 Douche/Irrigation 170
27 Sleep, Rest, and Relaxation 180
28 Exercising Your Patient 189
29 Pain Pills 195

30 Basics of Nutrition 197
31 Choosing Foods for Diets 206
32 The General Diet 212
33 The Liquid Diets 219
34 The Naturally Soft or Light Diet 222
35 The Mechanically Soft Diet 225
36 The Bland or Ulcer Diet 227
37 The Low-Residue Diet 228
38 The High-Calorie Diet 231
39 Low-Calorie Diets 233
40 The High-Protein Diet 238
41 The Low-Fat Diet 242
42 The Low-Cholesterol Diet 245
43 Low-Sodium Diets 259
44 Calcium, Low-Gluten, Phosphorous, and Potassium Diets 267
45 Diabetic Diets 268
46 Tube-Feeding Diets 278
47 Feeding Your Patient 280
48 Meals Can Be Fun 286
49 Keeping Track of Food Intake and Waste Output 290
50 Suggestions for the Working Nurse 294
51 Planning the Care of Your Patient 296
52 Visitors 304

Part Two: You—the Patient

53 So You're Going Home 311
54 So You're Home Now 312
55 On Suffering in Silence 315
56 Smile—It Could Be Worse 319
57 Give Your Nurse a Hand 320
58 Mealtime 322
59 Use Those Muscles! 325
60 Join the Family! 327
Glossary 331
General Index 333
Foods and Feeding Your Patient Index 341

Preface

Nursing at Home is not a text dealing with all the duties, chores, and responsibilities of the registered (or "trained") nurse or of the licensed vocational (or "practical") nurse on their daily rounds. Earning either of these degrees requires years of formal study at qualified schools and colleges, and supervised training in a hospital.

In an easy-to-read way, *Nursing at Home* covers the more or less routine work you must do to provide satisfactory nursing care for a patient at home. The work is not always easy, nor is it always difficult, nor will you find all parts of it pleasant. However, if you are willing and able to do it, you can give your patient excellent nursing care well seasoned with that priceless ingredient: TLC—Tender Loving Care.

Acknowledgments

With special thanks for their outstanding assistance in compiling illustrations for this book:

Ms. Paulette A. Leu
Abbey Medical
Los Angeles, California

Mr. Art Wyatt
Abbey Medical
Stockton, California

Mr. John Turner
Abbey Medical
Modesto, California

Illustration Credits

8-1 Vollrath, Sheboygan, Wisconsin 53081

8-2 Smith & Davis Manufacturing Co., St. Louis, Missouri 63110

8-3, see 8-2

8-4a Norwood, Janesville, Wisconsin 53545

8-4b Bio Clinic Co., Burbank, California 91502

8-5a Maddak, Inc., Pequannock, New Jersey 07440

8-5b Help Yourself Aids, Brookfield, Illinois 60513

8-6a, see 8-5a

8-7a Guardian Products Company, Inc., N. Hollywood, California 91605

8-7b J. T. Posey Company, Arcadia, California 91006

8-8a, b, see 8-1

8-9 Lumex Inc., Bay Shore, New York 11706

8-10 Wal-Jan Surgical Products, Inc., East Rockaway, New York 11518

8-11, see 8-9

8-12 Invacare Corporation, Elyria, Ohio 44036

8-13a Mah-Zell Precision Products Co., Inc., Brooklyn, New York 11238

8-13b, see 8-7a

8-13c ACTIVEaid, Inc., Redwood Falls, Minnesota 56283

8-14, see 8-9

8-15a, see 8-9

8-15b, see 8-12

8-16a Cove-Craft Industries Incorporated, Lakeport, New Hampshire 03246

8-16b, see 8-9

8-17a, see 8-4b

8-17b, see 8-7a

8-18 Authors

8-19, see 8-1

8-20, see 8-12

8-21a, see 8-9

8-21b Edco/Pasco, Passaic, New Jersey 07055

8-22, see 8-21b

8-23a, see 8-12

8-23b, see 8-9

8-24, see 8-1

8-25a, see 8-7a

8-25b, see 8-9

8-25c, d (patented), see 8-21b

8-26 Authors

8-27 Authors

8-28a, see 8-12

8-28b, c Everest & Jennings, Los Angeles, California 90025

8-29, see 8-28b

8-30 Palmco Engineering Co., Santa Fe Springs, California 90670

8-31, see 8-12

13-1 Authors

13-2 Authors

13-3 Authors

13-4 Authors

13-5 Authors

13-6 Authors

13-7 adapted with permission from *Being a Nursing Aide*, Copyright 1969 by the Hospital Research and Educational Trust, 840 North Lake Shore Drive, Chicago, Illinois 60611

14-1 Authors

14-2 Authors

14-3 Ted Hoyer & Company, Inc., Oshkosh, Wisconsin 54903

14-4 Chec Medical Products, Morristown, New Jersey 07960

14-5, see 14-3

14-6, see 8-12

15-1 Santyl, Knoll Pharmaceutical Company, Whippany, New Jersey 07981

16-1, see 8-5a

16-2, see 8-5a

16-3, see 8-5a

16-4, see 8-5a

16-5 Agricultural Extension Service, North Carolina University at Raleigh, Raleigh, North Carolina 27607

16-6, see 16-5

16-7, see 8-5a

16-8a, see 8-5a

16-8b, see 16-5

16-9, see 16-5

17-1, see 8-7b

17-2 Authors

17-3, see 8-5a

17-4, see 8-7b

17-5, see 8-7b

17-6 Authors

17-7, see 8-7b

17-8 Authors

17-9 Authors

18-1, see 13-7

19-1 Authors

19-2, see 13-7

19-3 Marshall Electronics, Inc., Skokie, Illinois 60077

19-4, see 13-7

20-1 Authors

21-1 Authors

22-1 Authors

22-2, see 19-3

22-3, see 19-3

22-4 Medical Products Division, Sybron Corporation, Rochester, New York 14692

23-1, see 8-5a

23-2a, see 8-9

23-2b Medi, Inc., Holbrook, Massachusetts 02343

23-2c, d Frohock Stewart, Inc., Northboro, Massachusetts 01532

23-3a E. F. Brewer Company, Menomonee Falls, Wisconsin 53051

23-3b Bollen Products Company, Cleveland, Ohio 44117

23-3c, see 8-9

23-4, see 8-9

23-5, see 13-7

24-1a Bard Home Health Division, C. R. Bard, Inc., Murray Hill, New Jersey 07081

24-1b, see 8-5a

25-1a Pharmaseal, Glendale, California 91209

25-1b Rexall Drug Co., St. Louis, Missouri 63115

25-1c Davol Inc., Cranston, Rhode Island 02920

25-2, see 13-7

26-1a Abbott Laboratories, Consumer Products Division, North Chicago, Illinois 60064

26-1b Eastern Medical Plastics Inc., Hingham, Massachusetts 02043

26-2, see 13-7

Tables 19-1, 21-1, 23-1, 23-2 Taber's Cyclopedic Medical Dictionary, 13th Edition, Copyright 1977 by F. A. Davis Co., Philadelphia, Pennsylvania 19103

PART ONE

You—the Nurse

What you, as an inexperienced nurse, can do to give your patient good nursing care at home.

The materials that you and your patient may need.

What you should not attempt to do for/to your patient without the guidance of the doctor or your visiting nurse.

How to establish good working relations with your patient, the doctor, and your visiting nurse.

Visitors, and how to handle them.

1 Just You Two Together

Most patients who can be taken home will usually respond better there to nursing care than they will if kept in an acute hospital or a convalescent or long-term hospital. There are several reasons for this. Sick people are more comfortable in their own environment. At home they are not bound by rigid hospital routine. They can relax and be themselves. And, being nursed by a member of the immediate family, or by a close personal friend, usually gives sick people a sense of security.

How much nursing experience you have is of minor importance. If you and your patient are willing, you can learn what is necessary.

Generally more important than the technical work of nursing is the special relationship that may develop between a patient and a home nurse. If you are not a trained, experienced nurse, as a rule your patient will not expect you to be perfect in your work, especially at the start. In fact, home patients often like to take it upon themselves, in a good-natured way, to help train their home nurses; and if they fail to remember some nursing task, they enjoy sharing the blame. This usually makes your work easier; and as you get deeper into the work of nursing you will deeply appreciate every person, every action, every article that lightens your work. At the same time, you want to give your patient the best possible care. As a result, you and your patient become a mutual-aid team working together to restore your patient to good health as quickly as possible, or to maintain whatever level of health that can be achieved.

The relationship between nurse and patient is different from the usual ones between spouses, parents and children, siblings, and close friends. As nurse, you will begin to notice certain facial expressions, tones of voice, body movements, and the like of your patient that you paid no attention to before. As your experience increases and you come to know your patient better as a patient, these signs will help you know how your patient is doing. And as you become more attuned or sensitive to your patient's condition and changes in it, your patient senses it and places more confidence in you.

Deciding to do it is often one of the more difficult steps in nursing a patient at home. There is so much to do, so much to learn, and your nursing experience may have been little more than providing aspirin and an icebag for a headache. But as long as medicine, meals, and other necessary nursing services are given as scheduled, it makes little difference whether you are an experienced nurse or just now learning "on the job." The doctor gave all this careful consideration before agreeing that you could care for your patient at home.

Do not worry about your inexperience. Your visiting nurse or someone at the doctor's office or at the hospital will teach you the special services that you may have to give your patient. Most of them will be glad to teach you, because the better the nursing care that your patient gets, the more time they can devote to less fortunate sick people. Do not hesitate to ask questions and seek instructions from any or all of these experts until you are sure that you can provide the proper care necessary.

2 Be Yourself

One of the hardest and most important tasks in the daily care of your patient is to "be yourself." The stronger the affection between you and your patient, the harder it may be for you to be the same person you were before illness or injury struck your patient. Of course, in some cases you and your patient may know and admit that this is utterly impossible. However, as a rule sick people want things around them to be the same as before they became disabled. Changes tend to upset them.

Changes in the behavior of family and friends may lead sick people to believe that they are worse off than they have been told. Some home patients tend to become quite suspicious . . . "Why do you say that?" . . . "What's this medicine for?" . . . "What did the doctor really tell you?" The sicker they are, the deeper their suspicions. They also tend to be more suspicious of members of the family and close friends than of casual friends and acquaintances. Unfortunately, your patient's strongest suspicions are usually of you—simply because you are the closest person in regular contact, the person most responsible for providing the proper care.

No matter how groundless your patient's suspicions are, to your patient they are real and normal, particularly if you are not an experienced nurse. Your patient does not distrust you as a person, but does have a natural fear that you may be more willing than able, that you do not know what to do in an emergency, and that you will try to hide bad news, just as your patient would if your roles were reversed. Because of these real fears, home patients usually pay as close attention as they can to the people around them, look for changes in behavior, and put their own meaning to them. As a rule the older a patient is, and the greater the difference between the levels of former good health and present disability, the stronger the sick suspicions are, and the greater is the attention given to the behavior of nurse, family, and friends. However, by maintaining as open and honest a relationship as possible with your patient, you may prevent some such fears or keep them from becoming serious.

Your emotional behavior, such as general worry about your patient, fear that recovery is not normal, dread of the progress of a terminal illness, and belief that you are unable to care properly for your patient are things that your patient, almost as a third person looking on, seeks out as definite signs of poor and worsening health. In an effort to conceal these and other normal worries and fears from your patient, you may try to create an extremely quiet home because, as "everyone knows," sound can be one of the most annoying things in life.

Whether you maintain normal household noise will depend entirely on the condition of your patient. To some patients, noise is extremely upsetting; therefore gauge your noise level to the degree that is comfortable to the patient. Whispers, or even mildly subdued tones instead of normal voices, arouse a sick person's suspicions. So does overly hearty laughter, particularly when the joke told is not very humorous. Tiptoeing instead of normal steps . . . unusual and perhaps unnecessary hush-hushing of children . . . extreme caution in handling dishes, shutting doors and drawers, and using the refrigerator and stove . . . unusually high or low volume of the TV and radio, all such obvious changes frequently make a patient ask, silently or aloud, "Am I really that sick?"

Changes in furniture arrangements and lighting also may upset a patient, although in most cases this can be explained in a way that the patient will accept, see Chapter 3. Patients should always be included in making decisions about such changes in order to support their role and feeling of importance in the family.

Next to changes in sound as possible signs of illness to your patient is the matter of discussion. Not so much discussions of health and sickness, see below, as talking over the more or less routine matters of household expenses, birthday and anniversary celebrations, upbringing of children, and other normal family affairs. This, of course, depends on your relationship to the patient and on the patient's health and attitude toward such matters; be sure to get the doctor's advice first. In most cases these family affair discussions, made just as if there was no sickness in the home, bring you and your patient closer together and, often even in terminal cases, give the patient a feeling of still being an important part of the normal life. Even a little worry over family matters can help by switching a patient's thinking away from problems of sickness.

Do not suddenly drop family problems into your patient's lap, so to speak, unless the doctor advises it. Instead introduce problems gradually, with the attitude that you need help and that your patient is able and willing to help you. Just saying that you need help is not enough; your patient probably will not believe you. But by showing, through discussing and asking advice, that you want help, you probably can convince your patient that you do need help and want it from one person only, your patient. Such discussions are not always easy to start or to keep going, particularly if in the past you avoided them or ignored your patient's advice.

In general, keep your relationship with your patient as near normal as possible, depending on your patient's ability and desire to do so.

Of course, whether or not you should discuss problems with your patient and maintain the home as it was before sickness entered depends on the individual patient and the nature and stage of the disability. Get definite instructions from the doctor, see Chapter 4. Ask specific questions, such as whether everything should be absolutely hush-hush around the home or is a little normal, healthy noise allowable.

Now one more, important word about whispers and subdued tones. If you must discuss your patient without his or her knowing about it, do not whisper or mutter about it in the next room. These tones often carry for an amazing distance. Get so far away that you cannot be heard in normal voice, and then talk it over quietly!

3 Home Not the Hospital

Even if your patient is confined to home for only a few days, you may have to make some temporary changes in your way of living. Depending on your patient's condition and the doctor's orders, these changes may range from simply fixing a comfortable place for your patient to rest in the living or family room to renting a modern hospital bed.

As a rule, there is no need to try to turn your home into a miniature hospital. Patients ill enough to actually require hospital care are, in most cases, kept in a hospital. This usually is because the patient needs surgical, medical, or therapeutic care requiring specialized equipment and highly skilled technicians available on short notice. As a rule, patients are sent home as soon as the doctor is confident that the normal home environment is appropriate for them. Also, most sick people are more comfortable and content at home than in the strange and sometimes frightening confines and routine of a hospital.

The changes you may have to make in your home are for the good of your patient and you, the nurse. Most people tend to put the good of the patient first and their own a poor second. But for the good of you both, you must make your home convenient for yourself and your patient. If you do not develop practical schedules for caring for your patient, for supervising or doing the necessary housework and meal preparation, and for tending to your personal needs, you may find yourself on a 24-hour treadmill. You may be able to keep going for a while, but for only a short while—and then who will care for your patient? So for the sake of your patient, think of your own good. If there are other family members to share in giving care, you as "chief nurse" can have time for rest as needed.

NEW LIVING QUARTERS

The development of practical schedules for you and your patient may involve moving your patient into new "living quarters" and rearranging the furnishings for greater convenience. Except in the case of bedfast patients, these changes generally are simple and easy to make.

If you live in a two-story or larger house, move your patient to the main floor. Constant trips up and down stairs will wear you out physically and emotionally in a short time. Also, to spare you some trips, your patient may not call you when you are needed.

FAMILY LIVING

Depending on the condition and desires of your patient, you may wish to move her or him into the living room or the family room. This will allow your patient more active participation in family life. However, such a move usually should not be made without consulting all other members of the family; in most homes these rooms are the center of family life and are meant to be used and enjoyed by all. Explain, if necessary, why you believe the move should be made.

Nurse From your standpoint as nurse, the fewer steps you must take in attending to the needs and desires of your patient, the less tired and more alert you will be. Also, if you are nearby you probably will feel that you can safely entrust some duties to other members of the family, even the children. Finally, and this can be very important when nursing patients who need almost continual care, in the family or living room you will have a convenient place to rest when you can.

Patient From your patient's standpoint, being in or near the mainstream of family life can be extremely important, especially for those who have had major responsibility and held dominant parts in family activities. Sick people who are isolated in a bedroom, even one close by with its door open to family life, often get feelings of being avoided and even rejected by family and friends. "Visits" may only strengthen the feeling of being some sort of outcast simply because they emphasize the idea that the patient is seen only when it is convenient for someone to do so. People who have happy dispositions often, after sickness strikes, become sullen and depressed; as a rule, being isolated from family life does not improve matters.

Moving your patient into the family or living room can do much to prevent or cure patient boredom. These rooms usually look out onto a garden or street, giving the patient welcome changes of scenery and things to talk about. Most often the television set is in one of these rooms and to most people, despite what they may say, TV is a good source of news and entertainment. Also, most telephones are located in either the family or the living room; as a rule it costs less to have an extension cord than to have an extension phone installed.

Family From the family's standpoint, the more they and your patient are in contact with each other the less the emotional strain on them, even in the case of terminal illness. Spells of sickness occur in most families, and the less they are treated as being distasteful and demanding hush-hush, tiptoe treatment the better. Also, the more nursing tasks you entrust to members of the family, the greater will be their understanding of your patient's sickness, needs, and possible changes of disposition and behavior, plus the demands placed on you as the nurse.

MAKING YOUR PATIENT COMFORTABLE

If a disability will be long-term and your patient confined to bed for most of the time, you should consider getting a hospital bed and other specialized equipment that the doctor or your visiting nurse recommends. These items are designed and built for proper care and safe comfort of a patient, and for convenience in nursing. Descriptions of professional equipment and suitable homemade substitutes commonly used in caring for the sick, and where they may be obtained, are in Chapter 8.

If most of your patient's time, including regular sleeping hours, will be spent in the family or living room, move in the patient's bed and other necessary bedroom furnishings.

If your patient will spend only normal waking hours in the family or living room, as a rule a comfortable chair or cot, depending on the patient's condition, should be placed to provide a clear view of the garden or street. Set a lamp so that the patient can easily turn it on and off. A hospital-type adjustable tray (Chapter 8), or a TV tray that adjusts over a patient's lap, is a very useful convenience. A water carafe and glass always should be on a sturdy table within easy reach of a patient. When using wooden bedside tables or other general furniture, protect the top from medicine or liquid spills with a sheet of heavy cardboard, several layers of newspaper, or plastic or household aluminum foil.

IN GENERAL

Not all the foregoing suggestions as to how to make over your home to suit the needs of a patient may apply to your home or patient. Aside from an illness being contagious, there are many good reasons why a doctor may want your patient to be kept more or less isolated. However, even under these conditions, as a rule the more you can combine the efficiency of a well-run hospital with the warmth and comfort of a pleasant home and family life, the better it is for your patient, the family, and you.

4 You and the Doctor

One of the more difficult duties for the average inexperienced home nurse is that of being a dependable go-between for patient and doctor. Since the doctor cannot be in constant attendance on your patient, it is up to you to represent each one to the other. You must find out what course the doctor believes the illness will take and what should be done, and carry out his instructions. You have to be able to report accurately how your patient responds to prescribed treatment. You must be trustworthy to both doctor and patient, even though sometimes it may be necessary to reveal the confidences of one to the other. All in all, being a good go-between is not easy.

YOU MUST BE ACCURATE

For most inexperienced home nurses, the hardest part of being a reliable go-between is learning to be accurate. As accurate as possible, at all times. Accurate in carrying out the doctor's orders, accurate in reporting your patient's response and condition.

Unfortunately, most people stray from the exact facts when making a report and relaying orders. They do not realize it at the time, but the results can be just as bad as if it had been done deliberately. Differences between the real and the reported facts or relayed orders may seem too small to be important. But what seems unimportant to the average layperson may be of utmost importance to the doctor and to your patient's health. For example, persons with some heart conditions normally have rapid respiration (Chapter 21); a change in their rate of breathing from that described as normal by the doctor can be of vital importance. Also, the doctor may tell you not to give a certain medicine if your patient's pulse (Chapter 20) is below a certain beat; if you do not measure the pulse accurately and give medication when it is too low, your patient may suffer a bad reaction.

As well as following the doctor's orders strictly, be careful to describe your patient's condition with accurate words and terms. If, for example, your patient was slightly restless during the night, describe it as just that. Do not make it more serious by describing your patient as having "twisted and turned" all night long. Nor should you report that your patient "didn't seem any more restless than usual." Your exaggeration either way can give the doctor a false impression of your patient's condition. Moreover, when it becomes obvious that you do exaggerate (the doctor can soon tell if your reports do not fit your patient's condition), your usefulness to patient and doctor is greatly lessened.

CAN YOU DO IT?

As soon as it is agreed that you are to be the nurse, tell the doctor. You will have to work together and rely on each other; you should know something about one another. Tell exactly what nursing experience or training you have had—school personal hygiene classes, group first aid, "I helped mom take care of us kids," and so forth. If you have had no experience or training, admit it. The doctor may suggest some books to read, or recommend that you ask the local Visiting Nurse Service for special instruction and assistance.

Be sure to tell the doctor if you have a fear of, or aversion to, sick people. Many of us are afraid of catching any disease or sickness, even those that are not contagious. Many people dislike being near, let alone actually touching, sick people regardless of their injury or illness. To people who have these fears or aversions, the feeling usually is quite strong and, to them, entirely natural and normal. If this is your problem, a thorough understanding of the disability, its cause, treatment, and likely outcome may help you accept and do the nursing with less fear and aversion to your patient.

Even though you are willing to at least attempt to do the nursing, the doctor and you may finally agree that you should not do it. Or that you may do some of it, and let someone else do the tasks that are beyond your ability or willingness. Either way, contact your local Visiting Nurse Service or Public Health Department. Professional nurses from either of these organizations can interpret the doctor's orders, teach you the necessary care of your patient, and help you dispel your fears of handling ill persons.

GET ALL THE FACTS FROM THE DOCTOR

When the doctor and you have agreed on how much nursing you will do, get as complete a prognosis as possible—all the information about your patient's present condition, the treatments and medication to be given, the patient's probable reactions or responses to them, and the duration, course, and likely outcome of your patient's debility. Do not feel that you are unnecessarily taking or wasting the doctor's time. The better you understand your patient's case, the more accurately you will be able to follow the doctor's instructions and the more reliable your nursing care and reports will be.

WRITE IT!

A basic rule of good nursing is—*do not rely on your memory*. Instead, write it! Here is a wise rule to follow: if anything is important enough to ask the doctor or your visiting nurse about, it is important enough to put in writing. Realizing the importance of written instructions, today more and more doctors write detailed *do*'s and *don't*'s for the patient and the home nurse. These instructions usually are in nontechnical language and cover the general care and diet, and the giving of medicines, probable reactions to them, and possible side effects. When necessary, the doctor writes special instructions.

Always read instructions carefully. Do not skip- or speed-read or form your own conclusions or opinions as to what the doctor means. If anything seems ambiguous or contrary, or you simply do not understand it, write it and the doctor's answer or explanation. Date all written instructions and explanations, and keep them in a notebook or a loose-leaf binder.

In addition to getting instructions for the more or less routine care of your patient, ask the doctor what special signs you should look for as indications of your patient's condition. Make a written list of such items as temperature, pulse, respiration, skin color, bleeding, swelling, shortness of breath, vomiting, loss of appetite, anxiety, restlessness, and other health indicators mentioned in Chapter 5. Write what conditions of each should be considered as normal for your patient, and what to do when there are changes from the norms. Consult this data sheet regularly; it can help you decide when to make a special call to the doctor.

If you are required to take your patient's temperature, pulse, respiration, or blood pressure, record the readings neatly on appropriate charts as in Figs. 19–1, 20–1, 21–1, and 22–1. Charting the readings, except in the case of blood pressure, makes it simpler for the doctor to analyze your patient's condition and for you to observe changes in it.

ANOTHER *MUST* FOR YOU

Almost without exception, today's doctor keeps detailed records of patients from first to last office visits and hospital, house, and phone calls. These records cover everything, from the most complicated surgery to little cold-relief pills for people who cannot tolerate over-the-counter remedies. However, parts of office records sometimes are lost. And people change doctors, usually just by starting with another without naming the previous one. Also, more and more people today buy patent medicines for the so-called simple ailments such as the common cold, arthritic aches and pains, sour stomach, sinus headaches, and so forth. The result of lost records, changes of doctors, etc., is that a doctor may unknowingly prescribe medicines that, taken in conjunction with others, can produce disastrous results.

So for the sakes of your patient and the doctor and yourself, put this *must* at the top of your list. Give the doctor written details of every medicine that your patient is taking or might take. Question the doctor about your patient's continuing with any over-the-counter medicine taken previously. Copy the ingredients of patent medicines. For prescription medicines, copy the ingredients and instructions from the label, the prescription date, number, and name and address of the pharmacy that filled it. Finally, do not give any of these medicines to your patient without the doctor's written approval.

5 When to Call the Doctor

Whether to make a special call to the doctor often is a bewildering problem for the inexperienced nurse. Has my patient's condition really changed? Is this change normal under the circumstances? What happens if I don't call the doctor right now? Should I wait a little longer and see what happens? How serious is it? What should I do?

First of all, it is important for you to calm yourself and remain calm. The calmer you are, the less apt your patient is to worry, become excited, even get hysterical. Also, the calmer you are, the more accurately you can observe your patient's condition and prepare yourself to give the doctor a clear, complete, concise description of it.

No two patients are identical, and each development and aftermath of a sickness, disease, or injury has its special problems. There are, however, certain changes in a patient that, regardless of the debility, should be reported to the doctor at once.

ANXIETY

Anxiety, apprehension, and fear are emotions commonly experienced by sick people in any stage of a debility. The usual signs of any form of anxiety restlessness by a patient are . . . continual twitching and twisting around . . . turning and shifting about in bed or elsewhere . . . frequently wanting the amount of bed covering changed . . . often asking that the pillows be plumped up, smoothed, placed higher or lower . . . inability to get and stay comfortable for more than a few minutes . . . continual picking and pinching up the bedding or clothing . . . unusual sensations in the hands and feet, and strong urges to scratch or rub them painfully hard.

Other anxiety signs, which sometimes are misunderstood as "sick-person fussiness," are as important as physical restlessness. The patient feels that something is wrong, but cannot tell you what it is. It may be a fear or dread of something, a dull ache, or just an indescribable feeling of something happening internally. Nonphysical restlessness commonly is accompanied by demands for extra attention . . . spoken or unspoken pleas of "do not leave me" . . . an obvious fear of being left alone or deserted for even a short time.

Carefully observe all the emotional and physical signs of anxiety, apprehension, fear, and restlessness, and report them in detail to the doctor. Be sure to report all details, even though some may seem far more important than others; let the doctor decide.

BLEEDING

Although any bleeding can be a serious matter, it is important that you do not panic at the sight of blood and frighten your patient. There are two types of bleeding: internal and external. Unless you have been ordered not to, report any bleeding to the doctor at once. But before reporting, examine the blood or bleeding and your patient so that you can give clear, prompt answers to the doctor.

Internal bleeding is indicated chiefly by blood in a patient's urine, stool, and vomit; see Bowel Movements, Vomit, below. Before reporting, examine the urine, stool, or vomit to determine . . . the color of the blood . . . the amount . . . its condition, such as fluid or clotted . . . and the color, condition, and odor of the urine, stool, or vomit. Is your patient in greater pain than usual? Flushed or feverish? Pale or chilled? What temperature (see Chapter 19)?

External bleeding is blood that comes from the body through a wound or sore, or from a ruptured blood vessel. The wound, sore, or rupture may or may not be on the surface of the body; if not, it flows directly from the source to the outer surface, as in the case of a nosebleed, oral surgery, etc. Before reporting, examine your patient to determine if the bleeding is steady or in spurts, heavy or slight, bright red or dark red. In the case of a bandaged wound or sore you may have only the show of blood on the surface of the bandage to report . . . how large the stain is . . . its color . . . approximately when you first saw it. Also, is your patient in greater pain than before? Unusually restless? Flushed or feverish? Pale or chilled? What temperature?

> NOTE: Unless you are experienced in first aid, you should not as a rule take the more drastic methods, such as applying a tourniquet, to halt bleeding. A large bandage or wad of sterile cotton, or a freshly laundered towel, pressed firmly against the body at the point of bleeding should protect your patient satisfactorily until you are instructed what to do by the doctor or your visiting nurse.

BREATHING

Two common conditions to watch for are shortness of breath and difficulty in breathing. Panting is the usual sign of shortness of breath, while gasping and wheezing indicate difficulty in breathing; see Chapter 21.

If there is shortness of breath, how many respirations does your patient have per minute? Count them. Is it a regular rate? Do the respirations vary in depth?

With difficulty in breathing, is it primarily when inhaling (inspiration), or exhaling (expiration)? Is there an unusual noise when your patient inhales or exhales? Describe the sound to the doctor.

BOWEL MOVEMENTS

Is your patient unable to control bowel movements or urination? Is there blood in the stool or urine? What is the color and condition of the stool and urine? See Chapter 49.

CHILLS

A chill is an extreme feeling of cold accompanied by shivering or trembling, chattering of the teeth, and, usually, pallor or whitening of the skin. Chills often are followed by an abrupt rise in temperature to above normal (37° C/98.6° F). Does your patient complain of almost freezing? How severe is your patient's shivering, chattering of teeth? How high does the temperature rise? How much time elapses between spells of chills-and-fever? How long do they last?

CONSCIOUSNESS

A loss of consciousness for any period of time other than for normal sleep can be of utmost importance. How deep does it seem to be? Can you rouse your patient at all? Did it come on suddenly, or did your patient seem to drift into a state of unconsciousness? Has your patient's breathing changed? Is your patient lying still? Or twitching? Or thrashing about? See Chapter 23.

CONTROL OF LIMBS

Does your patient show a gradual or sudden loss of control of an arm or a leg? See also Numbness, below.

CONVULSIONS

Convulsions are sudden spasms of uncontrollable contractions and relaxations of the muscles. Although they often are severe and affect the entire body, sometimes only the eyelids flicker. The doctor probably will want you to report your patient's convulsions in considerable detail. When did they start? Where did they start? Or did the entire body seem to be seized by convulsions at the same time? How long did they last? Did your patient froth or foam at the mouth? Lose consciousness? Lose control of bladder and bowels? Was there a rise in temperature shortly before the convulsions started? During convulsions did your patient's breath have an abnormal odor? Did your patient suffer any injury, especially a blow on the head, during the convulsions?

DRAINAGE

Describe in detail an increased amount or any change in the appearance (color, density, odor) of the drainage from a wound or sore.

ERUPTIONS, RASH

If eruptions or rashes appear on your patient, be prepared to describe them in detail to the doctor. Are they blotchy? Does the rash feel rough to the touch? Does it blanche (whiten) when you press on it? Are there bumps? What size are they? Does there seem to be fluid in the bumps? Where is the eruption or rash? On the face, neck, arms, legs, trunk, crotch? Does your patient look flushed, as though sunburned? The doctor will want to know.

NUMBNESS

Does your patient speak of a numbness or a tingling in the extremities—foot, ankle, leg, thigh, hip, hand, wrist, forearm, arm, shoulder? Is the sensation steady, or does it come and go? See also Control of Limbs, above.

SPEECH

If your patient's speech is slurred or there is difficulty in getting words out, test the strength of the hands by having your patient squeeze both of your hands at the same time. It will be easy for you to tell if there is a marked difference in the strengths of your patient's hands. It is important that you describe the difference to the doctor.

SWALLOWING

A difficulty in swallowing by your patient can be important, provided it is not due to food being given in too large bites, too much food at a meal, or food that your patient dislikes.

SWELLING

Swelling of the feet, ankles, and legs in particular, and swelling of any other part of the body in general, should be reported in detail. When did it start? How extensive is it? If swelling started with the feet, how high has it gone? Above the ankles? To mid-calf? To the knees? Above the knees? Does the swelling feel hot, feverish? Is the skin hard? Do swollen areas feel mushy? When you press on a swollen area, do your fingers leave a depression in it for a few minutes?

TEMPERATURE

Temperature is one of the most important indicators of a patient's condition (see Chapter 19). Unless you have been directly ordered not to, you should report to the doctor immediately when your patient's temperature is 1 degree or more above normal (37° C/98.6° F), or when it is more than 2 or 3 degrees higher than it was yesterday. As an extra precaution, take your patient's temperature again before calling the doctor.

URINATION

See **Bowel Movements**, above.

VOMIT

Vomit is the contents of the stomach ejected through the mouth. If you are to report your patient's vomiting to the doctor, examine the vomit first for . . . color . . . amount . . . odor . . . traces of blood . . . condition of blood . . . and unusual conditions such as the vomit looking like coffee grounds. Also, is your patient in greater pain than before vomiting? Flushed or feverish? What temperature (see Chapter 19)? Unusually restless? Thirsty?

IN ADDITION

In addition to the above conditions, which normally should be reported to the doctor at once, there may be special conditions that the doctor will tell you to watch for. As a rule, you will be told in detail which conditions are part of the normal course of your patient's sickness, disease, injury, and recovery, and which conditions indicate complications.

6 When the Doctor Visits

Whether the doctor's visit with your patient is at the office, the hospital, or in the home, there are certain things you should do and certain information you should get from the doctor. Depending on the nature of the information and instructions and the overall condition of your patient, the doctor may wish to speak with you privately. There is always good reason for this, and you make it easier for your patient and the doctor by obeying a quiet hint or suggestion instead of waiting for an outright statement that the doctor wishes to speak with you away from the patient. However, if after a private meeting with the doctor you feel that the patient should be given part or all of the information given you, explain this to the doctor. Possibly some facts you give will change the doctor's reason for secrecy, and in the majority of cases the more a patient is told by the doctor the better the patient's emotional condition will be.

NO MORE HOUSE CALLS?

Many people who are not familiar with problems of the medical profession wonder why so few house calls, even for an emergency, are made by doctors today.

There are three basic reasons for this, all of them working to your patient's advantage.

First, by seeing your patient at the office or the hospital, the doctor has immediate access to the technicians, special laboratory tests, X-ray, treatments, and equipment that may be needed, and consultation with other doctors and specialists if necessary. For emergency treatment, especially outside regular office hours, a doctor usually insists on meeting a patient at the hospital primarily for the good of the patient—hospital personnel are experienced in handling emergencies of all types, including the families and friends of injured people.

Second, by seeing a patient at the office or hospital a doctor can see more patients—including yours—more often and spend more time with each. In the hour that it might take a doctor just to travel from the office to your home and back, possibly four or five patients could be treated.

The third, and a truly distressing reason for doctors not making house calls, especially after dark, is that so many of them have been decoyed to a place and assaulted for the narcotics they are thought to carry. Wisely, most doctors will not make a house call unless they recognize the voice of the person calling.

Of course, there are conditions under which a doctor expects to make house calls; but these are exceptions to the rule and should be regarded as such.

Another point to consider is that the trip to and from the doctor's office or hospital can be a welcome change for your patient. Especially for fairly small children or somewhat elderly persons, by going one way and returning home a different way you may make the visit to the doctor a rather pleasant outing instead of a dreaded trip.

PREPARING FOR DOCTOR VISITS

An accurate, written history (Chapter 4) of what has happened to your patient since the last doctor visit is the most important preparation you can make for the next visit. Do not rely on your memory. Jot down the changes in your patient as soon as possible after they occur; let the doctor judge their importance. The more information you present, the better the doctor can judge the progress of your patient and plan for the future.

As another important aid to your patient and the doctor, list all medicines being given and the amounts of each on hand at the previous doctor visit and now. Make a note to ask whether to throw away or keep medicines that may not be needed at the present time.

WHAT TO DO AT DOCTOR VISITS

Whether you take your patient to the doctor or the doctor makes a house call, one of the first points to decide is if you should stay in the room with doctor and patient.

If the patient is your spouse, as a rule the doctor expects you to stay during examinations to learn firsthand what progress is being made, the prognosis, and the treatment to be given. This prevents deliberate or unintentional "misunderstandings" of what the doctor really told the patient or nurse.

However, when making examinations in the hospital or at the office following certain kinds of surgery, when changing complicated dressings, or when giving some special treatments, the doctor may ask you to leave the room. This is done primarily to ease the nervous strain on you and your patient. But if it is a house call, the doctor may need your assistance.

If the patient is not your spouse, be guided by the doctor and your own good common sense as to whether or not you should be present while the doctor treats your patient. Here are some suggestions. If you are not a member of the patient's immediate family and the patient is not a fairly young child, as a rule you should excuse yourself by saying something such as "I'll be back in a few minutes," or "If you want me, just call"; the doctor or patient will ask you to stay if they want you. But regardless of family relationship, if your patient is a fairly young child who looks to you for care and comforting, as a rule you should stay unless the doctor asks you to leave.

As a safeguard against false accusations, doctors generally will not examine a person of the opposite sex unless a third party is in the room. A professional nurse usually is present at an office or hospital examination. In the case of a home visit, you should stay in the room unless the doctor asks you to leave.

If you are present during an examination, change of dressing, or any treatment that exposes the patient's body, and if you are not asked to assist by the doctor, try to keep from embarrassing the patient by your presence. Go to a far part of the room. Turn your back on patient and doctor. Look at a book or magazine, or out the window.

However, all the above *do*'s and *don't*'s are guidelines at best, not hard and fast rules. In many cases, a patient needs the assurance and strength that you can give by being close and perhaps holding a hand. And there are people who truly enjoy, and perhaps benefit from, showing their family and friends their surgical scars and the treatment necessary to make them well.

THE DOCTOR'S INSTRUCTIONS

Except in rare circumstances, all the doctor's instructions for medicines, diet, exercise, and so forth should be given to you and your patient together. The importance of this to both of you cannot be overemphasized. A patient who does not care for an exercise, or wants a forbidden goodie to eat, or dislikes a necessary food or medicine often tries to win an argument by saying, "The doctor didn't tell me that!" And a just as natural tendency in an inexperienced nurse, who has only the patient's word that the doctor stopped a phase of treatment that the patient dislikes, is to say, "The doctor didn't tell me that!" By giving full instructions to both of you together, the doctor eliminates genuine misunderstandings and keeps both patient and nurse from adding their own *do*'s and *don't*'s.

Again, be sure to *write* all the doctor's instructions. If there are points that you do not understand, ask for a satisfactory explanation—and write it down! Before the doctor visit ends, read aloud in front of your patient what you have written so that all three of you agree as to what the doctor's instructions are.

There may be times when the doctor believes that you should be given additional information or instructions away from your patient. Be sure you go far enough away so that the patient cannot hear your voices. Do not just go into the next room and whisper. Even if your patient does not hear the hisses of whispers, the sudden halt of footsteps and normal voices will reveal that you and the doctor are trying to keep something secret. Also, do not be gone with the doctor for more than a very few minutes, if possible, or again your patient may become suspicious. Since this kind of suspicion can be quite harmful to a patient, ask the doctor how to pass on the additional information to the patient if necessary. Remember, the seriousness of "bad news" often can be lessened by the way the news is told.

7 The Visiting Nurse Program

For many years, there have been Visiting Nurse Services throughout the United States of America and Great Britain, whose business is to provide skilled nursing services in the home by registered nurses on a part-time basis. Originally most of these services were sponsored by nonprofit corporations or foundations, and some still are. But when Medicare and Medicaid were established in the United States by the federal government and public funding was made available by them, many city, county, and state Public Health Departments entered the home healthcare field.

Visiting Nurse Services are usually listed under that name or under Home Health Agencies in telephone directories. If they are not listed in your locality, ask the doctor or the local public health department how to obtain home nursing care.

Visiting Nurse Services charge for their services. Charges vary, but generally are based on an hourly rate. Medicare and/or Medicaid may pay for skilled nursing care, physical therapy, and speech therapy when ordered by a doctor, for qualified patients. Some private insurance policies also will pay for skilled nursing care and other services in the home.

Originally visiting nurse programs were limited to the services normally performed by a registered nurse. But in order to serve the public better and to release the registered nurse from tasks that can be done just as well by someone with less formal technical training, most Visiting Nurse Services added the services of Home Health Aides and Homemakers. These services also may be paid for by Medicare and/or Medicaid.

In many cases, having the services of the visiting nurse, Home Health Aide, and/or the Homemaker can mean that a patient may be kept at home and not have to go to a nursing home or the hospital.

REGISTERED NURSES

The key to the success of Visiting Nurse Service programs is that with your and your patient's cooperation a registered nurse can attend many cases on a part-time basis. Hypodermic injections, the changing of complicated dressings, certain kinds of irrigations, and other treatments that should be given only by skilled persons are done by the visiting nurse. There may be many other services that your patient needs, such as bed baths, enemas, body rubs, and so forth that the visiting nurse will teach you to do safely for your patient and you. If you cannot perform these services, the visiting nurse will do them or assign a Home Health Aide (see below), if available, to your case.

If you have little nursing experience, ask your visiting nurse to teach you how to do the various tasks expected of you. Very likely a nurse at the hospital or the doctor's office showed you what to do, but for most inexperienced nurses one "showing" is not enough. The visiting nurse will take you step by step through the work until you can do it safely and confidently.

If you have experience in nursing, be sure to tell your visiting nurse. It will save time for both of you. But do not take offense if the nurse asks you to show your ability. The good of the patient is more important than your momentarily hurt feelings, and the nurse cannot accurately judge your skill from words alone. Also, because of their experience, most visiting nurses have developed so-called tricks of the trade that may save you much time and hard work.

As well as treating your patient directly, the visiting nurse will gladly discuss and help you with other matters, such as special diets, schedules, rest periods, exercise, how to cope with patient boredom, etc. The visiting nurse will also advise you of, and may even bring you, literature that will help you and your patient.

In most sicknesses that last for more than a week or so, the nonprofessional nurse and patient usually come to think of the visiting nurse as the doctor's personal representative or assistant, or even as another doctor. Do not expect the nurse to prescribe treatment or medicines, or change a doctor's instructions without direct authorization; but in all other respects treat the nurse as you would the doctor (Chapters 4, 5, 6), except, of course, for emergency aid and advice.

> NOTE: If in an emergency you cannot contact your patient's regular doctor or appointed substitute, then by all means get in touch with your visiting nurse. Visiting Nurse Services have 24-hour telephone service.

Visiting nurse service is provided on a part-time basis. The frequency and length of visits are determined only by your patient's needs. If necessary, two, three, or more visits a day will be made to a patient.

HOME HEALTH AIDE

For all practical purposes, Home Health Aides are assistants to visiting nurses, and should be treated as such. If for any reason you cannot perform a service for your patient, the visiting nurse will either do it or call in a Home Health Aide.

Home Health Aides usually have little, if any, formal training in nursing. As a rule, their work is limited to giving bed baths, enemas, body rubs, changing simple dressings, and other services that do not require extensive training. Be assured, however, that your visiting nurse knows the abilities and limitations of the Home Health Aide assigned your patient, and will provide special extra training and supervision as necessary.

HOMEMAKERS

Homemakers is an important part of a Visiting Nurse Service program, but these people are not trained in nor allowed to practice any phase of nursing. Homemakers is essentially a support service designed to do only the most urgent day-in day-out housework. However, in certain circumstances Homemakers service may be done on an essentially permanent basis. This is particularly true where both patient and nurse are elderly and the nurse cannot assume the total care of patient and household.

Although the duties of a Homemaker are not the same everywhere, they are in general limited to light housework and cleaning. Exactly what chores may and may not be done will be clearly defined by the supervisor at the beginning of the service. However, here are some fairly reasonable guidelines.

A Homemaker may wash the dishes but cannot be expected to scour the stove. A Homemaker usually will put clothing through a washing machine and dryer, but cannot be expected to do a wash by hand. A Homemaker may sweep the floor or even wet-mop it, but cannot be expected to scrub it on hands and knees. Heavy cleaning, such as washing windows and cleaning walls and woodwork, is not included in a Homemaker's duties.

IT IS IMPORTANT TO REMEMBER THAT—

Visiting nurses, Home Health Aides, and Homemakers are valuable helpers for you and your patient. They are not servants or "hired help," and never should be treated as such. Do not embarrass them by offering tips.

8 Sickroom Equipment You'll Need

An early worry for most inexperienced nurses is, "What sickroom equipment do we need and where do I get it?"

First of all, do not panic. You actually may need nothing more than your regular household furnishings . . . and even the more highly specialized sickroom needs usually are readily available . . . and often you have a choice of buying, renting, borrowing, or using low-cost substitutes.

Your sickroom needs will depend, of course, on the condition of your patient and the care and treatment required. But in most sicknesses except long-term or terminal, the bedding, dishes, and other usual household furnishings are satisfactory. However, it may be to everyone's advantage to increase the supply of some items; for example, have several extra sheets for your patient's bed to reduce the number of washings and to have one or more clean sets on hand for an emergency.

When special sickroom equipment is needed, as well as asking the doctor, discuss it with a nurse—hospital, office, or visiting—who is well aware of your patient's condition. Due to the nature of their work, and knowing of other people with problems similar to yours, experienced nurses usually know what sickroom equipment is really necessary . . . what can be done without . . . and money-saving substitutes.

WHERE AND HOW TO OBTAIN SICKROOM EQUIPMENT

Most communities of more than about 50,000 population have one or more hospital supply stores, usually listed in the telephone or city directory under Hospital Equipment & Supplies. As a rule, they stock all the common and many of the specialized items of sickroom and convalescent equipment, and can get others for you in a few days at most. In smaller communities, drugstores and hospitals usually have what you need or will get it for you in a short time.

Other good sources of sickroom equipment are the Visiting Nurse Service, Heart Association, American Cancer Society, Veterans of Foreign Wars, women's clubs, and service clubs. These and similar groups usually have fairly extensive "loan closets" of much specialized as well as commonplace sickroom equipment to be loaned free of charge. All you need do is go get it and return it. If you lose or damage anything you are, of course, expected to replace it or have it repaired satisfactorily.

In addition, there often are friends or relatives who no longer need equipment that your patient must have. It is amazing how often people buy something, such as crutches, and when finished with it hide it away in a closet.

Many commercial dealers in sickroom equipment sell or rent their wares. Choose the plan that is better for you, based on cost and the probable length of your patient's needs; rental equipment is thoroughly cleaned before you get it. After the need is gone, you may be able to sell equipment back to a dealer. Or you may prefer to donate it to a "loan closet," which will put it to good use.

Sickroom equipment is listed below in alphabetical order; cross-reference is given for items that may be known commonly by more than one name. Practical substitutes, with instructions for selecting or making them, are described where pertinent.

Most Important! The most important part of planning and getting sickroom equipment is, DO IT EARLY! Find out exactly what you will need—make every effort to have it ready for use before your patient comes home. Especially after major surgery, or severe illness or injury, your patient probably will be quite tired just from the trip home, and want only to rest quietly without the hustle and bustle of someone's getting the sickroom ready.

SICKROOM EQUIPMENT

The equipment listed in this chapter is primarily for general sickroom needs and patient care. Specialized equipment, such as for care of the feet, taking temperature, giving enemas, etc., are treated in the chapters dealing with those topics.

Most of the sickroom equipment described and shown in this book are examples of the types of articles, not necessarily the exact items, that your patient may need. A major reason for this is that designs are continually being changed in keeping with new medical treatments and to utilize new materials, especially in the field of plastics. Another reason for dealing with basic kinds instead of exact pieces of equipment is that often there are many similar but importantly different articles made for the same general purpose; for example, there are many designs of canes, each made to help a patient cope with a particular problem in walking. Your patient's doctor or therapist, or your visiting nurse, will advise you as to the particular design of item that is best for your patient, and what other designs or substitutes may be satisfactory as second or third choices.

As well as describing various pieces of sickroom equipment and practical substitutes for them, in many cases their recommended use and care is given. In other cases, this information is contained in the chapter or chapters dealing with its use; for example, the use of a draw sheet is given in Chapter 13, Making the Bed, and in Chapter 14, How to Move Your Patient Safely—for Both of You!

Note! Although manufacturers are listed in connection with many of the commercial articles depicted in this and other chapters of *Nursing at Home*, the authors thank them but do not endorse or recommend any brand of merchandise. Your patient's doctor or therapist, or your visiting nurse, are the people best qualified to advise you as to the particular equipment that is best suited to your patient's needs.

B

Bath Basin Several sizes, up to 20–23 cm./8–9 in. deep, of plastic basins in two basic shapes are made for bathing patients in bed (Chapter 23). Whether to get a basin with sloping sides, as in Fig. 8–1, or with fairly straight sides, as in Fig. 23–5, in most cases is a matter of personal choice. However, for giving a complete bed bath the bottom of the basin should be large enough to hold your patient's foot, flat. An ordinary oblong plastic dishpan is an excellent bath basin. A metal or enamel pan is satisfactory, but weighs more than a plastic one the same size and may be difficult to handle.

Patients at most modern hospitals receive, and are charged for, a disposable (plastic) bedside aid kit that usually contains a bath basin. It belongs to the patient and should be taken home.

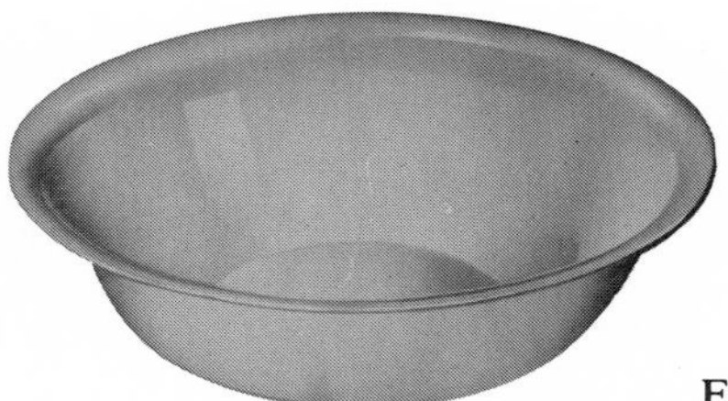

Fig. 8–1 *Commercial bath basin*

Bath Blanket You should have at least one bath blanket for covering your patient for modesty and for protection against chills while the bed is being made (Chapter 13) and while being bathed in bed (Chapter 23). Hospital bath blankets usually are twin-bed-size cotton flannel sheets. A large beach towel is an excellent substitute bath blanket.

Bed If your patient will be confined to bed for more than 2 weeks, get an electrically operated hospital bed if at all possible. It will save you and your patient more effort, and probably contribute more to your patient's well-being than any other sickroom equipment. A typical semielectric bed, as in Fig. 8–2, usually is designed so that:

The mattress can be set anywhere between its highest and lowest levels, Figs. 8–2*a, c, d,* to make it easier and safer for your patient to enter and leave the bed, and to make your work of tending your patient in bed simpler and less tiring.

The height of the bed and the many positions of the frame and mattress are easily controlled, Fig. 8–2*b*, by the patient if so desired. In a fully electric bed, all positions are electrically operated. In semielectric beds, some positions are manually controlled by cranks and adjustable bars.

Various parts of the bed (head, thigh, and leg and foot areas) may be elevated to desired degrees of slant separately or together, Figs. 8–2*e–j*, as required by your patient's condition or simply for reasons of comfort.

Manually operated hospital beds may or may not have all the position adjustments of electrical beds. Most adjustments are made with a crank, Fig. 8–3; some adjustments commonly are made by setting a swinging bar into a notch or slot.

If you do not have a hospital-type bed, you may need extra regular pillows or Bed Wedge Pillows to make your patient comfortable by building up parts of the bed to slant as in Figs. 8–2*e, g,* and *h*.

If the springs of your patient's bed are more than about 2 years old, it may be advisable to place a bedboard between the springs and mattress.

Guardrails Ask the doctor or your visiting nurse if bed guardrails, as in Fig. 8–2*k*, are needed for your patient, what type is best, and when they are to be used. The ends of standard guardrails slide up and down, and may be locked at various heights, in metal tubes that are secured to the bed. There are several designs of bed guardrails; all are easy to install and remove. Those for hospital-type beds usually are fastened to the metal side rails of the bed frame; some, however, fasten to the spring frame. For other beds, guardrails as in Fig. 8–2*k* usually are held in place by metal bars crossing the bed between mattress and spring at the head and foot. A temporary substitute for regular guardrails is to set one side of the bed against a wall, and to the other side tie backs of chairs that are high enough to keep the patient from rolling or falling out of bed.

Bed Padding If your patient is thin, elderly, or has very tender skin, and will be confined to bed for even a day or so, you should get special bed padding, Fig. 8–4, to prevent pressure ulcers or bedsores (Chapter 15). These sores develop over bony parts of the body, particularly the heels, lower back, shoulders, and elbows. Two

Fig. 8–2 *Semielectric hospital bed, bed guardrails*

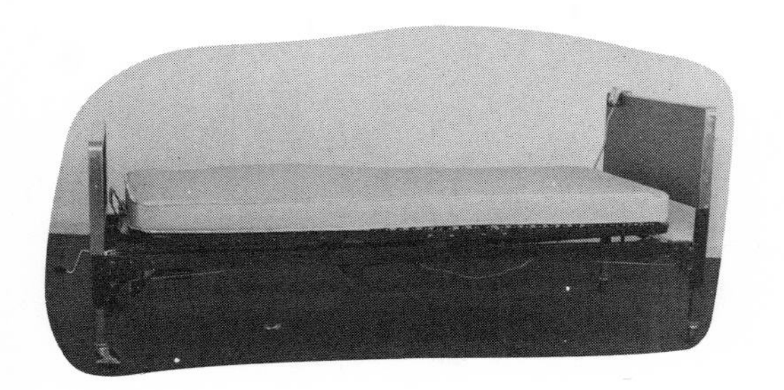

Fig. 8–2*a* *Mattress at medium level*

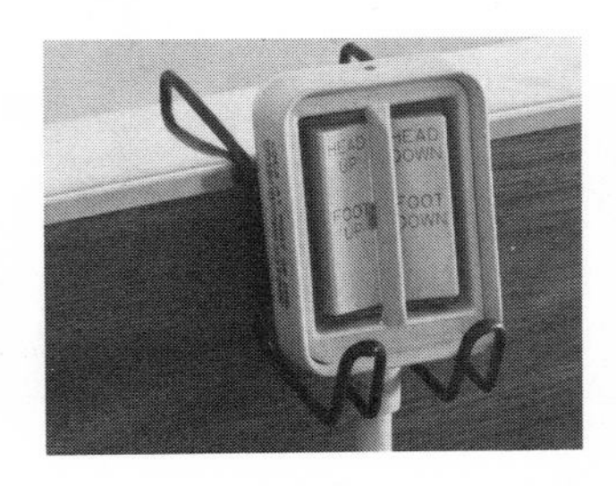

Fig. 8–2*b* *Electric control box*

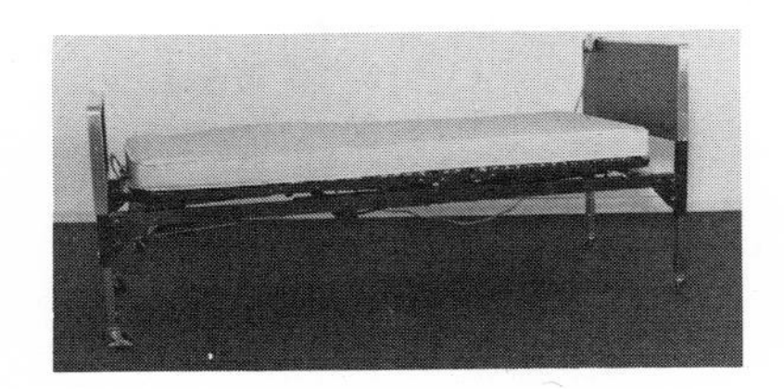

Fig. 8–2*c* *Mattress at highest level*

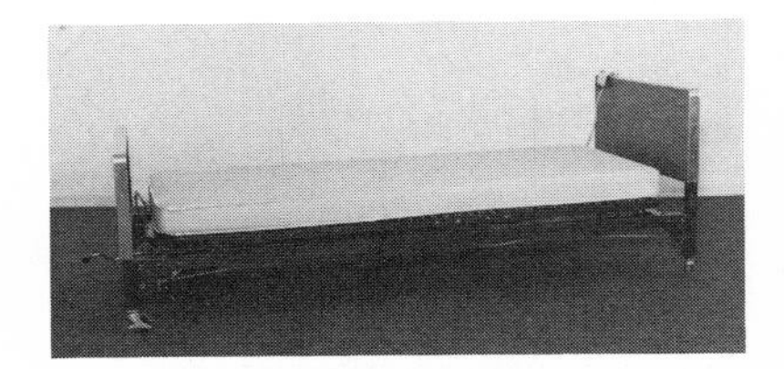

Fig. 8–2*d* *Mattress at lowest level*

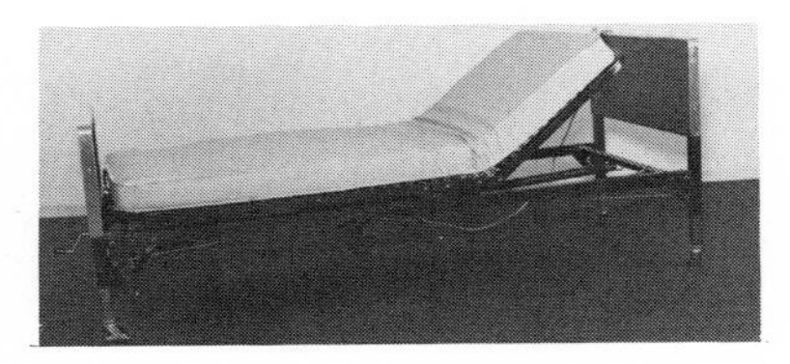

Fig. 8–2*e* *Head of bed partly elevated*

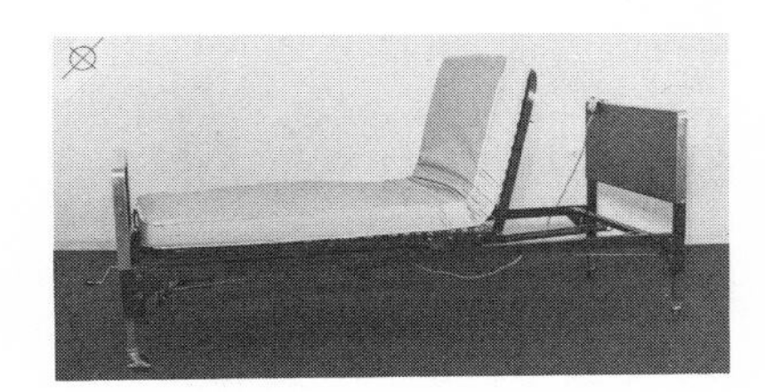

Fig. 8–2*f* *Head of bed fully elevated*

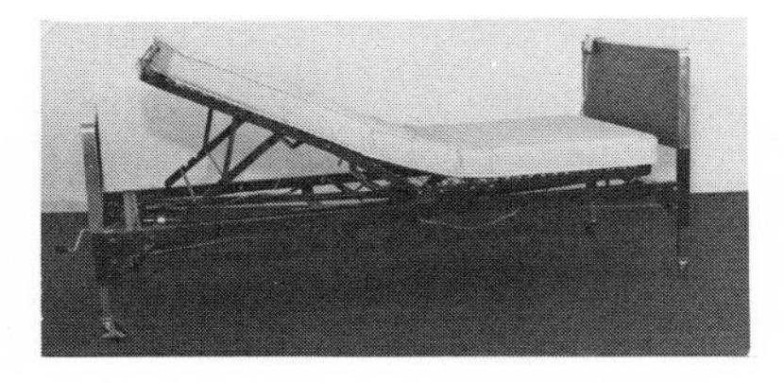

Fig. 8–2*g* *Leg and foot area elevated*

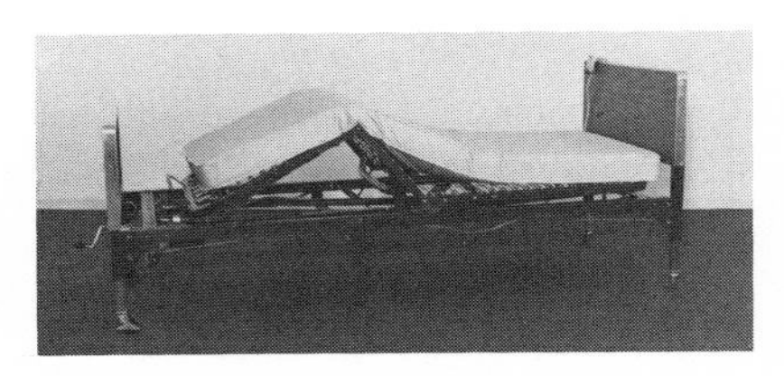

Fig. 8–2*h* *Thigh area elevated, head flat*

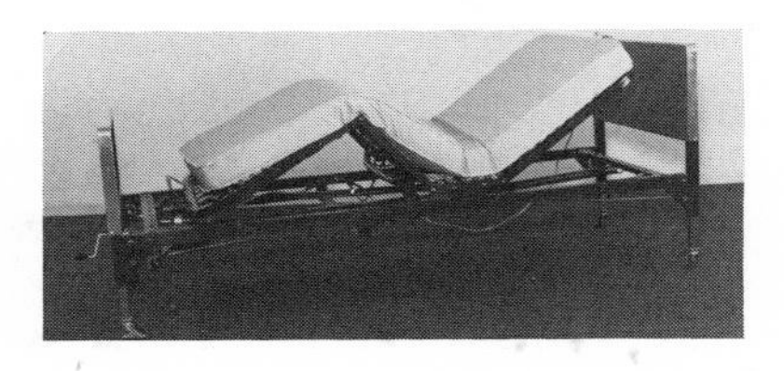

Fig. 8–2*i* *Thigh area and head of bed elevated*

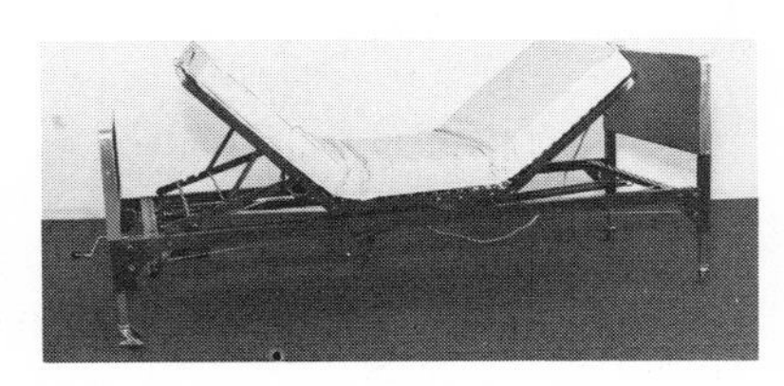

Fig. 8–2*j* *Leg and foot area and head of bed elevated*

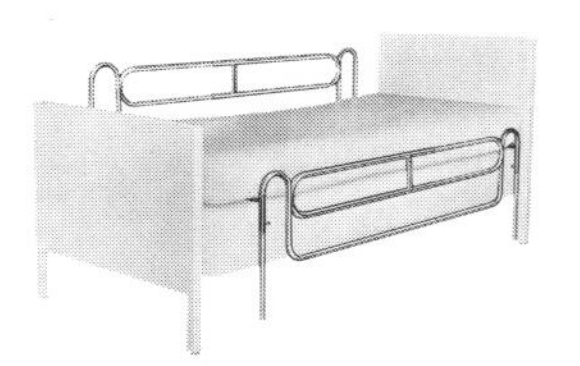

Fig. 8–2*k* *A bed guardrail*

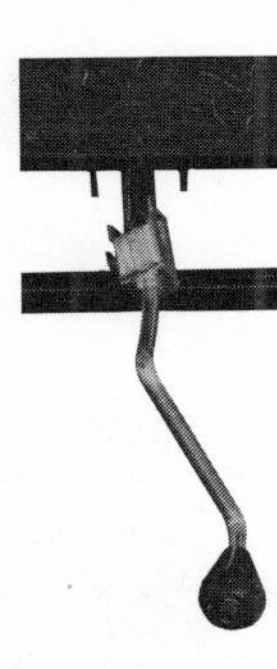

Fig. 8–3 *Crank adjustment for bed*

common types of bed padding are artificial sheepskin and Eggcrate® pads. Paddings usually are available in sheets ranging from about 61 x 76 to 76 x 152 cm./24 x 30 to 30 x 60 in. As a rule, you should have at least two, preferably three, sheepskin pads: one in use on the bed, one in the laundry, and the third ready for use in case the bedding unexpectedly must be changed. Two Eggcrate® pads usually are sufficient, although one may be enough if your patient will need it for only a week or so.

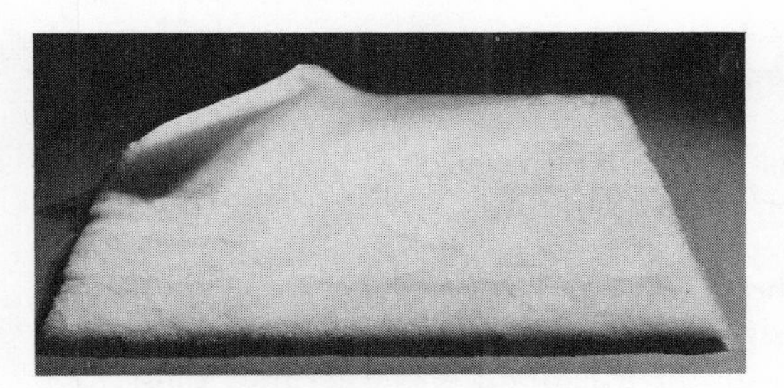

Fig. 8–4*a* *Artificial sheepskin padding*

Fig. 8–4*b* *Eggcrate® bed padding*

Sheepskin Bed Padding Artificial sheepskin padding, Fig. 8–4*a*, resembles a moderately thick rug. The patient lies directly on it, no sheet, and is supported by the furlike fibers. These mat down under body protuberances or bony parts, spreading the patient's weight over a wide enough area to prevent the small concentrations of weight that cause pressure ulcers or bedsores.

In use, first make the bed the usual way (Chapter 13) with mattress pad and bottom and draw sheets. Then set the sheepskin padding neatly in place, pile surface up; be sure the pad extends to beyond all the points of the bed that your patient's body will touch. If your patient uses a pillow, place the pad on top of it. After settling your patient on the pad, smooth away wrinkles or folds that may have developed.

Artificial or synthetic sheepskin, generally a polyester pile, does not require special laundering. Treat it the same as any other heavy, synthetic-fiber fabric; ample laundry instructions by the manufacturer usually come with it. Since the soiling of a sheepskin bed pad depends on a patient's bodily functions and condition, and external medication if any, ask your visiting nurse how often it should be changed.

Genuine sheepskin may be used instead of the artificial, but its shape usually makes it unsatisfactory except for fairly small children. It also costs more than the artificial, is more difficult to launder, and tends to become hard and stiff from laundering.

Eggcrate® Bed Padding The Eggcrate® plastic bed padding shown in Fig. 8–4*b* is chosen by many experienced nurses because it is easy to use, highly effective, and low in cost. It is excellent for management and treatment of bedsores. The deep, soft, wave-cut plastic foam is cool, durable, and also lightweight ... nontoxic and will not support bacterial growth ... easy to install and does not twist, wrinkle, or slide in use. Despite its sturdy qualities, Eggcrate® bed padding is inexpensive enough for practical single-patient use, for which it is recommended. If your patient has a pad at a hospital or other institution, ask to take it for use at home.

Washing Eggcrate® padding is not recommended; it is a costly, time-consuming process and decreases the quality of the plastic. Since the soiling of a pad usually is due to excessive moisture or medication on a patient penetrating the cover sheet, or to a patient's being incontinent, it may be advisable to get a protective "sleeve" to keep the uppermost pad clean and dry.

After making the bed the usual way (Chapter 13) with mattress pad and waterproof sheet, if any, set the Eggcrate® padding in place, smooth side down; as a rule it completely covers the top surface of a standard hospital bed mattress. One pad generally is enough for the prevention of bedsores; two are recommended for patients who have relatively simple bedsores; and three pads for those with serious multiple sores. Place each successive pad smooth side down on top of the preceding one. Cover the top pad with the usual bottom sheet, draw sheet, and incontinent pad, if any. But DO NOT tuck in the sheet too tightly, as it may then hammock the patient up out of the natural softness of the padding; instead, work the sheet just tight enough to the sides of the bed to smooth away any wrinkles. Rather than tucking the sheet under the mattress, many nurses just let it drape down over the sides.

Eggcrate® padding often is used in wheelchairs to guard against bedsores for patients who have little ability to move about. Spread the padding, smooth side down, over the seat, back, arm and leg rests, cover it loosely with a bed sheet, and assist your patient into the chair. If a patient must sit still for long periods of time but otherwise can move about, instead of a large sheet of padding an Eggcrate® seat cushion, Fig. 8–17*a*, may be used.

The polyfoam padding commonly used for upholstery and mattresses generally is not a satisfactory substitute for Eggcrate® padding. The continuous solid surface of the upholstery-type padding does not distribute body weight as well as the wave-cut cones do; and since the solid surface offers little ventilation it makes a much "hotter" surface.

Auxiliary Pads Instead of sheepskin or Eggcrate® padding, fairly thin water- or air-filled mattresses or auxiliary pads often are used to protect patients against bedsores. They are not, however, as flexible as bed padding in adapting to bed or patient. Of course, if they are deemed best for your patient, the doctor or your visiting nurse will advise you what kind of auxiliary pad to get and how to use it. In an emergency, a camper's tubular air mattress may be used.

Bed Rinse/Shampoo Tray A rinse/shampoo tray, Fig. 8–5, is almost essential for washing a patient's hair in bed (Chapter 23), giving ear irrigations (Chapter 26), or a wet scalp treatment. Both the rigid-type tray, Fig. 8–5*a*, and the soft, inflatable, *b*, have drain hoses for emptying liquids into a bucket or basin, and shut-off clamps to keep liquid in the tray. The air ring of the inflatable tray is easily blown up by mouth; a clamp seals the air in.

As a rule, prior to starting a shampoo or other treatment you should remove the bed pillows and get your patient into a comfortable supine position. However, if your patient must lie on a side instead of the back, you may need some pillows or slabs of fairly thick polyfoam plastic to hold the tray at a comfortable level. To protect the bedding, before starting a shampoo or other wet treatment place a small sheet of waterproof material, or eight or ten sheets of newspaper, and a medium-size, thick-pile or fluffy towel under the tray. Work the towel fairly snug around the neck niche of the rigid tray (against the air ring of an inflatable one) and your patient's neck and shoulders. Give the shampoo, irrigation, or other treatment the usual way.

There are many excellent dry shampoos. They do not require shampoo trays.

Fig. 8–5 *Bed Rinse/Shampoo Trays*

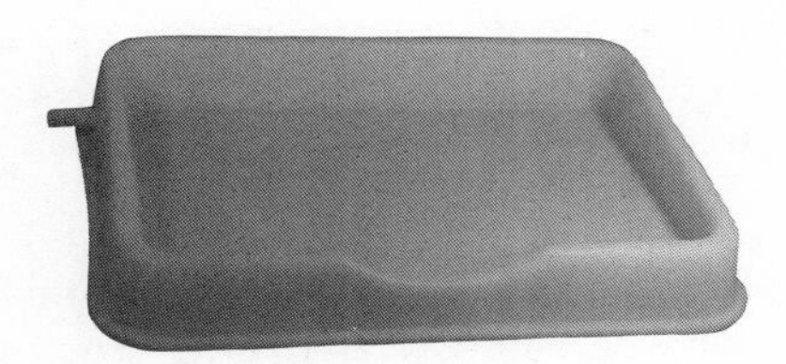

Fig. 8–5*a* *Rigid tray*

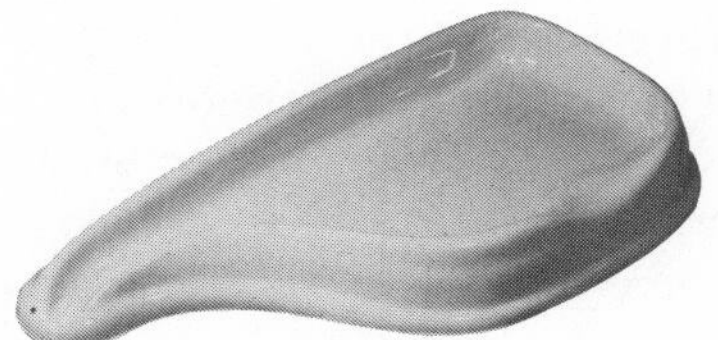

Fig. 8–5*b* *Inflatable tray*

Bed Sheets Depending on the length of time your patient will be confined to bed, you should have at least three sets of bed sheets—six flat sheets, or three flat and three fitted bottom sheets. When sheets must be changed daily, or even only three or four times a week, the more you have, the lower your laundry costs usually are. Also, the better prepared you are for an emergency.

In addition to the usual bottom and top bed sheets, draw and waterproof sheets may be needed. For a draw sheet, you may use a full or twin-size flat sheet folded in half the long way, Fig. 8–18.

Flat and Fitted Sheets Some nurses prefer flat to fitted sheets, particularly for the bottom sheet, if they are long enough and wide enough for ample tuck-in. Flat sheets are more versatile than the fitted types; they can be used for bottom, top, and draw sheets.

Fitted bottom sheets are easier than flat sheets to put on a mattress, but cannot be kept tight enough crosswise to prevent wrinkles that can annoy and even harm a patient. However, such wrinkling can be overcome by use of a draw sheet. On the other hand, fitted bottom sheets usually stay tight enough from top to bottom. Fitted bottom sheets are excellent for use with mattresses that have slick, plasticized tickings.

Fitted top sheets often cannot be loosened enough for good care of the feet (Chapter 17). If your patient will be confined to bed for more than 3 or 4 days, do not use fitted top sheets. They can induce the pressure that commonly causes bedsores on toes and heels, and they may help cause foot drop.

The "right" side or surface of a bed sheet is the same as the smooth side of the seams at the ends. The other surface of the seams is relatively rough and can irritate a bed patient. Always fold bedding so that the "right" side or surface will go on the bed properly:

Bottom Sheet. Right side up, to keep the patient's feet off the rough seam at the end of the bed if the sheet is too short or comes out from under the mattress.

Top Sheet. Right side down, so that when the top sheet is folded back near the head of the bed, the patient's arms and hands will rub on a smooth, not a rough, seam surface.

Changing Sheets Sheets should be changed daily for patients who are confined to bed for most of the time, or who perspire freely in bed. For other patients, sheets usually may be changed only once or twice a week. Soiled sheets should, of course, be changed as soon as possible. If your patient is bedfast and soiled sheets cannot be changed at once, cover the soiled area with a large enough bath or beach towel. In order to reduce laundering costs, it is fairly common practice when remaking a bed to use the old top sheet, if clean, for the new bottom sheet.

Electric Sheet Electric sheets are preferred by many people who want warmth without the weight of blankets. Most electric sheets have controls offering a wide range of heats. Electric sheets are placed on top of the top bed sheet. For safety, follow the manufacturer's instructions for the use, care, cleaning, and storage of an electric sheet.

> NOTE: Do not use an electric sheet for a child, or for an irrational, unconscious, or unreliable patient.

Bed Springs In most cases, the bed springs that your patient is accustomed to—hook-in link, open coil, box springs, etc.—will be satisfactory. Under certain conditions, your patient's doctor or physical therapist will recommend a bedboard.

Bed Wedge Pillow Polyfoam bed wedge pillows, as in Fig. 8–6, often are used in conventional beds to elevate and support parts of a patient's body much the same way as by a hospital bed, Fig. 8–2. Wedge pillows usually are encased by cotton slipcovers or tickings; change and launder these the same as you would bed sheets or pillow cases.

Regular pillows can be used with or instead of wedge pillows. This may not, however, be practical or comfortable for your patient. For example, you may need many pillows placed in careful arrangement to build a gentle elevation for your patient's back and shoulders—and if the pillows get out of place, the "elevation" may become quite uncomfortable.

Fig. 8–6 *Bed wedge pillows*

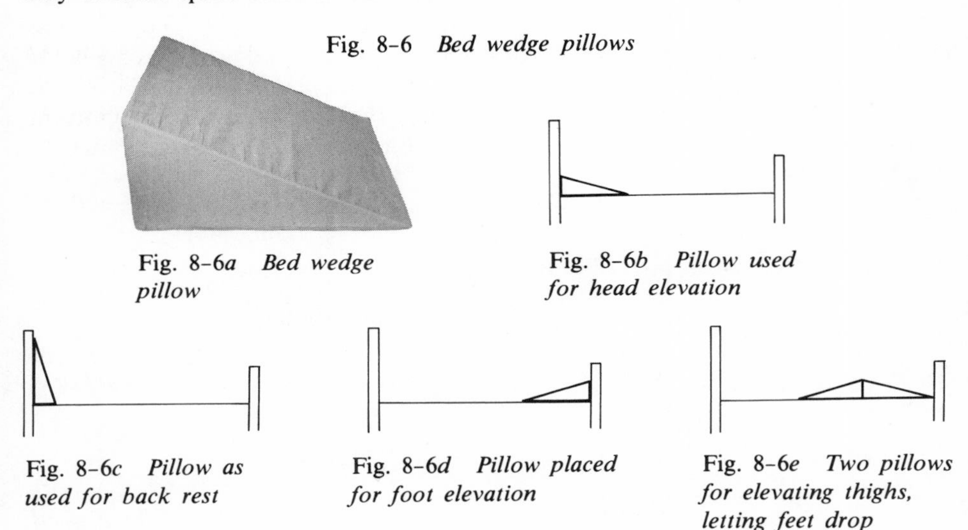

Fig. 8–6*a* *Bed wedge pillow*

Fig. 8–6*b* *Pillow used for head elevation*

Fig. 8–6*c* *Pillow as used for back rest*

Fig. 8–6*d* *Pillow placed for foot elevation*

Fig. 8–6*e* *Two pillows for elevating thighs, letting feet drop*

Bedboard A bedboard placed between the bed spring and mattress strengthens the springs, makes a polyfoam mattress firmer, prevents sagging of the mattress between the ends of a bed, and helps distribute body weight evenly for greater comfort. Bedboards often relieve backaches, and frequently are recommended for long-term invalids and for fracture patients.

Commercial one-piece bedboards often are about 1 cm./$^{5}/_{16}$-in. or thicker plywood lightly padded with cotton and encased by a ticking. As a rule, they are made in bed sizes:

Cot: 61 x 153 cm./24 x 60 in.
Cot: 61 x 153 cm./24 x 60 in.
Twin: 77 x 153 cm./36 x 60 in.
Three-quarter: 92 x 153 cm./36 x 60 in.
Double: 122 x 153 cm./48 x 60 in.

Homemade bedboards can be cut from 1.25 cm./½-in. hard plywood, Grade #2 or Sound or better. Sand smooth and paint or varnish all surfaces to keep the board from snagging the mattress or spring ticking.

Bedding Frames Often the weight or just the touch of even the lightest-weight bedding can be very uncomfortable or downright painful for a sick person. In this case a bedding frame, cover support, or cradle, Fig. 8–7, is a must. There are many good designs of bedding frames; most of them can be used singly to support the bedding in a fairly small area, as across a patient's feet, or in pairs to hold the bedding up off a large area of the body. Bedding frames are also used to improve air circulation in bed and lessen perspiration, especially of the feet.

The type of support in Fig. 8–7*a* easily adjusts to any desired height, fits all beds, and is held in place by the mattress. Commonly a single frame is used at the end of a bed to benefit the patient's feet. Two supports, placed on either side of a bed, act as a complete cradle to support the bedding for a fairly large area.

The support frame in Fig. 8–7*b* extends completely across a bed, clamps onto the mattress at any desired point, is not height adjustable, and usually is available only for standard hospital or twin-size beds. It is used mainly for foot benefit; it may be used with a foot support band, stretching from side to side, to help prevent foot drop (Chapter 17). Two or more of these frames may be used to make a bedding cradle for a large area of the bed.

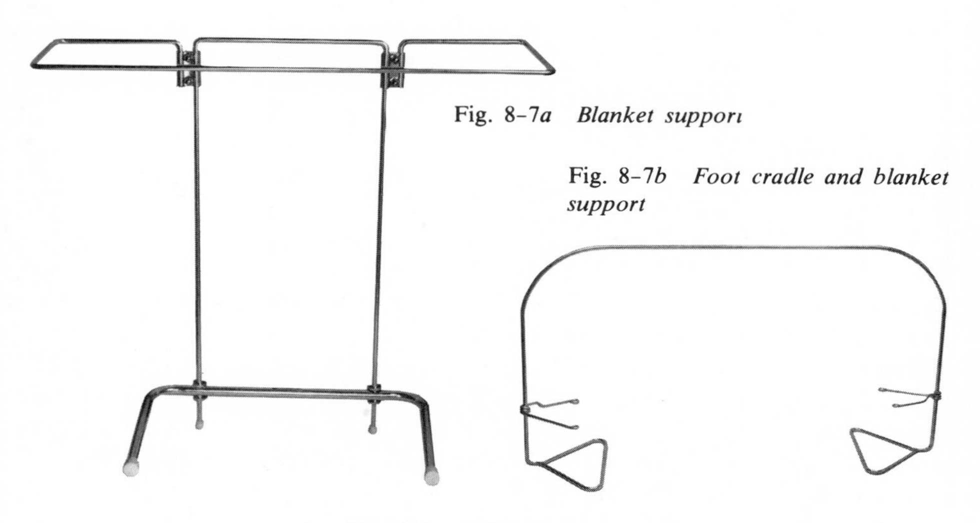

Fig. 8–7*a* *Blanket support*

Fig. 8–7*b* *Foot cradle and blanket support*

Fig. 8–7 *Bedding frames*

Homemade bedding frames or cradles may be cut from fairly heavy corrugated cardboard cartons, as in Figs. 8–7*c* and *d*. When using separate supports, as in *c*, it may be necessary to fasten the outer edges with adhesive tape to the bottom sheet to keep them upright.

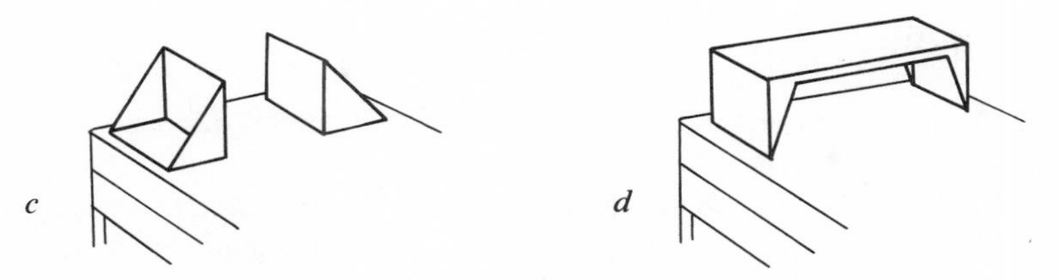

Fig. 8–7*c, d* *Homemade bedding supports*

Foot Protection Bedding pressing on a patient's toes can cause pressure ulcers or bedsores (Chapter 15) that are painful and slow to heal. As well as bedding frames, other devices are used to protect the feet (Chapter 17).

Bedlamp The kind of bedlamp to get depends on the patient's mobility. For bedfast patients who have very little ability to move about, a lamp that attaches to the headboard may be the most practical. For a patient who can move about freely in bed, a conventional floor or bridge lamp, or a lamp on a bedside table or nightstand, may be satisfactory. Whatever type is used, it should be one that your patient can turn on and off without assistance. If the light switch is in the socket, as often happens, it may be advisable to install a press-switch in the electric cord within easy reach of your patient.

Bedpans As with most other sickroom equipment, there is variety in bedpans and the one to select is that which is best suited to your patient. Bedpans usually are available in stainless steel, baked enamel, and plastic, the latter often being part of a bedside aid kit. An emergency bedpan can be made from newspapers. As to basic kinds or designs of bedpans:

Contour, Fig. 8–8*a*, the style of bedpan most commonly used, generally is available in adult and child sizes.

Fracture or "slipper" bedpans, Fig. 8–8*b*, are smaller and flatter than contour pans and usually are slid or "slipped" under a patient. Fracture pans are easier to use and more comfortable than the contour for immobilized patients, such as those in body casts, and patients who have unusual difficulty in getting on a bedpan.

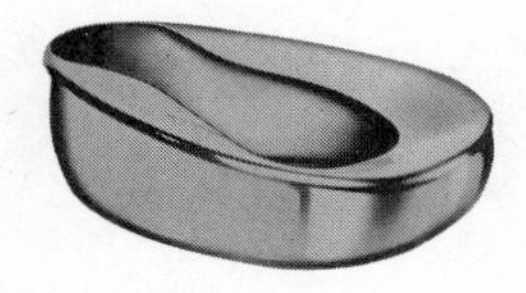

Fig. 8–8*a* *Stainless steel contour bedpan*

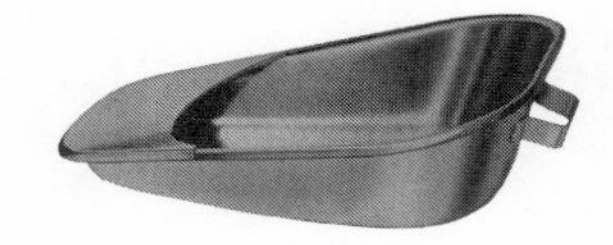

Fig. 8–8*b* *Stainless steel fracture bedpan*

Fig. 8–8 *Bedpans*

NOTE: Fracture bedpans also serve as female urinals.

Giving a bedpan may be somewhat difficult for you and your patient the first few times. Here are some ways to make it easier:

1. If using a stainless steel, enamel, or other metal bedpan, warm it with hot water before placing it, empty, under your patient.
2. To protect the bedding, place four or five sheets of fully opened newspaper under your patient extending downward from the waist. Then set the bedpan in place on the papers and draw the free end of them up between your patient's legs to act as a "splatter" board or shield. Draw them over the bedpan as a cover when carrying it to the bathroom; it helps confine odors to the bedpan.
3. To simplify emptying and cleaning a bedpan, just before giving it to your patient put some water in it, slosh it around to wet the bottom and sides, then empty it. This would, of course, be part of warming a metal bedpan, 1 above.
4. When your patient has finished with a bedpan, empty it into the toilet and rinse it thoroughly with *cold* water; use a regular toilet brush to loosen feces not readily rinsed out. A disinfectant or toilet bowl cleaner may then be used to eliminate disagreeable odors.

Emergency Bedpan In an emergency—it should not be done otherwise—you can make a newspaper bedpan, Figs. 8–8*c* and *d*, as follows:

1. *Center a piece of waterproof* sheeting at least 92 cm./26 in. square under the patient's buttocks.
2. *Arrange a pile* of twelve or more fully opened sheets of newspaper to form a large circle as in Fig. 8–8*c*.
3. *Crush and roll* the piled newspapers into "walls" about 5 cm./2 in. high all around, as in Fig. 8–8*d*, to help contain liquids or soft feces that your patient may excrete.
4. *Make a "splatter"* board or shield by folding one or two standard-size sheets of newspaper into a pad about 58 cm./32 in. long by 18 cm./7 in. wide.
5. *Place the newspaper* bedpan under the patient's buttocks. Work about

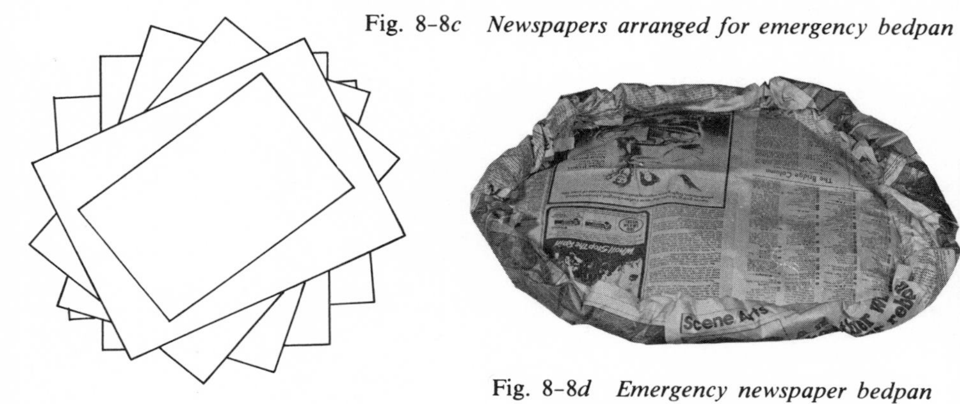

Fig. 8–8*c* *Newspapers arranged for emergency bedpan*

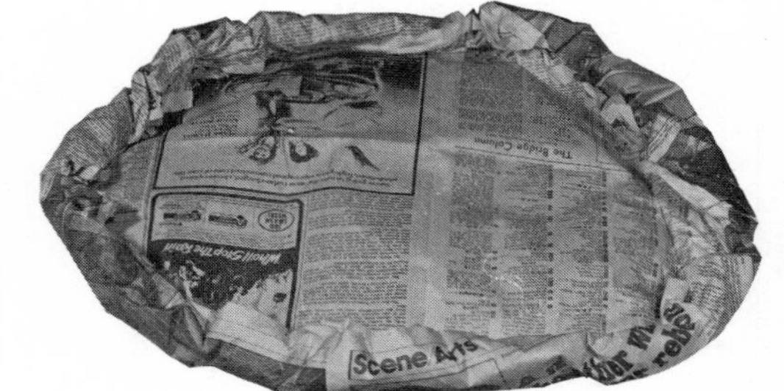

Fig. 8–8*d* *Emergency newspaper bedpan*

25 cm./10 in. of the newspaper splatter board under the bedpan between the patient's legs, and draw the free end up between the legs as far as necessary for the board to fit snugly but not tightly over the genital area.

6. *When your patient is off the bedpan*, gather up the sides of it to make a "bag." If the contents are soft or liquid, draw the waterproof sheeting up around the bedpan bag while removing it.

7. *If your patient cannot get off* the emergency bedpan after using it, slide it, the splatter board, and the waterproof sheeting downward until the upper end of the bedpan is just free of your patient. Then proceed as in 6 above.

Bedside Aid Kits To reduce the chance of passing infection from one patient to another, most modern hospitals provide, and charge for, plastic "one-patient use" bedside aid kits. The smallest is a simple three-piece kit consisting of a drinking tumbler, small tray, and a covered water pitcher or carafe. Larger kits, made up to fit a patient's needs, may include a bath basin, emesis or kidney basin, soap dish, bedpan, enema set, douche or irrigation set, and urinal. The kit belongs to the patient and should be taken home. If left at the hospital it will be destroyed.

Bedside Tables If your patient will be confined to bed for more than 4 or 5 days, as a rule you should get a hospital-type bedside table, Fig. 8–9. These tables are built to be moved about with little effort, yet are quite difficult to tip over. They easily adjust to fit over the bed at a convenient height for the patient. The tray can be tilted to comfortable angles for reading, writing letters, and so forth.

An over-the-lap bedtray or breakfast tray may be used if a hospital-type bedside table is not available.

In addition to the hospital bedside table, there should generally be a conventional bedside table or large nightstand for holding a lamp, books, water tumbler and carafe or pitcher, box of facial tissue, etc.

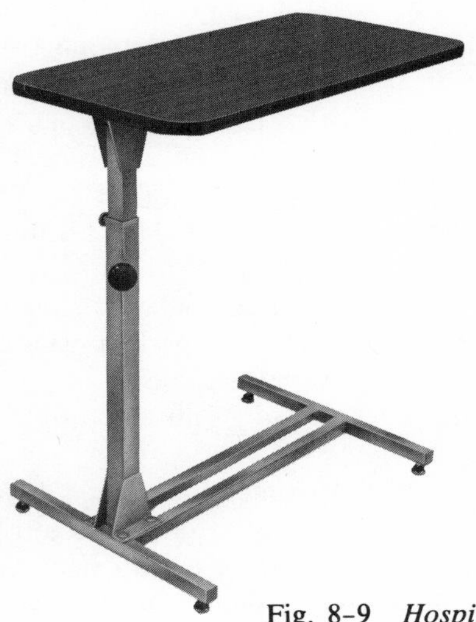

Fig. 8–9 *Hospital-type bedside table*

Bedspread A bedspread is not essential, but does offer worthwhile advantages to you and your patient. It protects a patient to some extent against drafts and sudden brief changes of temperature in a room, and shields blankets from minor soil. A bedspread can also bring a welcome change in the color of a room. If it is a color other than white, a spread may reduce annoying reflections and glare of lights.

Flat bed sheets, blanket covers, and lightweight washable bedspreads are commonly used. All usually are available in a variety of colors, and with floral and other designs.

Pile, brocaded, quilted, and other decorator bedspreads are not advisable for sickroom use. Most of them are too heavy for patient comfort, and too costly to risk being ruined by spilled food or medicine.

Bell A handbell or other device for summoning aid always should be within easy reach of a patient who cannot call or shout loudly enough to be heard by you any place in the home or just outside it. Instead of a bell, a police or other shrill whistle may be used—if your patient can blow it loudly enough.

If your patient probably will be bedfast for more than 2 weeks or so, it may be practical to install an electric call system. One can easily be made at home with light-duty extension cord, an entrance or bell button, an electric buzzer or bell, and suitable batteries or a transformer.

Under certain conditions, it may be best for your patient and you to install a simple intercom.

Blankets Unless patients are allergic to their regular blankets, as a rule it is not necessary to replace them with special blankets. If you are replacing blankets, keep these points in mind:

Artificial or synthetic fiber washable blankets are recommended for most patients because of their warmth, light weight, and almost zero allergy factor.

Cotton usually is satisfactory in warm and hot weather. But in cool and cold weather the number of cotton blankets needed to keep a patient warm may weigh too much for comfort. Do not confuse cotton bed blankets with bath blankets; they are not the same.

Electric blankets may be used if a patient is accustomed to them, and is mentally and physically able to manage the controls. However:

Never put an electric blanket on a child . . . on a paralyzed or an unconscious person . . . on an irrational or an unreliable patient.

Never use a connected or "plugged in" electric blanket as a bath blanket.

Weight. The less the blankets weigh, the more comfortable a patient usually is. Of course, there are people who insist on having heavy blankets.

Wool usually is satisfactory for patients not allergic to it. This also applies to blankets made of wool blended with other fibers.

Unless your patient's illness will be for a fairly short time, you should have at least two, preferably three, sets of blankets: one set on the bed, one in the laundry, and the third set in the bedding cupboard or closet ready for use in an emergency. A "set" of blankets may be one or more, whatever your patient wants on the bed.

Blenders. See Food Blenders.

Blood Pressure Cuff A blood pressure cuff is part of a medical instrument (Chapter 22), not of normal sickroom equipment.

C

Canes There are many types of canes, each made to meet a particular need. Get the kind that your patient's doctor or physical therapist prescribes; a different style could be highly impractical or completely inadequate.

Traditional Wooden Canes Special advantages of traditional wooden canes, as in Fig. 8–10, are that they are the most readily available of all and that they are made in a wide variety of woods, colors, and designs. Most of them can easily be cut short to fit a patient.

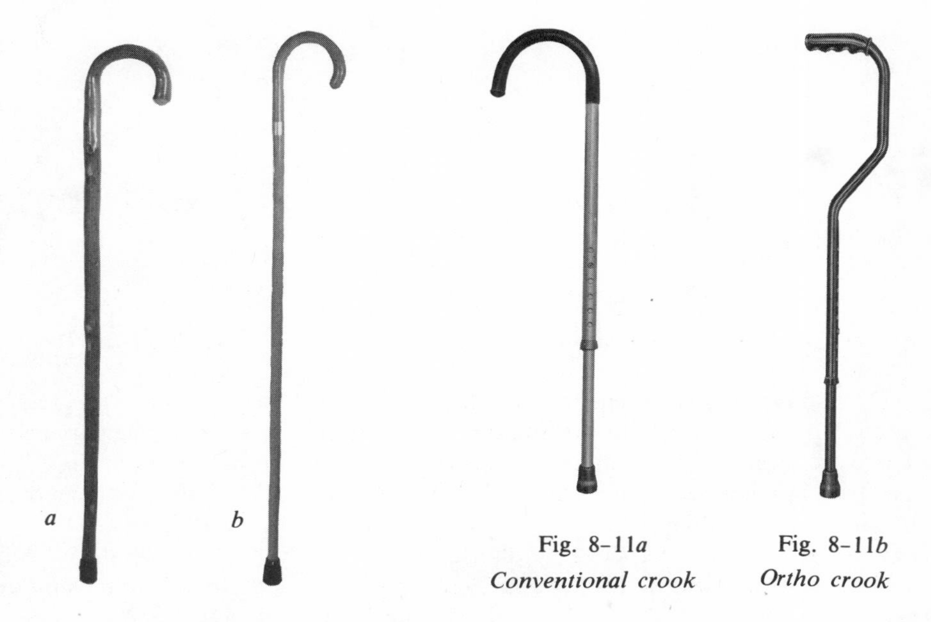

a *b*

Fig. 8–11*a* *Conventional crook*

Fig. 8–11*b* *Ortho crook*

Fig. 8–10*a, b* *Traditional wooden canes*

Fig. 8–11 *Modern unipod metal canes*

Modern Unipod Canes Modern metal unipod canes, as in Fig. 8–11, feature vinyl-coated crooks or handles, adjustable aluminum shafts or support tubes, and extra-large safety-tread tips. The conventional design, Fig. 8–11*a*, features a full hand grasp that reduces wrist fatigue. The Ortho design, Fig. 8–11*b*, places the patient's weight directly downward, in line with the shaft, and prevents off-center leverage. Both types of canes usually are available in regular and long sizes, and have approximately 23-cm./9-in. push-button adjustments to fit them to the patient.

Forearm Cane The forearm cane, Fig. 8–12, also known as Canadian cane, supports body weight on a patient's forearm when the hand cannot be used for weight bearing. The padded, formed-steel trough has a Velcro® fastener to secure it to the forearm. The hand grip adjusts forward and backward and rotates to either side to lock in a position comfortable for the patient. The aluminum support shaft has a push-button height adjustment.

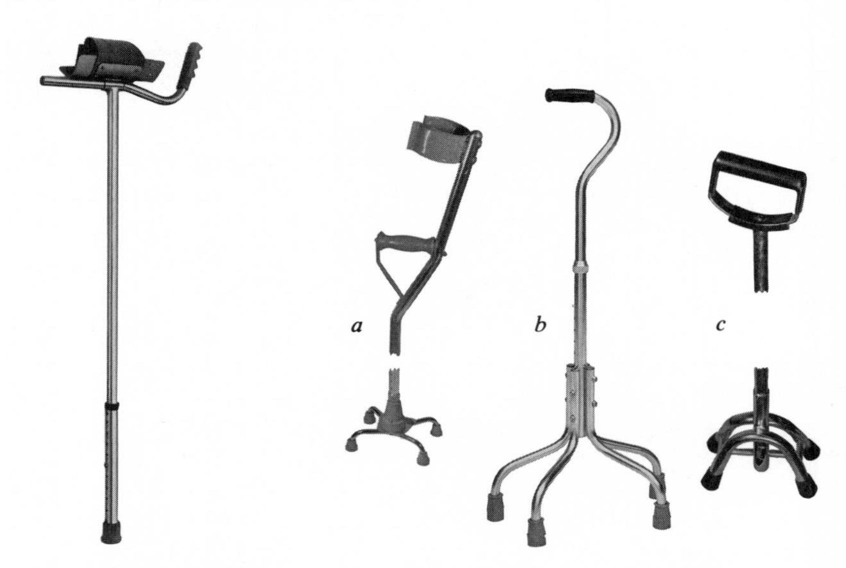

Fig. 8–12 *Forearm cane*

Fig. 8–13*a, b, c* *Quad canes*

Quad Canes Quad canes, Fig. 8–13, provide broad-base stability with greater safety, and help patients in making the transition from crutches to regular canes. There are several styles of quad cane bases in addition to those shown in Fig 8–13. The base in *b* is attached to the shaft by a rubber collar that allows shaft and base to move slightly in relation to each other, thus making walking easier for the patient; the collar also acts as a shock absorber. A variety of handles also is available, such as the Ortho-type in Fig. 8–13*a* . . . a forearm grip, *b* . . . and an active grip, *c*, with a 30-degree tilt adjustment to right and left. Quad canes have push-button and other locking height adjustments; some makes are available in child, adult, and large adult sizes.

Walkane The hemiwalker quad cane, Fig. 8–14, is lighter than a walker, stable than a cane. Both height and angle of the legs have push-button adjustments. The unit folds flat for storage and transportation. Walkanes usually are available in standard-height and extra-long sizes.

Tips As well as safety-tread tips, ice-gripper tips with tempered-steel spikes imbedded in steel plates are available for most canes and crutches. A special steel-reinforced rubber adapter tip may be needed.

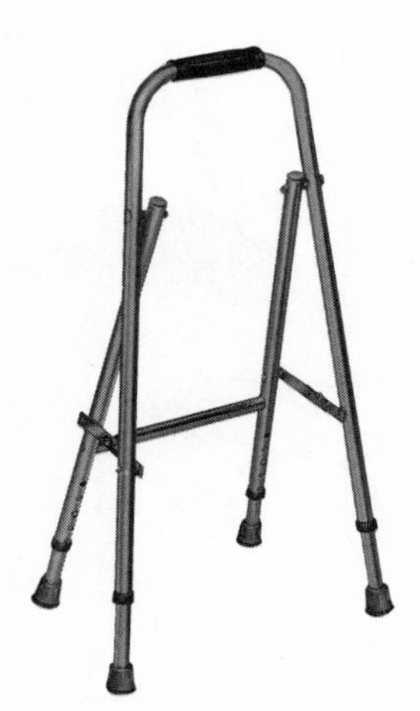

Fig. 8–14 *Walkane*

Carafe or Water Pitcher Unless the doctor has restricted it, a covered carafe or pitcher of clean drinking water should be convenient to the patient at all times. Fill with fresh water several times during the day, as well as the first thing in the morning and the last at night. Ice water may or may not be allowed; ask the doctor.

A one-liter/-quart-size carafe or pitcher usually is adequate; it may have come with your patient's bedside aid kit. A larger one, especially if glass or metal, may be too heavy for your patient to handle safely.

If the carafe or pitcher does not have a lid, press a piece of paper toweling down over the sides of the open top. Or cover it with a cloth napkin. Poke a corner of the napkin through the handle and flip the rest of it over the open top.

Clock A traditional or a digital clock or watch with a second hand or indicator is needed if you are to count your patient's pulse or respiration (Chapters 20, 21). Large sweep-second hands are recommended if using traditional clocks or watches.

If your patient wants a bedside clock, by all means provide it. Even though they are not going anywhere, bedfast patients often are more relaxed and content if they know what time it is.

Commode A commercial commode or portable toilet should be available for the patient who is allowed out of bed but cannot go or be taken to the bathroom. For best results in the use and care of a commode, follow the manufacturer's instructions to the smallest detail.

The multipurpose all-steel commode, Fig. 8–15*a*, can be used as a separate standing commode, or you can remove the Poly/Pro pail and use as a safety toilet frame. It has a conventional toilet seat and lid. The pail and cover are autoclavable, leakproof, and have no enclosures or attachments to trap soil. Legs have push-button height adjustments.

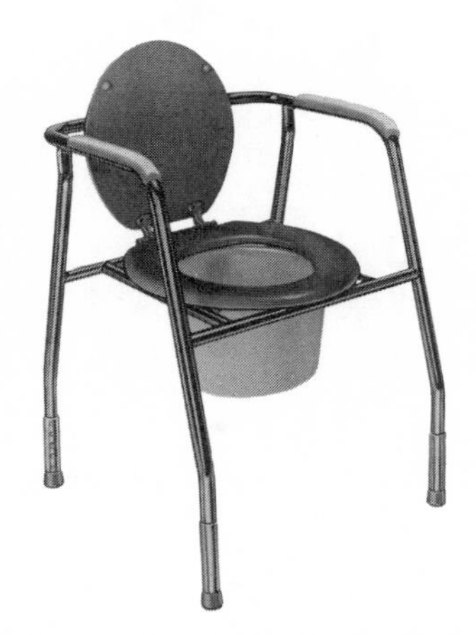

Fig. 8–15*a* *Multipurpose all-steel commode*

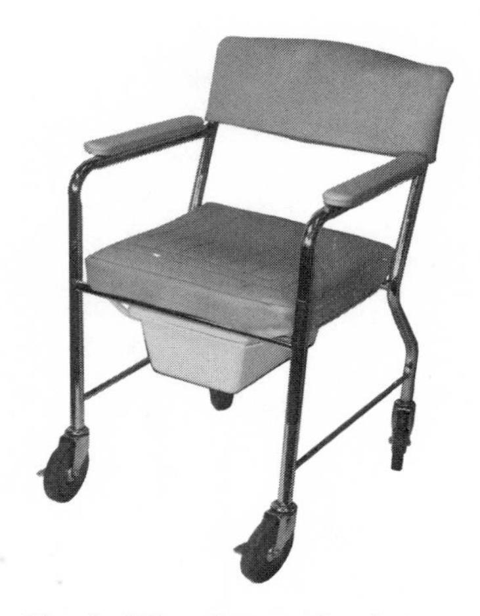

Fig. 8–15*b* *Commode chair*

The commode chair, Fig. 8–15*b*, has an upholstered seat that lifts to expose a comfortable toilet seat. Seat and lid are hinged, finished in white baked enamel with a plastic coating. The white polypropylene plastic receptacle is autoclavable, acid resistant, and stainproof. The arms swing out and lock behind the commode. Front casters lock to hold the unit securely in place.

Cover for Bathing Patient. See Bath Blanket.

Crutches There are several styles of crutches, each planned to fill a particular need and make walking easier for the user. Most modern crutches are made in three or more sizes—infant, child, youth, adult, and tall adult or extra-long—and have height adjustments of about 23 cm./9 in.

Traditional adjustable crutches, as in Fig. 8–16*a*, are available in wood and aluminum models. The aluminums weigh less than wooden crutches of the same size, and are less tiring when used for long periods of time.

The Ortho forearm or Canadian crutch, Fig. 8–16*b*, is designed to direct a patient's weight straight downward along the shaft, thus eliminating to a great extent the pressures that can cause shoulder separations. This type of crutch is commonly recommended for long-term use.

> NOTE: If your patient needs crutches for long-term or permanent use, get the type recommended by the doctor or therapist—but have your patient try each of the available designs for 2 weeks or longer before buying.

Tips. See under Canes.

Cushions Special seat cushions or pads often are needed for comfort, to help prevent bedsores, and to keep a patient from sliding out of a chair.

The Eggcrate® cushion or pad, Fig. 8–17*a*, puts an end to sliding out of a chair

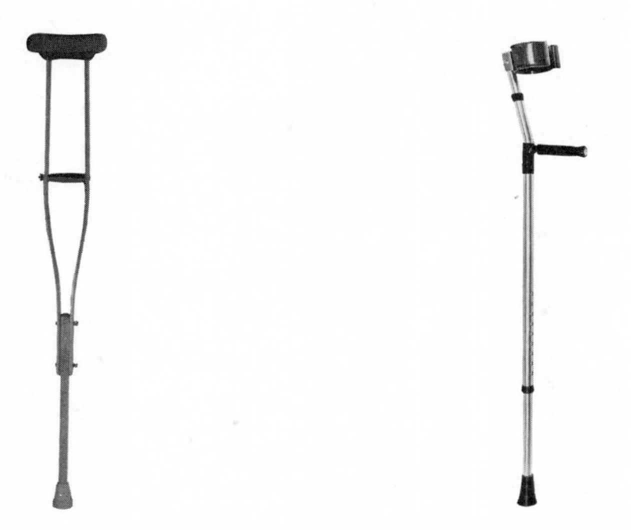

Fig. 8–16*a* *Traditional crutch*

Fig. 8–16*b* *Ortho forearm crutch*

by insuring vertical patient positioning with no effort and no discomfort. It also provides air circulation and helps prevent pressure ulcers or bedsores; see under Bed Padding.

Ring cushions, of which there are many kinds, have a "comfort well" to suspend and cradle sensitive lower areas of the body, especially the rectal. The latex foam ring cushion in Fig. 8–17*b* has a flat top contact area to eliminate pressure ridges and distribute body weight over a greater area for even, soft support. In use it is covered by a cotton twill casing that is easily removed for laundering. Latex cushions or pads usually are made in several sizes.

NOTE: Ring cushions often are used when tub bathing patients who have recently had rectal surgery, and for sitz baths (Chapters 23, 24). Do not use latex or other cushions that will be ruined by immersion in water.

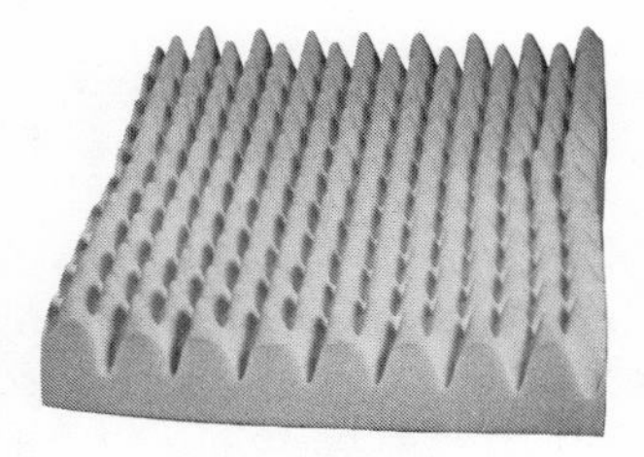

Fig. 8–17*a* *Eggcrate® cushion*

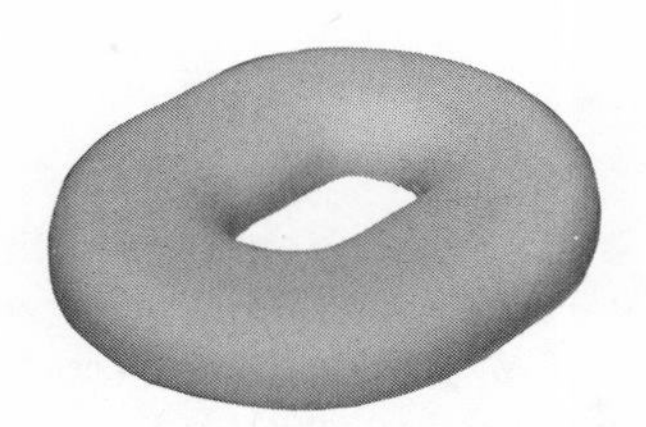

Fig. 8–17*b* *Ring cushion*

D

Draw Sheet A draw sheet is a special sheet, or a flat sheet folded in half lengthwise, Fig. 8–18, stretched across a bed from side to side to provide a smooth, wrinklefree surface for a patient to lie on . . . to protect the bottom sheet if there is no waterproof sheet . . . and to help you turn or move a weak or helpless patient (Chapter 14).

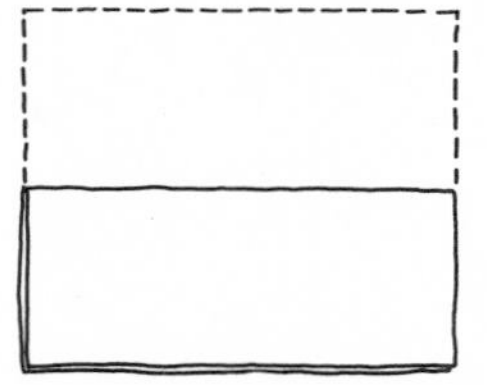

Fig. 8–18 *Sheet folded the long way*

> NOTE: The draw sheet completely covers a waterproof sheet, usually overlapping it by about 2.5 cm./1 in. toward the head and the foot of a bed. A draw sheet may be used without a waterproof sheet, but the waterproof always must be covered by a draw sheet.

Draw sheets manufactured for hospital-type and standard-size twin beds are available at most places dealing in hospital equipment. Flat sheets, double-bed size and larger, often are used for draw sheets at home. They are folded once the long way and placed across the bed with the fold about 30 cm./12 in. from the headboard. A draw sheet may extend toward the foot of a bed as far as its width permits, as long as it covers the waterproof sheet. Change and launder draw sheets as often as you do bottom sheets.

Drinking Glass, Tumbler, or Cup A clean glass or tumbler for drinking should be convenient to your patient at all times. Because of its handle, a cup may be better for some patients. In dusty areas, turn the tumbler, glass, or cup upside-down on a small plate or saucer to keep it clean. A plastic tumbler usually is part of a bedside aid kit.

Drinking Straw Plastic or paper drinking straws are needed by patients who cannot drink satisfactorily from a tumbler, glass, or cup. Flexible, disposable straws are generally the most practical. Nonflexible straws are not as easy to drink through as the flexible. A drinking straw is the easiest, most convenient way to drink for anyone who is lying down.

E

Emesis Basin The primary purpose of an emesis or kidney basin, Fig. 8–19, is to receive vomit from a bedfast patient. These basins, which are curved to fit around the side of a person's face when lying down, are available in stainless steel, enamelware, and plastic, and in a few sizes. A plastic emesis basin often is part of a bedside aid kit.

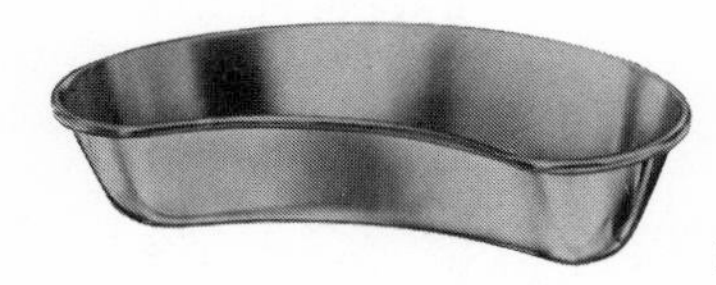

Fig. 8–19 *Emesis basin*

Patients who can sit up in bed may use any kind of large enough bowl or basin instead of an emesis basin.

Food Blender An electric food blender, grinder, or similar machine is almost essential to have if your patient is on a mechanically soft diet (Chapter 35). As well as for preparing a wide variety of special diet and regular foods, use a blender for making fruit and vegetable drinks, ice snow or "slush" novelties, milkshakes, and other extras.

Frames for Bedding. See Bedding Frames.

Frame for over Bed. See Trapeze Bar.

G

Gloves Rubber or plastic nursing gloves may or may not be needed or advisable for the care of your patient:

1. If you must touch or nearly touch (as when applying an ointment) an open wound or cut, sore, or deep rash, you should wear sterile gloves as a safeguard against infecting your patient.
2. If your patient's illness or infection can be transmitted by direct contact (Chapter 12), protect yourself by wearing gloves while touching your patient or dressings, clothing, bedding, and other articles that have been exposed to the disease or infection. Sterile gloves are advisable but not required.
3. Gloves are often worn by home nurses to reduce a patient's embarrassment at having to be touched, especially in the perineal area, while being bathed, given an enema, douche, or irrigation. Patient embarrassment tends to be greatest when patient and nurse are different sexes, and when the patient is many years older than the nurse. Clean, not necessarily sterile, gloves should be worn.

Gloves satisfactory for nursing care usually are available in small, medium, large, and extra-large sizes. Surgical gloves may be used, but generally are too costly to be practical for home nursing.

Rubber gloves are satisfactory if they need not be sterilized. They can be washed and rinsed with an adequate disinfectant at home, but sterilizing them to meet hospital standards seldom can be done.

Plastic gloves, both sterile and nonsterile, usually are available in sealed packages at hospital supply stores, drugstores, or pharmacies. They may be cleaned and reused a few times, the same way you clean rubber gloves, when sterile gloves are not required. When sterile gloves are required they should, for the protection of your patient and you, be destroyed immediately after use.

Gowns. For patients, see Hospital Gown. For nurse protection see Chapter 12.

H

Hospital Bed. See Bed.

Hospital Gown The traditional hospital patient gown or Nightingale, open down the back and seldom reaching below the knees, is highly practical. The open back makes it easy and quick to put on or take off a patient under almost all circumstances. The gown's short length eliminates unnecessary bulk bunching up under the bedding.

Satisfactory patient gowns can easily be made from a men's dress-type (not pullover) shirt. Since the front of the shirt will become the back of the gown, remove all buttons and frills or trim on the shirt front. Sew tie tapes on the shirt front, a pair up near the collar, the other pair about halfway toward the bottom of the shirt front; handy tape lengths are approximately 10 cm./4 in. Remove the shirt collar. Remake the top of the shirt into an opening to fit comfortably around your patient's throat and neck. Long sleeves may be left long, although gowns usually are more comfortable with sleeves reaching to just above the elbows. Use various colors of shirts to get away from the white that so often becomes tiresome.

I

Intercom Depending on your patient's condition, the dwelling, and your workload, it may be highly advisable to install an intercom or intercommunications system enabling you and your patient to call one another and talk back and forth. It also can be used to monitor or listen for sounds in your patient's room.

Intercom systems generally are sold by the larger radio stores and departments in a fairly wide range of prices, installations, voice quality, and operations. A system that is simple to install and use is the type that works on the standard household electric wiring system. The units transmit and receive. Use as many as you wish, no special equipment is needed; simply plug the units into the regular household electric outlets.

M

Mattress The bed mattress that your patient is accustomed to—air, innerspring, polyfoam or foam rubber, hair, feather, water, etc.—usually is satisfactory in time of sickness or injury. However, patients facing long-term confinement to bed, or who tend to develop pressure ulcers or bedsores (Chapter 15), need some type of bed padding. Under certain conditions a bedboard may be required.

Mattresses seldom need to be replaced unless they wear out or become permanently depressed, or a different density (degree of firmness) or type is required for a patient. Some mattresses, usually the polyfoam and foam rubber, have removable tickings; launder these as often as you change blankets. Mattresses with nonglazed fabric covers should be vacuum cleaned about once a year regardless of use. But do not vacuum clean feather mattresses, as the suction may pull fine quills through the ticking; once this starts, usually a new ticking is soon needed.

For the longest and most comfortable use, all mattresses except water, air, and polyfoam or foam rubber with exposed core holes on the lower surface, should be "turned" once a week or every 10 days. There are two kinds of turning, and they should be alternated. One time turn the mattress over from side to side, the next time from end to end. If your patient often sits on the edge of a mattress for much longer than it takes to get in or out of bed, more frequent turning of a mattress may be advisable. Also, to protect the sides of a mattress against packing or losing shape where a patient sits, hit the mattress hard several times with your fists every day or so.

If you are replacing another type of mattress with a polyfoam or foam rubber, it may be to your patient's advantage to place it on a solid wood base instead of a spring surface. The wooden base serves, of course, as a bedboard. For best results, a foam mattress generally should be medium to firm stock, and no less than about 13 cm./5 in. thick.

Mattress Cover If your patient's mattress casing or ticking is not waterproof, a waterproof mattress cover should be used. A fitted cover is the easiest to keep tight and smooth. A sheet of medium or heavy plastic large enough for a 61-cm./2-ft. tuck-under all around a mattress usually is satisfactory. It may need tightening and smoothing from time to time while making the bed.

Mattress Pad A mattress pad provides greater comfort for a patient and protects the mattress against soil. The pad usually is a quilted material approximately the size and shape of the upper surface of the mattress; it may or may not have boxing. Boxing helps hold a pad in place; it extends from the outer edges of the pad and fits under the mattress. Plain or unboxed pads are available with and without elastic loops at the corners to pass under the mattress and hold the pad in place. Most mattress pads are reversible; some have a side covered by waterproof material.

Mattress pads should be changed frequently, but once a week usually is adequate for patients who are confined to bed for most of the time. For those who are out of bed for at least half of each day, mattress pads need be changed only about once a month. Of course, when soiled, a pad should be changed and laundered immediately.

Measuring Cups, Pitchers, and Spoons If your patient is on a strict diet or must take medicine any way except by pills or capsules, you need an ample supply of measuring cups, pitchers, or spoons. You should have at least one 1-l./1-qt. pitcher, three 250-ml./8-oz./1-cup pouring cups, several 30-ml./1-oz./1-tbsp. pouring containers, and two or three sets of standard measuring spoons. The larger containers usually are graduated or marked in units of 25 or 50 ml./2 or 4 oz., and halves, thirds, and quarters of a cup. The smaller containers generally are graduated in 5-ml. units, tbsp., tsp., and fractions of them. Sets of measuring spoons commonly are 1 tbsp., 1-, ½-, and ¼-tsp. The largest containers generally are glass, the smaller ones glass or a clear plastic, and the spoons either plastic or metal.

Since measuring cups and spoons should not be used for eating or drinking, as a rule there is no need to buy ones that safely can be boiled or otherwise heat sterilized.

P

Pillow When sick or injured, people generally may use and will be more comfortable with the same kind of pillow—down- or feather-filled, molded or shredded polyfoam or foam rubber, polyester fiber, cotton, etc.—they had when well.

Better-quality pillows usually are encased by a ticking that can be removed for laundering. Do not vacuum clean a pillow containing down or feathers; the air suction probably will pull the fine quills through the pillow's internal downproof ticking and external casing, and it soon will be necessary to replace the downproof ticking. It is not advisable to vacuum clean cotton- or kapok-filled pillows; the air suction may pack the broken fibers or break them into dustlike particles.

Pillows seldom need to be replaced unless a different type (probably due to patient allergy), density or degree of firmness, or shape is needed.

Under normal conditions, pillow tickings should be laundered about as often as a patient's blankets are changed. If your patient perspires freely, pillow tickings should be laundered frequently; it may be advisable to have several spare pillows, and a waterproof cover under the pillowcase may be necessary. If you must dry a pillow, not just the removable ticking, hang it up to air as long as necessary, but not in direct sunlight. Direct sunlight and other kinds of excessive heat can damage many of the common pillow fillings.

Pillows should be plumped up as often as needed for patient comfort and, by rearranging the areas of contact with the patient's head and neck, to help prevent bedsores (Chapter 15). Plumping up is most effective with loose-fill pillows such as down, feather, and those made with shredded polyfoam or foam rubber. Plumping up is least effective with molded polyfoam and foam rubber, and polyester pillows; these, however, often are so soft that they tend to distribute pressure fairly evenly on a patient's head and neck instead of concentrating it on a few points. Although plumping up pillows nearly always is advisable for the good of a patient, it should be done somewhat sparingly to cotton- and kapok-filled pillows; cotton tends to mat into hard lumps from being plumped up, and kapok tends to break into dustlike particles.

Pillowcases If your patient will be bedfast for more than a few days, use a variety of colored or decorated pillowcases if possible. They break part of the monotony of being in bed and help make the room more cheerful.

Pillowcases should be changed daily, unless soiled. Then they should be changed as soon as you can, and the soiled areas should be covered with towels until you can make the change. If a patient perspires freely, change a pillowcase as soon as it becomes noticeably damp. However, in severe cases of perspiration it may be more practical to cover the pillow with fairly thick bath or beach towels, and change them when damp to the touch.

Q

Quilts If your patient prefers quilts to blankets on a bed, usually there is no reason to change. However, often it is more difficult to make a bed with quilts than with blankets.

S

Scales If your patient is on a diet requiring foods to be measured by weight, you need an accurate kitchen scale. Since some diet weights are specified in grams and others in ounces, you will save time and work by getting a scale that is marked for both systems.

Seat Pads. See Cushions.

Shampoo Tray. See Bed Rinse/Shampoo Tray.

Shaving Equipment Unless the doctor orders that a change be made, as a rule the kind of shaving that your patient did before his disability is all right now, particularly if he shaves himself. But if you must do it, it probably will be to your mutual benefit to use an electric shaver. If he is not conditioned to one, it may be a week or so before he feels that he is getting a clean, close shave. Instead of an electric shaver, you and your patient may prefer a spring-driven one; except for having to be wound like a clock, they operate much like electric shavers.

There are many reliable, easy-to-use electric shavers. For bed or invalid use, one with a rechargeable battery generally is best; an electric cord can be a nuisance when shaving in bed. Arrange, if possible, for your patient to try several makes of shavers, each for a week or so, before deciding which to get.

Sheepskin. See Bed Padding.

Sheets. See Bed Sheets, Draw Sheet, Waterproof Sheeting.

Sliding Board or Transfer Board Under certain conditions a sliding board, Fig. 8–20, can greatly assist a patient in moving or being moved from one stationary article to another, such as from bed to a locked wheelchair, from locked wheelchair to the toilet, and so forth. Properly used, a sliding board can be of great help; IMPROPERLY used, it can be very dangerous. Do not use or let your patient use a sliding board without your visiting nurse's positive approval.

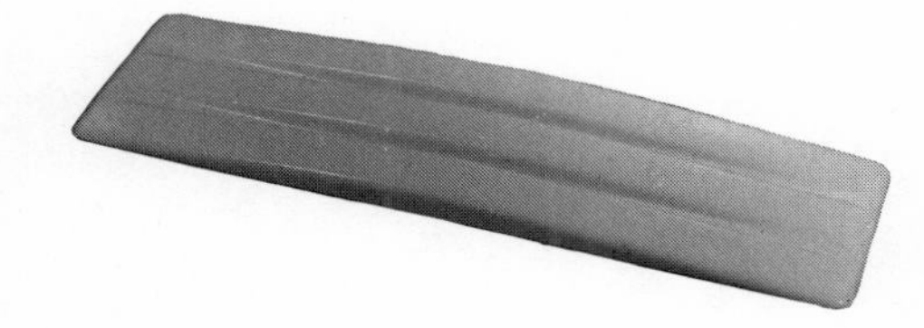

Fig. 8–20 *Sliding board*

Soap Dish Keep bar soap not in use in a soap dish or container at all times; one usually is part of a hospitalized patient's bedside aid kit.

The drier you keep a bar of soap when not in use, the longer it generally lasts. Before putting a bar away, shake all water off it to prevent a slippery scum forming on the bottom of the bar and the dish.

Sphygmomanometer The sphygmomanometer, a medical instrument for measuring blood pressure (Chapter 22), is not a regular part of sickroom equipment. It should be used only when ordered by a patient's doctor.

Stethoscope The stethoscope is a medical instrument for listening to heartbeat and other sounds of the body. In nursing a patient at home, it is used chiefly as part of the equipment for measuring blood pressure (Chapter 22).

T

Thermometers A thermometer should be in every home at all times, as a change in body temperature (Chapter 19) can be extremely important in many minor as well as major illnesses.

Toilet Seats and Safety Frames Auxiliary seats to raise the height of a toilet seat are ideal aids for arthritics, geriatrics, postoperative patients, fracture convalescents, and other persons who have difficulty in sitting down on and arising from standard-height toilet seats. Most auxiliary seats have easy-to-set height adjustments, Fig. 8–21 . . . are available plain, as in *a*, or with an assistance frame, *b* . . . have splash guards . . . do not readily accumulate foreign matter . . . have bowl brackets that will not scrape or mar the fixture . . . and can be attached and removed without tools. There are several kinds of auxiliary seats, including cushioned, front-opening, and portable models. Ask the patient's doctor or your visiting nurse what style of seat to get and how high to set it.

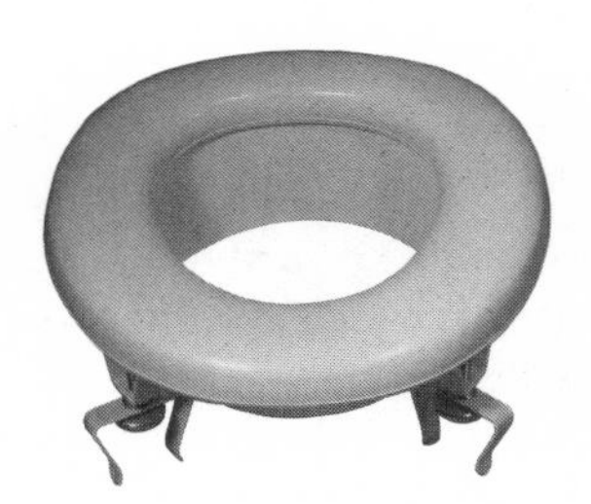

Fig. 8–21*a* *Plain*

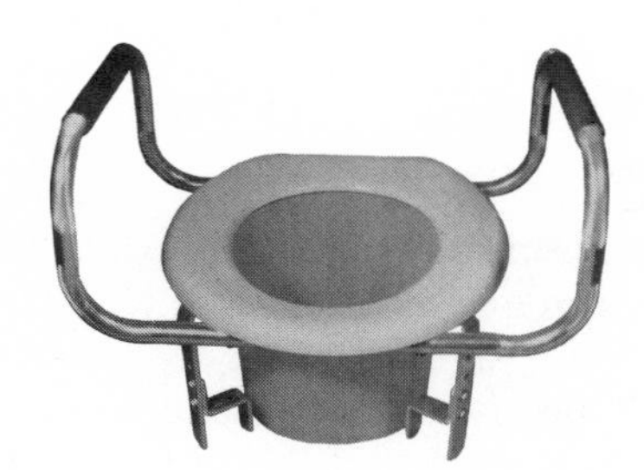

Fig. 8–21*b* *With assistance frame*

Fig. 8–21 *Adjustable-height toilet seats*

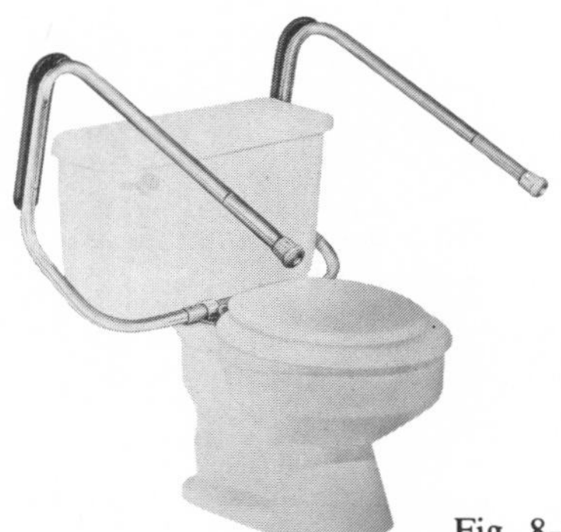

Fig. 8–22 *Toilet safety frame*

Toilet safety frames, as in Fig. 8–22, attach easily and quickly to most toilets by means of a mounting bracket. Depending on the make and model of frame, either or both arms may be removed and replaced as needed or swung up out of the way, and width between arms and height of the legs is adjustable.

Toothbrush In most cases, there is no need to change from the dentifrice and toothbrush that your patient is accustomed to. For brushing in bed, you also need a tumbler of water for washing and rinsing, and an emesis basin for emptying the mouth.

There are handicap aids (Chapter 16) that may be practical for patients who want to brush their teeth themselves but have disabled hands, arms, or shoulders. In some of these cases an electric toothbrush may be needed. There are several excellent makes. Ask your visiting nurse which electric toothbrush is best for your patient.

Towels An ample supply of medium to large thick-pile (terrycloth) clean towels should be readily available at all times. A few guest-size towels are handy for quick cleanup jobs, such as washing before meals. Beach towels are an excellent substitute for hospital-type bath blankets.

NOTE: Towels can easily become contaminated and spread an infection. Do not allow anyone in the home to use any other person's towels.

Transfer Board. See Sliding Board.

Trapeze Bars Trapeze bars, as in Fig. 8–23, give physically disabled patients a practical means for helping themselves in changing position in bed, moving from

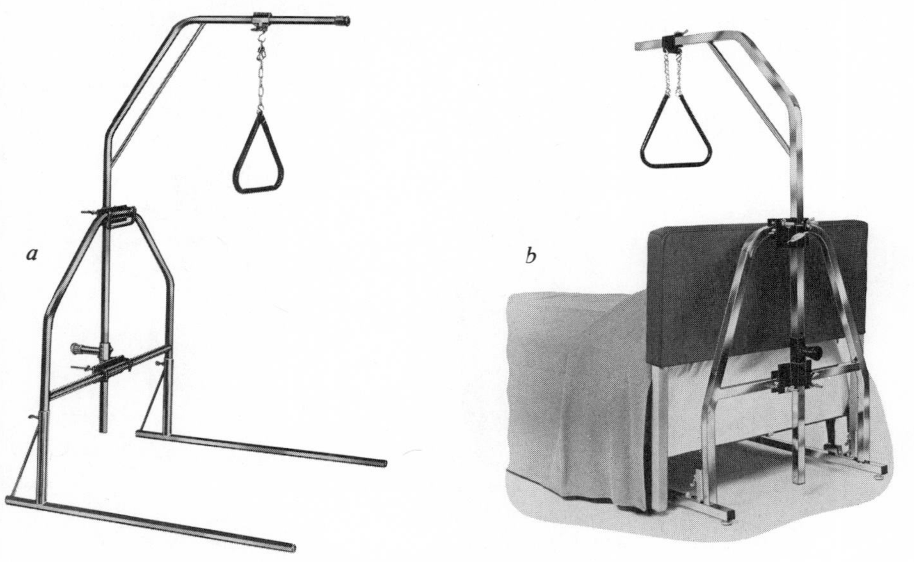

Fig. 8–23*a, b* *Trapeze bars*

bed to commode or wheelchair, and so forth. Trapeze bars are also excellent for exercising the hands, wrists, arms, shoulders, and possibly other parts of the body. There are several good makes of trapeze bars and most are similar in design. There are, however, differences in how they function, so be sure to ask your patient's doctor or therapist, or your visiting nurse, which one will best meet your patient's needs.

The trapeze bars in Fig. 8–23*a* basically consist of the bars, complete with grab bars, mounted on floor stands. The basic parts are available separately; often the bar is attached to the back of a bed headboard. The floor stand makes the trapeze bar more useful, as it can be set over a bed, Fig. 8–23*b*, or chair, or in some other place that a patient wants. Regardless of their mounting, trapeze bars may be in fixed position or they may swivel or turn, usually up to 90 degrees to right and to left. Height of the basic bar is easily adjusted, and the grab bar (the suspended triangle) can be moved inward and outward along the horizontal bar and locked in place. Grab bars have a chain height adjustment.

Tumbler. See Bedside Aid Kit; Drinking Glass.

U

Urinals Urinals, receptacles for collecting and transporting urine, are for use by bedfast patients and by others who cannot use a commode or a toilet. There are two basic kinds of urinals, those for use "as needed" and those that are worn by persons who have no or impaired bladder control (incontinence). Common as-needed male urinals are shown in Fig. 8–24; the generally preferred as-needed urinal for females is the fracture bedpan, Fig. 8–8*b*. There is so much variety in urinals for incontinent patients that you should have the doctor prescribe one. Regarding the as-needed male urinals in Fig. 8–24:

a The plastic urinal with cover has a dual-purpose handle for hanging on bed when not in use. The tight-fitting cover, marked "Urinal" to avoid other

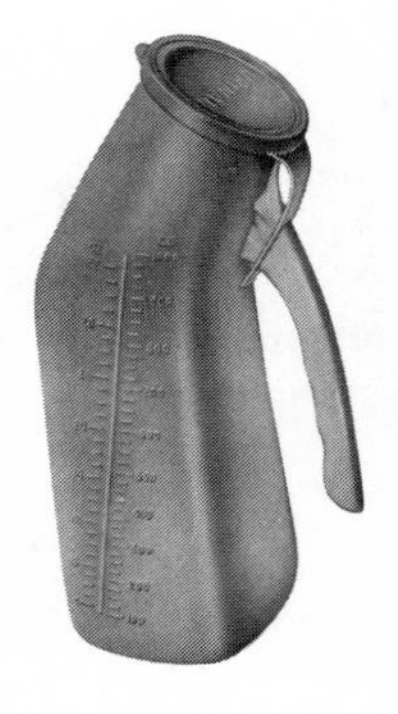

Fig. 8–24*a* *Capped urinal, as needed*

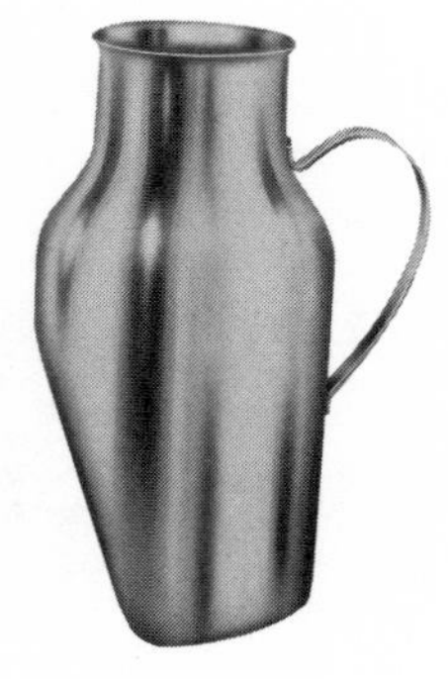

Fig. 8–24*b* *All-position urinal, as needed*

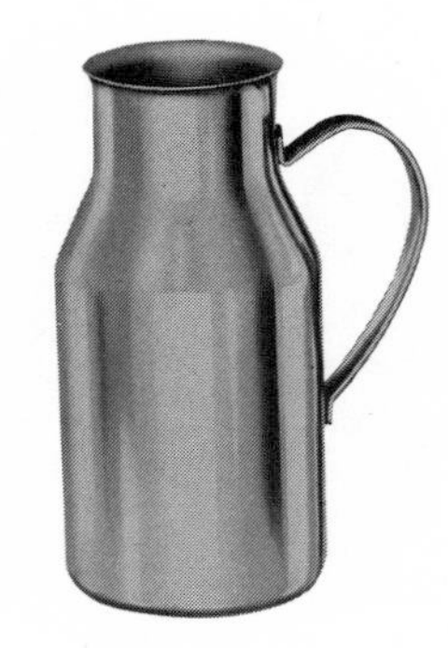

Fig. 8–24*c* *Upright urinal, as needed*

Fig. 8–24 *Male urinals*

uses, helps prevent spillage and confines odor. The container has accurate, easy-to-read cc./oz. graduations, a great convenience if you have to measure your patient's excretions (Chapter 49). The urinal can be used by a patient when lying, sitting, or standing.

b The long-lasting stainless steel common male urinal, also available in plastic, has a large loop handle for easier handling by patient and nurse. This model urinal also can be used by a patient when lying, sitting, or standing.

c The upright stainless steel male urinal can only be used vertically or at a very slight angle with, in most cases, the patient standing or sitting. Because it stands vertically instead of on a side, as in Fig. 8–24*b*, the upright urinal may be more practical in certain cases.

NOTE: Some patients want bedpans instead of urinals. Ask your visiting nurse how to get your patient to use a urinal; it will simplify your work and in the long run probably be more comfortable for your patient.

Use No matter how careful patient and nurse are with urinals, there always is a chance that urine may leak out or spill. To protect the bed, before giving a urinal spread a few sheets of newspaper, a towel, or a piece of waterproof material under your patient's perineal area.

Unless very elderly or ill, males usually can manage an as-needed urinal without assistance. Make sure that the penis is well inside the opening of the urinal.

Cleaning Rinse urinals thoroughly with *cold* water immediately after emptying. Clean them with soap, warm water, and a toilet brush at least once a day.

If a strong odor persists in a urinal, soak it in a pine-scented household deodorant for an hour or so. Be sure the deodorant is completely rinsed out before giving a urinal to a patient.

V

Vomit Dish. See Emesis Basin.

W

Walkers There are many types of walkers, in adult and child sizes, each made to help a patient cope with or overcome a certain disability or move about more readily and independently. There are walkers designed especially for cerebral palsy, polio, and spastic paralysis cases . . . for arthritic and newly ambulatory patients . . . for persons who can walk only a short distance and then must stop and rest. To assist patients make the transition from crutches to canes there is the Walkane, Fig. 8–14. Even the simpler walkers, which often are quite similar, as in Fig. 8–25, have features that can make one better than another for a particular person. For example, the walkers in Figs. 8–25*a* and *b* are sturdy, are available with wheels for easier maneuvering and without wheels, and fold flat for convenient transportation—yet most people will find one easier to manage than the other. For persons who must go up and down stairs as well as walk on the level, the simple-appearing walker in Figs. 8–25*c*, *d* was designed.

As well as many kinds of walkers, there are special attachments, such as forearm

Fig. 8–25 *Walkers*

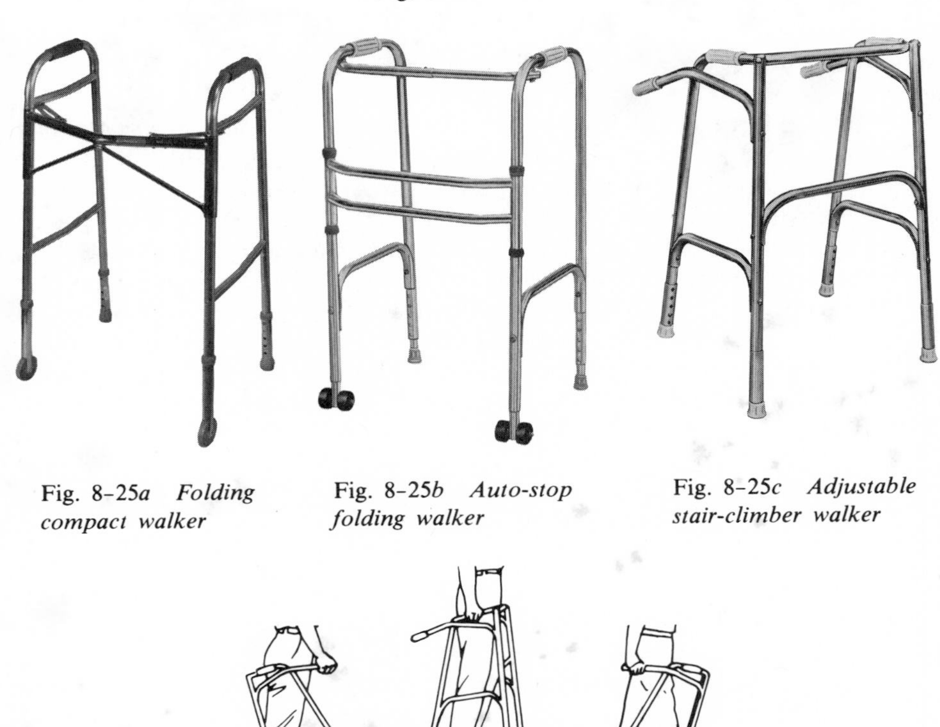

Fig. 8–25*a* *Folding compact walker*

Fig. 8–25*b* *Auto-stop folding walker*

Fig. 8–25*c* *Adjustable stair-climber walker*

Fig. 8–25*d* *Stair-climber walker in use*

holders for patients with weak or arthritic hands and wrists . . . accessories such as sling seats, and crutch-type arm rests as in Fig. 8–16*b* . . . and utility pouches, trays, and baskets for carrying personal articles.

If a walker is needed, get complete written specifications as to the size, weight, type, attachments, and accessories that your patient should have. When there is a choice of models, arrange for your patient to try them all for a reasonable time to find out which works best.

Washbasin. See Bath Basin; Bedside Aid Kit.

Washcloth Fairly large, thick, terrycloth-type washcloths are the most practical for all washing and bathing of a patient. For best results, choose cloths that absorb water readily; they are the easiest to rinse clean of soap while bathing a patient.

> NOTE: Do not under any circumstances use or allow anyone around you to use somebody else's washcloth. A "community" washcloth is a sure way to spread infections throughout a household.

Wastebasket and -Bag A wastebasket should at all times be within convenient reach of most patients who have any mobility. It need only be large enough for facial tissues, paper towels, and other fairly small articles to be dropped into. Lining a wastebasket with newspapers or a paper bag keeps the inside of the basket clean and makes it less disagreeable to empty—simply wrap the liner around the waste while removing it.

Instead of a wastebasket, a paper bag of suitable size may be pinned to the side of the bed at a convenient height. Before pinning the bag, fold the top edge down about 5 cm./2 in. inside the bag; pin through the folded-down area. Folding the bag this way strengthens it against tearing, simplifies dropping papers into it, and tends to keep them from coming out.

A wastebag can easily be made from a sheet of newspaper. Fold it as in steps *a, b, c,* and *d*, Fig. 8–26. Pin the bag to the bed near the top of the several thicknesses as shown in *d*.

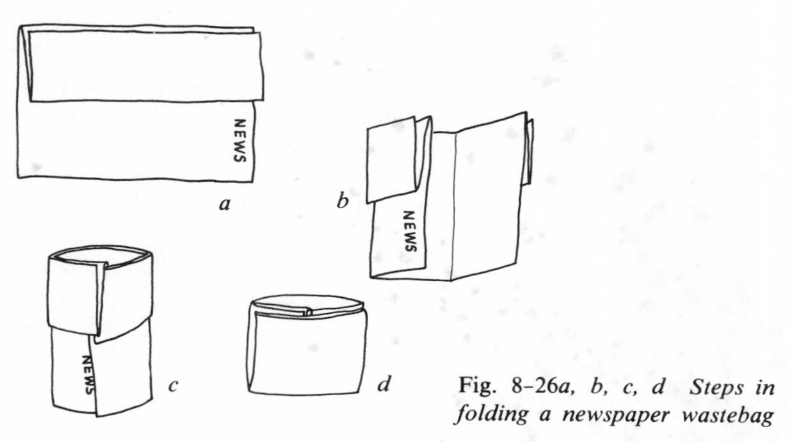

Fig. 8–26*a, b, c, d* *Steps in folding a newspaper wastebag*

Watch. See Clock.

Water Beds, Mattresses, and Pads Many hospitals and convalescent homes use water beds, mattresses, and pads to help keep patients from developing pressure ulcers or bedsores (Chapter 15). Although highly effective, they are not necessarily the complete solution to the bedsore problem in all cases. Before deciding for or against a water flotation device for your patient, consult the doctor or therapist, and your visiting nurse.

> NOTE: If a water bed or mattress seems worthwhile from a medical standpoint, find out if the sickroom is strong enough to withstand its weight. Weight seldom is a problem with water pads, as they are considerably smaller than the beds and mattresses.

Water Glass, Pitcher, and Tumbler. See Bedside Aid Kit; Drinking Glass.

Waterproof Sheeting A waterproof sheet, as in Fig. 8–27, covers a bed from side to side directly under the draw sheet. Its purpose is to protect the bottom sheet, bed padding if any, mattress pad and cover, and mattress, especially one that does not have a waterproof ticking. As a rule, waterproof sheeting is used only for as long as it is necessary. Throughout their use, waterproof sheets should be changed and laundered on the same basis as the bottom bed sheet.

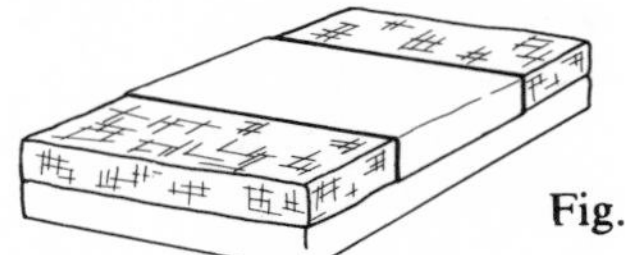

Fig. 8–27 *Waterproof sheet on bed mattress*

As a rule, any waterproof sheeting may be used. Some, however, tend to become brittle and may crack and leak in a relatively short time. Ask your visiting nurse what sheeting will be best for your patient's needs. There are two basic kinds of waterproof sheeting:

Rubberized Sheeting. There are two types of rubberized waterproof sheeting. One is a cloth base with rubber coating on both sides. The other is a rubber-cloth base with both sides covered by an absorbent cotton flannel.

Plastic Sheeting. Medium or heavy or thick plastic is commonly used for waterproof sheeting; very thin or lightweight plastic does not stay in place well as a rule. The plastics used for automobile shelters, and house painters' heavy-duty dropcloths usually are adequate for bed use. Do not use the plastic clothes bags given by many dry cleaning shops; the plastic is too light to stay in place well. Also, many localities require breather holes in plastic clothes bags.

A waterproof sheet should be long enough to cover a mattress from one lower side edge to the other, plus about 46 cm./18 in. at each side for tucking under the mattress, as in Fig. 8–27, and wide enough to reach from just above the patient's shoulders to the knees. Narrower or wider sheeting may be used, if it will be completely covered by the draw sheet.

Wheelchairs Except for the traditional wooden type, Fig. 8–28*a*, modern wheelchairs are made up of various components selected to meet the individual patient's needs. "Components" include such items as back and leg extensions, adjustable foot rests, removable arms, holding straps, deep reclining backs, commodes, and so forth—almost any- and everything that can make a wheelchair more comfortable, practical, and useful for a patient.

There are several basic kinds of wheelchairs, each with certain features or advantages. The traditional wooden chair, Fig. 8–28*a*, with large front and small back swivel wheels, is exceptionally easy for a patient to move and steer; it is, however, somewhat bulky. The modern manual wheelchair in Fig. 8–28*b* readily folds into a fairly flat package that takes up little space and easily can be stowed for traveling. The recliner wheelchair in Fig. 8–28*c* actually is a regular modern manual chair with a back extension, removable arms, and special leg rests; wheelchairs of this modification often are used for patients in body casts.

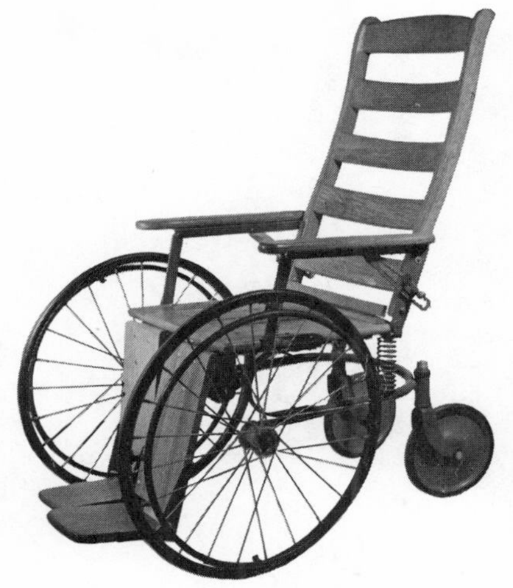

Fig. 8–28*a* *Traditional wooden wheelchair*

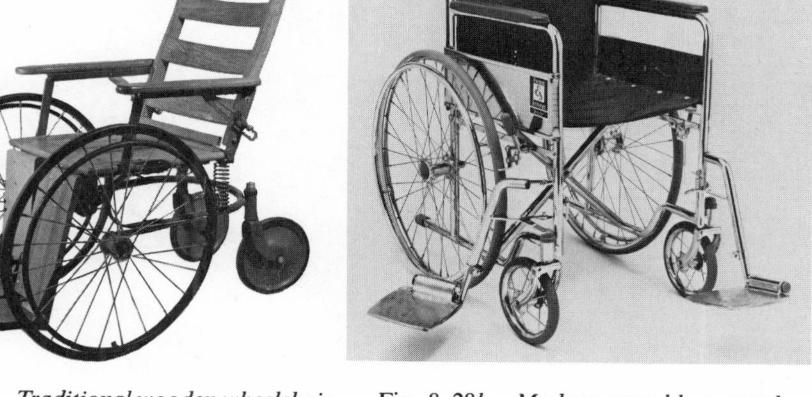

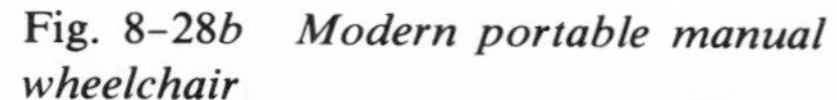

Fig. 8–28*b* *Modern portable manual wheelchair*

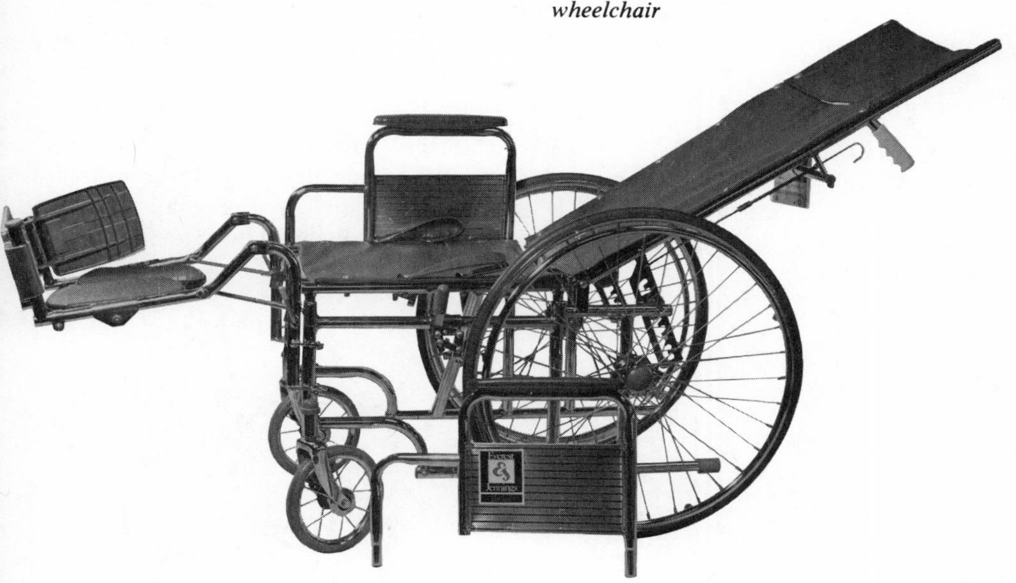

Fig. 8–28*c* *Recliner-converted modern wheelchair*

Fig. 8–28 *Manual wheelchairs*

Powered Wheelchairs The electric-battery-powered wheelchairs in Fig. 8–29 are built for different conditions of travel, hence the large rear-drive wheel in *a* and the small wheels in *b*. Powered wheelchairs are available in foldable models, and there are special cases for transporting batteries.

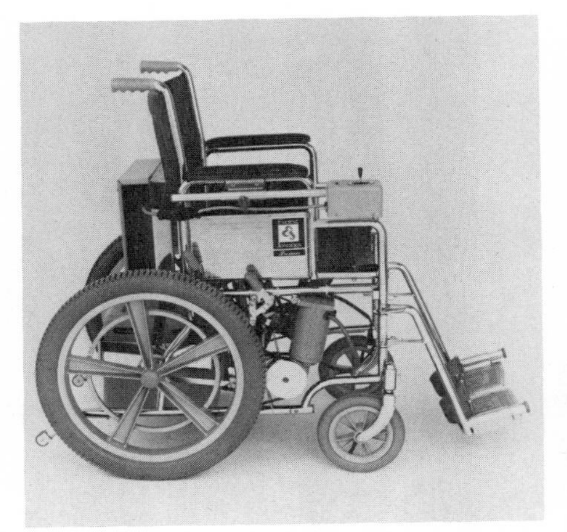

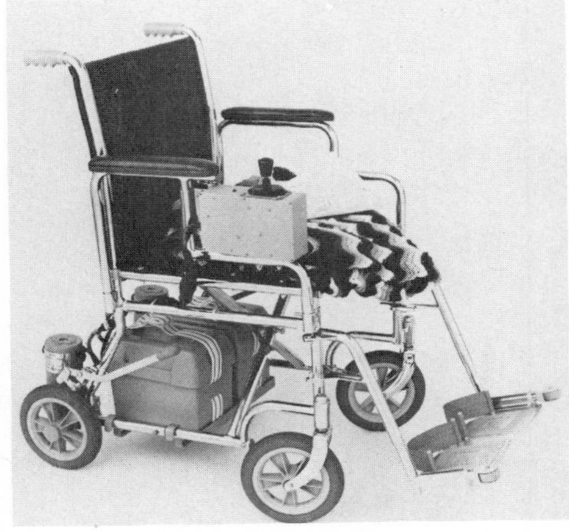

a Fig. 8–29*a, b* *Electric-powered wheelchairs* *b*

The wheelchairs in Fig. 8–29 show a simple electric control box, just in front of the right arm rest, for driving forward and backward, stopping, and steering by making one wheel revolve faster than the other. There are similar controls for a patient to operate by chin, even by the tongue and mouth.

Special Child's Wheelchair A special wheelchair to accommodate a child who cannot sit with head up is shown in Fig. 8–30. The chair has padded supports to hold the child safely upright in a comfortable position. The chair and its attachments are easily adjusted to accommodate a growing child. Similar chairs are made for adults.

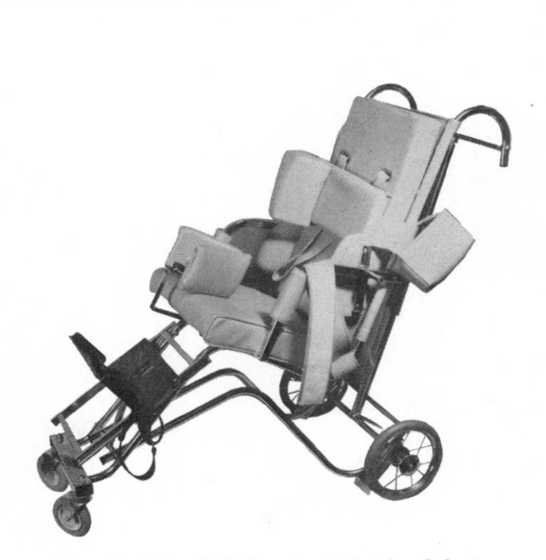

Fig. 8–30 *Child's special wheelchair*

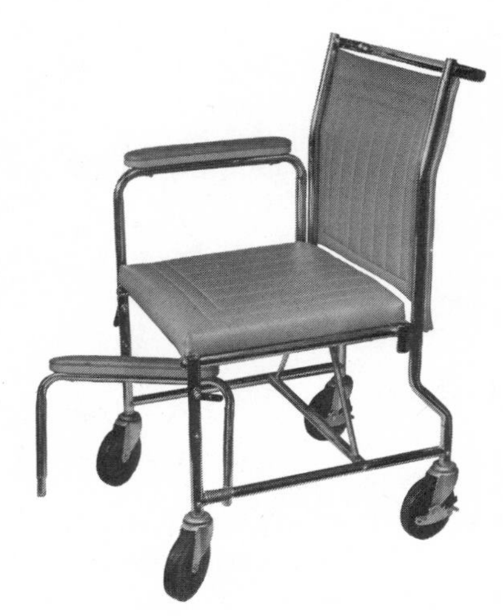

Fig. 8–31 *Wheel-mounted chair*

Wheel-Mounted Chair Although technically a wheelchair, the type in Fig. 8–31 actually is a somewhat regular chair mounted on wheels for the patient who does not require the more complicated, and costly, models. This style of chair takes up relatively little space, can be moved up close to a table for eating, has removable arms for easy entry and exit, has locking wheels, and is light enough to be moved with little effort.

Wheelchair Accessories There are numerous accessories to make a wheelchair patient's life more comfortable, safe, and complete . . . cane and crutch holders, desk arms, headrests, roller bumpers, special rims for hand-powered chairs, antitip devices, utility trays, special cushions, seat pads for incontinent persons, back supports, cushions, beverage holders, pushing cuffs, safety belts, and so on.

9 The Supplies You'll Need

Most of the supplies other than medicinals (Chapter 10) needed for a patient are those usually found in the average home. Unless the doctor specifies a particular brand or kind of item, such as soap, or prescribes a medicated one, use the one that your patient is accustomed to and likes. Just as it is with equipment (Chapter 8) you should have all the necessary supplies on hand before your patient arrives.

PATIENT SENSITIVITY

Commercial lotions, dentifrices, powders, etc., that bear a seal of medical acceptance are formulated and prepared to be free of irritants. However, there is always the chance that someone may be allergic or sensitive to one or more of the ingredients. If a skin irritation, rash, or other possible sign of an allergy or sensitivity appears anytime after your patient starts using a substance, discontinue it immediately and report the condition to the doctor or your visiting nurse. Be sure to keep the part of the label or container listing the ingredients of the product; without that information the doctor or nurse may not be able to readily determine why the product is not suitable for your patient.

A

Air Deodorant and Freshener Some medicines, medical treatments, and sicknesses have odors that are disagreeable to the average person. It may be advisable to deodorize all rooms occupied by your patient for more than a few hours with an air deodorant or freshener. Use one that has an aroma that your patient likes and is strong enough to overcome the disagreeable odors. In an emergency or when quick deodorizing is wanted, dab a few drops of cologne on a hot electric light bulb. Burning a scented candle in the room also can mask disagreeable odors.

Alcohol Denatured or rubbing alcohol (a poison if taken internally) may be used in and for body and hand lotions (below).

B

Body Deodorant A body deodorant is applied directly to a person's body either to neutralize a disagreeable odor or to inhibit the growth of bacteria that produce odors. Commercial deodorants generally are suitable, although some will be more effective than others in certain conditions. Instead of a deodorant as such, a patient may prefer bathing with a deodorant soap.

Body Lotions Body lotions generally soothe a patient's skin, help reduce or even prevent minor skin irritations and rashes caused by being in bed for a long time, and help neutralize the body odor so often given off by bedfast patients. Lotions generally are more acceptable than body powders (below) as they are less apt to dry a patient's skin. Use the body lotion your patient wants unless, of course, there are medical reasons for not using it. See Patient Sensitivity.

If no commercial body or hand lotion appeals to your patient, here is the recipe for an easy-to-make rubbing solution that was popular in the nursing profession many years ago. It consists of 2 parts rubbing alcohol, 2 parts witch hazel, and 1 part bay rum; stir or shake lightly together to mix. Store in a glass container at room temperature. Before using the solution in cold weather, warm it by placing the container in a pan of warm water.

Back Rub One of the most soothing services for a patient confined to bed is a back rub (Chapter 18). It is also an important part of good skin care. Rubbing alcohol and body or hand lotions are all acceptable as rubbing solutions, although alcohol by itself may dry the skin too much. Do not use a lotion that leaves a sticky or gummy residue on the skin.

Body Powder Body and dusting powders are used for the same purposes as body lotions (above), and despite their drying effect on the skin are preferred by some patients. Body powder also makes it easier for a patient to move about in bed.

As a rule, body or dusting powder is applied as the last or final step in bathing a patient (Chapter 23). But apply it whenever it may make your patient more comfortable.

Unless your patient is allergic to certain perfumes, or the doctor prescribes a medicated powder, use any body or dusting powder she likes. Baby powder and unscented talcum usually are preferred by men. See Patient Sensitivity.

Cornstarch Old-fashioned cornstarch, lightly rubbed in creases where skin surfaces touch, will help prevent raw, irritated areas from developing due to moisture.

C

Cornstarch. See Body Powder.

Cotton Absorbent cotton is excellent for applying and removing dry and liquid products, and for general touching of sensitive areas. Use sterile cotton when working on or close to open sores or wounds, and raw or inflamed skin rashes and irritations. Cotton swabs are excellent for cleaning ears, nostrils, and mouth, and for dabbing medicine onto small, sensitive areas.

D

Dental Floss Use for conventional cleaning between teeth.

Dentifrice Unless there has been recent oral surgery, or there are open sores on the lips or in a patient's mouth, any dentifrice that a patient likes is usually satisfactory. See Patient Sensitivity.

Brushing teeth after every meal is an important part of good dental care for well persons; it is of extra importance for sick persons because of their general lack of activity. Some patients may wish to brush their teeth or at least rinse out the mouth *before* eating breakfast. This is especially true of people who wake up with a bad taste in the mouth; food tastes better if the bad mouth taste is eliminated before eating.

H

Hand Lotion. See Body Lotion.

L

Lotion. See Body Lotion.

M

Mouthwash Unless your patient has had recent oral surgery, or has open sores on the lips or in the mouth, any commercial mouthwash usually is satisfactory. Unless used for medication, a mouthwash is purely for patient comfort; it is not a substitute dentifrice, although it may be used instead of a dentifrice before eating breakfast. A glass of warm water with a teaspoon of table salt dissolved in it may be a satisfactory mouthwash for some people, but for most it is not as refreshing as a typical commercial wash. See Patient Sensitivity.

Medicated mouthwashes can be important in the treatment of a patient and should not be discontinued without the doctor's permission.

Special Mouthwash Under certain conditions a patient may develop an annoying, sometimes painful scale on the lips and in the mouth. Unless the doctor prescribes a different treatment, you can remove the scale, with minor patient discomfort, with a mixture of 5 ml./1 tsp. baking soda and the juice of 1 lemon. Mix them together and while the mixture is fizzing, brush it on the affected areas of the lips and mouth with a cotton swab, such as a Q-Tip® (which see). As scale is loosened, gently work it free with the swab. It may be necessary to increase the size of the swab tip by wrapping it with sterile absorbent cotton (which see).

P

Paper Facial Tissue One of the most all-round useful supplies for both patient and nurse is paper facial tissue. An open container of tissues, preferably the pop-up type, should be within easy reach of a patient at all times. The small, half-size tissues may be less wasteful than the large ones.

Paper Towels Because paper towels are heavier and stronger than paper facial tissue, many people prefer them for wiping up liquid, drying sweaty skin, etc. A generous supply always should be convenient to your patient.

Powder. See Body Powder.

Q

Q-Tips® and Swabs Q-Tips®, a popular commercial cotton swab, are excellent for cleaning in and around the ears, nostrils, and mouth, and applying medicines in those places and on and near open sores, cuts, and raw rashes.

Double-tipped Q-Tip® safety swabs consist of a short "stick" with cotton wrapped around each end; sometimes it may be necessary to build up an end with additional absorbent cotton. Q-Tips® usually are available with a choice of sticks: wooden, which make a rigid, strong swab; and plastic, which are somewhat flexible. The flexible-stick Q-Tips® are particularly recommended for use with infants and young children, and with patients who cannot hold still in a positon for several minutes.

R

Rubbing Alcohol. See Alcohol, Body Lotion.

S

Shampoo How often hair should be shampooed usually depends to great extent on what your patient wants. Some people like to have their hair washed daily, others may want it done once a week or even less often. Unless a medicated shampoo is prescribed by the doctor, a commercial or homemade one that a patient likes is usually satisfactory. See Patient Sensitivity.

Soap Any soap that your patient likes is satisfactory for all washing. However, some deodorant soaps have ingredients that may irritate the skin of a person who has been confined to bed for a long time. Ask the doctor or your visiting nurse about soaps that may not be suitable for your patient. See Patient Sensitivity.

If medicated soap is prescribed, it should not be discontinued without the doctor's permission.

The drier you keep a bar of soap when it is not in use, the longer it generally lasts. Before putting a bar away, shake all water off to prevent a slippery scum forming on the bottom of the soap and the soap dish. Some thrifty homemakers buy bars of soap several months before their probable use, remove the wrappers, and stand them on end in a closet or other dry place for excess moisture to evaporate.

Swabs Q-Tips® (which see) are the cotton swabs most often used in home nursing. If a different kind of swab is needed for your patient, the doctor or your visiting nurse will provide it or tell you where to get it.

T

Toilet Paper Usually any brand of toilet paper that a patient is accustomed to is satisfactory. If a paper seems too rough or scratchy for your patient, try using Paper Facial Tissue (which see).

Toothpaste and Powder. See Dentifrice.

U

Unguents A lubricant, such as petroleum jelly or Vaseline®, or an ointment or salve may be used to reduce friction between parts of the body that rub against one another, or against an irritating foreign substance, as they move. Both oil-base and water-soluble lubricants are available; use the type that the doctor or your visiting nurse recommends. Water-soluble lubricants are easier to wash off a patient and your hands.

V

Vaseline®. See Unguents.

10 The Medicinals Your Patient Needs

Two basic kinds of medicines, *prescription* and *patent*, are needed by most patients. Through wise buying you can often make worthwhile savings on the high cost of sickness. But do not under any circumstances try to save money by giving a medicine prescribed for one person to another unless that person's doctor gives you direct permission to do so. Remember, what can help one person may kill another.

PRESCRIPTION MEDICINE

A prescription medicine is one prepared by a pharmacist or druggist according to a doctor's written and signed order or prescription, which must contain the name and address of the patient. A prescription tells the pharmacist to provide an exact amount of a specific drug or medicine, and gives the directions or instructions for use of the preparation. These must be copied by the pharmacist and placed on the container in which the medicine is delivered to the patient. If a prescription label comes off a container, do not replace it unless you are absolutely certain that it is the proper label for that container. If there is any doubt in your mind, either throw the medicine away or ask the pharmacist who prepared the medicine if the label and contents belong together.

Many prescriptions specify a drug or medicine by its trade name instead of its generic or "chemical ingredient" name. Trade name items usually cost more than the same products sold under their generic names. So when having a prescription filled, ask if it allows for use of generic products. Most pharmacists will gladly make the substitution. It often happens that the pharmacist knows of a suitable substitution and will ask the doctor if it is permissible.

NOTE: In certain localities a pharmacist is allowed, without consulting the doctor who issued a prescription, to substitute generic for trade name products.

Some prescriptions can be refilled by a pharmacist one or more times without consulting the doctor. Others can be refilled with the doctor's verbal permission, a phone call from the pharmacist being sufficient. But in many cases a prescription cannot be refilled without a new written order or prescription from the doctor; a pharmacist is legally bound to obey all of a doctor's order, and *non repetat* (do not repeat) may have been written on the prescription.

It is fairly common for prescription medicines to deteriorate with age. As a rule, they merely lose potency; but it is possible that through chemical changes due to aging a medicine could become harmful to your patient. There is also the fact that the doctor may wish to reevaluate your patient's need for a medicine after a given time. For these reasons you often find on the labels of prescription medicines the warning "Do not use after" and a date. If a label has no expiration or cutoff date and the medicine is more than 3 months old, play it safe and ask the pharmacist whether to keep or throw it away.

Depending on the condition of your patient and the instructions for use of a prescription medicine, it may be kept within easy reach of a patient for self-dosage, or it should be stored in a medicine chest. When having a prescription filled, ask if it may be harmful or hazardous if taken, especially internally, by anyone other than your patient. If so, mark it clearly, preferably with a red marking pen, as being hazardous or harmful; place it in the most difficult to reach corner of a medicine chest or, better, lock it in a drawer. A wise rule of thumb is to keep all medicines and drugs out of the reach of small children and of patients who are not mentally alert.

PATENT MEDICINES

Patent or over-the-counter medicines are the manufacturer-packaged pain-killers, headache remedies, skin treatments, sleeping tablets, antihistamine sprays, etc., that can be purchased without a prescription. Patent medicines usually are much less expensive than similar prescription medicines, but contain a lower dose of some ingredients. When a patent medicine is adequate for your patient, the doctor usually will tell you so. If a prescription calls for a common patent medicine by name, the pharmacist generally will sell it to you at the lower, patent medicine price, but will not label it with the specific directions the doctor ordered.

Although most patent medicines do deteriorate with age, they are not as a rule marked with an expiration or "do not use after" date. However, they usually have a coded or plainly printed date indicating safe shelf life, such as "do not sell after." Generally a patent medicine will be satisfactory for at least a couple of months after the shelf-life date, but fresher buys are preferable.

SOME DON'T'S

Don't keep medicines of any kind within the reach of small children or of patients who are not mentally alert.

Don't get and administer medicines in the dark.

Don't give a patient any more or less of a prescription or patent medicine than the doctor ordered.

Don't rely on your memory for the proper dosage of a medicine. Read the label, preferably twice.

Don't keep a medicine after the doctor has permanently discontinued its use. Discard it down the toilet.

Don't leave medicines for an extended period of time in direct sunlight. Sunlight, even coming through window glass, can be very detrimental to certain drugs and medicines.

Don't leave or store medicines in places having higher than normal room temperature. Excessive heat can adversely affect certain drugs and medicines.

Don't leave or store medicines in areas having higher than normal humidity, such as the bathroom or the ledge over the kitchen sink.

Don't use the unfinished portion of a medicine for a previous illness to treat a new, similar illness without *specific* authorization from the doctor.

Don't guess! When in doubt, always ask the doctor, nurse, or pharmacist.

SOME DO'S

Always read the label—carefully!—before giving a medicine.

Always keep the cap on a container except when you are actually removing medicine from it.

Always measure medicine in light bright enough for you to see clearly what you are doing.

Always measure medicines accurately. "Close enough" can be a long and serious way off!

When measuring liquid medicines, always hold the measuring spoon, cup, etc., at eye level.

When measuring dry medicines, always use a *level* spoon- or cupful.

Always thoroughly clean a measuring spoon, cup, etc., immediately after use.

11 Germs, Viruses, and Bacteria

Our world is full of microorganisms, minute living bodies both beneficial and harmful which cannot be seen by the naked eye. The harmful ones are commonly called germs. Scientists such as Pasteur, Koch, and Lister spent many years studying the causes and effects of the various microorganisms in our world, and how to avoid the undesirable results of their presence.

Disease is a departure from the normal. In the medical world, disease is considered to be any visible, harmful departure from the normal condition of the body. Infectious disease results from the entrance of organisms into the body that can multiply in or on body tissues and damage them. Your patient is in a weakened condition and has less resistance to these organisms and their effects. A major part of your duty as nurse is to try to protect your patient from disease-producing organisms. This is done by cleanliness and by keeping your patient away from people or animals who have diseases, or people, animals, plants, or things that have been exposed to sicknesses, such as the common cold, flu, fevers, and so forth.

WHAT THEY ARE

The disease-producing organisms are called *pathogenic*, and often are classed as parasites. They may be *macro*scopic, such as various insects and worms large enough to be seen by the naked eye; or they may be *micro*scopic, such as bacteria, yeast and mold spores, rickettsiae, viruses, and protozoa, which can be seen only by use of a microscope. Classified by "size," they are:

Microbes: The smallest microbes can be seen only through electron microscopes that magnify 20,000 diameters or more. Many microbes have been identified as germs causing disease in man and animals; but in comparison to the total known number of microbes, only a few are disease-producing or pathogenic.

Viruses: The smallest of the disease-producing microbes, and responsible for such diseases as smallpox, the common cold, and poliomyelitis. A virus is a tiny parasite that lives, grows, and reproduces its kind inside a host cell. When viruses damage or destroy the cells they invade, they produce virus diseases (smallpox, common cold, rabies, polio, etc.). Viruses are spread in a variety of ways. Some virus diseases, such as chickenpox and measles, are spread by contact or by droplets in the air. Some are transmitted only through a wound; for example, by the bite of a rabid animal. Many virus diseases are spread by insects. Rarely, they are spread by water, milk, or food that has been contaminated by a virus.

Bacteria: Larger than viruses, bacteria are tiny, one-celled plants without green coloring matter (chlorophyll) that can be seen through microscopes that magnify them 600 diameters or more. There are many kinds of bacteria, and they are classified in many ways. Not all bacteria produce disease; some, such as those that normally inhabit the lower intestinal tracts, are almost essential to our good health. There are numerous sizes of bacteria, but only three principal shapes:

1. Rod- or pencil-shaped: the bacilli. They produce diseases like tuberculosis and Hansen's Disease.
2. Spherical or dot-shaped: the cocci. They exist in pairs (diplococci), in strings or chains (streptococci), and in grapelike clusters (staphylococci). Typical diplococci are the gonococcus, cause of gonorrhea, and the pneumococcus, cause of pneumonia. Streptococci are responsible for "strep" infections such as scarlet fever, and the sore throat that often is a forerunner of rheumatic fever. Staphylococci are present in boils.
3. Spiral or comma-shaped: such as the corkscrew spirochete of syphilis and of cholera vibrio, which frequently causes death.

HOW MICROORGANISMS ATTACK

Normally the body defends itself well against invading microorganisms. But when, for some reason such as overfatigue or improper diet, the body's resistance is lowered, then the invading microorganisms multiply faster than the body can fight them, and a disease occurs. Other factors that influence the occurrence of infection or disease are:

1. *The portal of entry*, or means by which an organism enters the body;
2. *Virulence*, or the organism's power to produce infection or disease; and
3. *Dosage*, or numbers of invading organisms.

Portal of Entry The portal of entry through which invading microorganisms enter the body is important in determining the occurrence and kind of disease.

Ordinary microorganisms cannot penetrate unbroken skin. A scratch or cut, however small, will allow them to enter the body.

The thin mucus membranes surrounding the eye, in the nose, throat, and lungs, and in the genitourinary tract (kidneys, urinary bladder, organs of generation and their accessories) are less able than the body's outer skin to withstand the invasion of microorganisms.

There are certain microorganisms that, under ordinary circumstances, can enter the body only by contact with the respiratory tract.

Some microorganisms, such as Shigella (a species that causes digestive disturbances ranging from mild diarrhea to severe, often fatal dysentery), can invade the body or host only through contact with the alimentary or digestive tract.

Virulence Virulence of microorganisms is a property that combines:

1. *Infectiousness*, or the ability of a microorganism to start and maintain an infection in a host or body by evading or overcoming local defense measures, such as normal antibodies.
2. *Invasiveness*, or the power of a microorganism to advance into the host or body from the portal of entry, or initial site of infection, and grow in other tissues. The invasion of blood and tissues may or may not result in obvious

disease; it depends on the strength of the organism and the resistance of the host. Organisms that invade the blood can be carried to other parts of the body, such as the spleen, liver, bone marrow, and lymph nodes, especially those of the intestine.

3. *Pathogenicity*, or the ability of a microorganism to injure the host (cause a disease) once an infection is established.

MICROORGANISMS OUTSIDE THE BODY

Many microorganisms cannot tolerate conditions outside a body, and in fairly short time will die. For example, "drying" is fatal to meningococci (the cause of meningitis), gonococci (gonorrhea), and syphilis spirochetes. Other organisms cannot tolerate sunlight, and some cannot live in natural bodies of water, soil, or in feces. Those that can exist outside the body depend on extraneous or unrelated moving agents to transport them any distance. Such agents may be dust, water, food . . . droplets of saliva from sneezing and coughing . . . saliva-contaminated hands . . . articles contaminated with oral, nasal, or intestinal matter . . . plants and parts of plants . . . insects and animals. All these disease-transmitting agents are called *vectors*. Vectors are classified as animate and inanimate.

Animate vectors include vertebrate animals, people, insects such as flies, mosquitoes, fleas, and lice, and arachnids (a class of Arthropoda) such as spiders, mites, and ticks. Examples of insect-transmitted diseases are malaria, spread by the anopheles mosquito . . . epidemic typhus, spread by lice . . . and bubonic plague, spread by fleas. Mites are common transmitters of mange and scabies, and ticks spread a variety of rickettsial diseases of the spotted fever group. Some diseases are spread by the bite of an animate vector . . . some by its feces, urine, body hairs, or feet . . . and some by direct contact with its saliva, nasal secretion, blood, or parts of blood such as plasma, serum, and hemoglobin.

Inanimate vectors are:

1. *Fomites*: Any inanimate object or substance that serves to transfer infectious microorganisms from one host (person, animal, plant) to another. Typical fomites are soiled bed linen and clothing, eating and drinking utensils, toys, pencils, and so forth. These are dangerous after being in contact with infected hosts harboring microorganisms, especially those causing respiratory and intestinal diseases that can be transmitted by such means.

2. *Foods*: Milk, water, moist foods (soup, pudding, etc.) that are not very acid may be excellent substances for the growth of many microorganisms such as typhoid bacillus . . . dysentery bacilli . . . *Staphylococcus aureus* and *Clostridium botulinum*, which cause food poisoning . . . hemolytic streptococcus, which causes "strep" throat and scarlet fever . . . diphtheria bacillus, and many others.

3. *Dust*: Common dust-borne diseases are coccidioidomycosis or valley fever, parrot fever, and respiratory infections.

4. *Sewage*: Feces and urine from infected people can transmit disease if sewage is not properly handled, and if persons handling bedpans, etc., do not thoroughly wash their hands after such handling.

PREVENTIONS

When the route or method of disease transmission is known, effective preventive action can be taken. For example, if cholera is endemic (usually present in a locality), it is necessary to cook all foods and boil all drinking water. And it is important to keep people who have contagious diseases isolated from all others. But the all-round best way to prevent the spread of disease-producing microorganisms is cleanliness.

Washing One of the best ways to protect yourself and your patient against the spread of disease is to wash your hands with a rich lather of soap and water immediately after handling anything—dishes, clothing, bedpans, urinals, bedding, etc.—contaminated or used by your patient. Always wash your hands with soap and plenty of water after going to the toilet yourself. Before handling anything that goes in the mouth, wash your hands!

> NOTE: It is not necessary to use a special germicidal soap for washing your hands unless the doctor or your visiting nurse so orders. It is more important to use enough soap and water, preferably warm to hot, to work up a thick, rich lather. Rub it in between your fingers and up your arms well above the wrists, then rinse thoroughly with warm water. Instead of trying to "kill" the organisms, we wash them off. Our skin could not withstand repeated use of materials that are strong enough to kill many germs or microorganisms.

Wash your patient's dishes, silverware, and cooking utensils in soap or detergent with as hot water as possible, and rinse with boiling water. Most mechanical dishwashers are satisfactory for this work.

Towels See that each person in the family, including your patient and you, has individual, private, no-one-else-use towels and washcloths. Do not under any circumstances allow a "community" hand towel.

Utensils Unless they have been thoroughly washed, never drink from a glass or cup, eat from a dish or with cutlery that someone else has used.

Cuts and Scratches If you have a cut or open wound, or deep scratch, on your hands, wear rubber or plastic gloves when handling your patient or unwashed dishes, cutlery, etc., used by your patient.

House Cleaning When cleaning your patient's room, vacuum the floor—do not use a broom. Broom sweeping stirs the dust, and spreads it and its microorganisms through the air.

If you use a dust mop, make sure it is either damp or has an oily base to hold the dust instead of spreading it through the air.

Dust the furniture with either a damp cloth or one containing a dust-absorbing or holding material.

REMEMBER

Microorganisms are all around us. There are beneficial and there are harmful microorganisms. Unfortunately, we cannot separate them. But with reasonable care and precautions, and good hygienic health habits, we usually can make it extremely difficult, and often impossible, for the disease-producing microorganisms to do their dirty work. Just keep in mind that they won't quit trying, so neither should you!

12 If It's Catching

No matter how mild it seems, if your patient has a disease or sickness (as opposed to surgery, broken bones, burns, etc.), keep in mind that it may be "catching," or communicable to other people, including you. There is no safe disease. Oftentimes the germs (Chapter 11) that cause a mild discomfort in one person may bring serious sickness or even death to another, just as some people can take penicillin safely while others react violently to it. Also, unless you have permanent immunity to a disease there is always the chance that even though you do not get it from one exposure or contact, you may from another. Fortunately, transmission (below) of disease usually can be prevented by taking fairly simple precautions. Different diseases usually have different periods of communicability; some may be a few hours, others much longer periods—days, weeks.

A major basic step in nursing is to find out, if possible, from the doctor (Chapter 4) exactly what disease your patient has, how it is usually transmitted, generally how susceptible other people may be to it, and the precautions to take.

Doctors throughout the United States and many other countries are required by law to report certain diseases to the local, state, or national public health service. Certain diseases must be reported by telephone as soon as the diagnosis is made. Depending on the disease, the degree of danger to the public health, and the number of suspected or proven cases in a community, a representative of the public health department may visit your patient to observe and report the course of the disease and give instructions on how to prevent further transmission of it. When a public health nurse calls, do not feel that you or your patient are being singled out as "spreaders of disease." The calls are made to help protect you and everyone else from getting the disease. Also, these representatives usually are experienced nurses and will gladly give you practical advice on how to make your patient more comfortable, as well as how to prevent spread of the disease.

The most serious aspect of some communicable diseases is that they are commonly in their most infectious state shortly *before* noticeable symptoms appear. Always consult your doctor if someone you have been in close contact with comes down with an infectious disease within 2 or 3 days.

TRANSMISSION

The sooner a patient's symptoms are diagnosed and treatment of a disease is started, the sooner the patient becomes noncommunicable; that is, cannot transmit the disease. In areas having modern medical practices it is seldom necessary to isolate a diseased patient for more than a few days. Antibiotics, vaccines, and immune serums reduce the potency of germs given off by a patient. Today it is the disease itself, rather than the patient, that is isolated. Despite this, diseases still are commonly transmitted by: (1) the air; (2) direct contact; (3) contaminated objects; (4) the fecal-and-oral route; and (5) bites. Many diseases are spread or transmitted by more than one way.

Airborne Transmission Some germs (Chapter 11), such as those causing colds, chickenpox, and flu, travel through the air from infected persons. Fortunately, most airborne germs usually have a fairly short active life; if they do not find a receptive "host" within a few hours, they lose their ability to infect.

> NOTE: Ask the doctor or your visiting nurse if there are certain persons, such as pregnant women, who should be especially careful to avoid exposure to your patient's disease.

The most common airborne transmission of disease is by spreading secretions from the nose and mouth when an infected person sneezes or coughs. The best preventive against transmission is for the infected person to sneeze or cough into a disposable facial tissue held tight against the nostrils and mouth; after use, fold the outer edges of the tissue in over the middle portion to cover it, and deposit in a wastebasket or bedside sack (Chapter 8). If instead of a tissue a patient sneezes or coughs into a handkerchief, there is a chance that the germs may live in it and later infect whoever prepares it for laundering. Holding a hand instead of a tissue or a handkerchief over the nose or mouth when sneezing or coughing merely deflects the flow of germs from the nose or mouth to a different direction.

Most wise people try to avoid the direct blast of a patient's cough or sneeze. But they do not realize that airborne germs may be given off by normal breathing. For this reason, you should keep all unnecessary persons away from your patient during the communicable period.

The only sure defense against most airborne diseases is to keep away from an infected person during the contagious or communicable period. Since you, the nurse, cannot do this, be sure to ask the doctor or your visiting nurse what special protective steps you should take, such as immune serum, antibiotics, gamma globulin, etc.

Transmission by Direct Contact Some diseases are transmitted by direct contact or touch with the mucous membrane of an infected person. Gonorrhea and syphilis usually are transmitted by some sort of sexual contact. However, they and many other infectious diseases can be transmitted through an open cut, scratch, or sore in the recipient's body; in some cases infected mucous fluid or blood has inadvertently been rubbed or brushed into a doctor's eye or cut and transmitted a disease.

As a rule, as long as your hands have no open scratches, cuts, or sores you can touch your patient safely, regardless of an infectious disease. Under certain conditions you should wear disposable plastic gloves (Chapter 8), and discard them after one use. Ask the doctor or your visiting nurse what steps to take to prevent transmission of your patient's disease.

Transmission by Contaminated Objects It is a generally accepted fact that a great number of diseases can be—and are!—transmitted by contaminated objects, such as articles freshly soiled by discharges or the saliva of an infected person.

Why so many people, those in the medical profession as well as others, are so careless is hard to understand. But they will drink from the same glass or cup . . . use the same towel, washcloth, or bar of soap . . . eat with the same utensils and from the same dishes used by someone with a communicable disease. In many cases, thorough cleansing with soap or detergent and hot water removes contamination from an object. But because even the most expert cleansing cannot be fully trusted, reusable hypodermic needles have been abandoned by modern medical practice; instead, disposable needles and syringes are used.

> NOTE: Serum hepatitis is most commonly transmitted by dirty hypodermic needles, common household needles and pins, small eye droppers, and syringes and other items used to cut into a vein and inject narcotics.

As well as objects, certain insects can become contaminated and transmit disease. The household fly is notorious for spreading germs. However, unless it settles on an open sore, scratch, cut, or other wound shortly after becoming contaminated, it cannot spread most of the diseases transmitted by direct contact (above).

Satisfactory cleansing and, in certain cases, destruction are the ways to prevent transmission of disease by contaminated objects. The ideal method is to burn all objects—utensils, towels, bedding, etc.—that a patient has used, and in some cases it may be necessary. But as a rule thorough washing with hot water (60° C / 140° F), a strong soap or detergent, and a bleach is sufficient. Modern home laundry and dishwashing machines usually are adequate for the work.

If bed linen is stained with blood or body secretions, soak it first in cold water for about 30 minutes to prevent setting the stain by washing in hot water. Before washing, work soap or detergent into stains that remain after the soaking.

If bed linen is heavily soiled, soak it for 10 minutes in hot water containing approximately 300 cu. cc./1 fl. oz./2 tbsp. of bleach per l./gal. of water. Then launder the usual way.

For best results in thorough cleaning with the least damage to perishable articles, such as bedding, ask an experienced nurse. Be specific as to the materials involved, such as cotton, wool, or acrylic blankets, and plastic or ceramic dishes. A method of cleaning that might not harm an acrylic blanket, for example, possibly could ruin a woolen one.

Fecal-and-Oral Transmission The fecal-and-oral transmission of sickness is the easiest one to prevent, yet happens far too often. In nearly all cases it is due to carelessness.

In a hurry to finish a disagreeable task, or perhaps tired from unaccustomed work, the nurse takes the bedpan from a patient, empties and cleans it (Chapter 8), and rinses hands to mark the end of the job. *Rinses*, not washes. If there were infectious germs on the bedpan, which is always a probability, some of them quite likely spread to the nurse's hands to be transmitted to everything the nurse touches—clothing, dishes, food, and so forth. Since foods in general stimulate the growth and reproduction of germs, shortly after infection by the germs coming from the patient feces, the food becomes essentially a poison that may cause a fatal sickness. Yet all this could have been prevented by the nurse's spending a few minutes at the washbasin (below).

Whether you have to clean a patient after using a bedpan is not an important point. The simple act of handling a bedpan, of touching it, is enough for germs in the patient's feces to spread to your hands. True, it does not always happen, even with the most contagious diseases. But it can happen at any time. So never take a chance! The moment you have finished cleaning a bedpan, wash your hands.

NOTE: For general safety everyone, sick or not, should wash their hands thoroughly with warm water and soap or detergent after each urination or bowel movement.

Washing Hands No special brand or type of soap or detergent is needed for good, preventive washing of hands. The amount of soap lather and scrubbing used is more important than the kind of soap. The warmer the water is, the better, but it should not be uncomfortably hot. To wash, wet the hands well, then work up a good lather with soap or detergent. Work it in between all the fingers, on the front and back of both hands, and up the arms to above the wrists, spending at least 1 minute in this process. Then rinse off all lather and dry hands carefully with a clean, or your own, towel. *Make it a strict rule in your home or wherever you are nursing a patient that no one ever uses anybody else's towels*!

Strict observance of the above method of washing and drying hands by all members of a family or household will do much to prevent the spread of disease there.

Transmission by Bite Diseases that are classed as being transmitted by bite are not contagious except by a bite or through a break in the skin.

DON'T BE A TRANSMITTER!

Depending on how a disease may be transmitted, the simple act of being with and handling someone having a communicable disease makes you, the nurse, a potential transmitter. By practicing the ways of preventing transmission of germs (above), you can greatly reduce the chance of spreading disease. However, you have been exposed to it and generally should avoid close contact with other people during the first 3 or 4 days of your patient's sickness. During the time that your patient's sickness is known to be communicable:

1. If you must mingle with other people, dress and groom yourself after you have completed the handling of your patient for the time being.
2. Wear a nurse's gown, such as a smock, cobbler's apron, or coverall apron over your clothes while caring for your patient. After washing your hands and before leaving your patient's room, remove the gown and hang it on a hanger inside the room. The gown protects your clothing and lessens the chance of carrying your patient's disease germs to other people in the household.

13 Making the Bed

Making a bed while a patient occupies it is not necessarily difficult, and usually may be done by one person unassisted. However, if your patient is able to help with the task, encourage it in every way.

The main difference between regular home beds and those made for sick people is that the latter usually have waterproof sheets and draw sheets.

When selecting bedding for your patient, use a variety of colored or decorated sheets, pillowcases, and bedspreads when possible. They break the monotony of seeing one color day after day, and create a more cheerful atmosphere. Also, bright white bedding can cause tiring light glare and reflection.

BEDDING AND MATTRESSES

The items most commonly used for sickbeds are listed below and described in Chapter 8. Articles that usually are needed only in special cases are treated in chapters relating to those cases, or you will be given all the necessary information by your patient's doctor, physical therapist, or visiting nurse.

In Chapter 8 see:

Bed
Bed Padding
Bed Sheets
Bed Springs
Bedboard
Bedding Frames
Bedspread
Blankets
Draw Sheet
Mattress
Mattress Cover
Mattress Pad
Pillow
Pillowcases
Quilts
Water Beds, Mattresses, and Pads
Waterproof Sheeting

GENERAL PREPARATION FOR MAKING BEDS

A bed is made basically the same way whether it is empty or occupied. It is, of course, much easier to do when empty; and if allowed by the doctor, a patient should be out of the bed, even for a short time.

Patients who can take tub or shower baths unassisted should do so now. Those who must be bathed in bed usually are bathed after you have removed the bedspread and blankets. Others, depending on their condition, should be made comfortable in a chair or on a cot or couch either in the bedroom or, preferably, in a nearby room. The change of scenery, even if only for a short time, usually is beneficial. Be sure your patient is comfortably warm during this time.

Room Temperature Bring the bedroom to a comfortable temperature, 22°–24° C/72°–76° F, either by heating or by air conditioning. It may be slightly warmer than normal for your home. Depending on the time of year, weather, and your home, a bed patient may become accustomed to a "body and bed" heat that is well above room temperature; an abrupt change to a lower temperature could make the patient quite uncomfortable and perhaps cause a chill. For extra safeguard against low room heat, help your patient into a warm bathrobe or dressing gown while getting out of bed. If your patient sits in a chair, drape a lightweight blanket around the legs. If your patient lies on a sofa or couch, cover with a light blanket or quilt.

Cleaning Room cleaning should be done after the bed has been changed, as the process of remaking a bed always creates some dust.

As a rule it is best to dust, vacuum clean, sweep, and do any other cleaning, changing of flowers, or watering of plants, while your patient is out of the room. But if your daily time with your patient is limited and your patient enjoys your company, making the clean-up time into a sort of special visit will be good for both of you.

Bedding Place two chairs, or a chair and a laundry bag, convenient to the bed for holding bedding. The less walking and reaching you need do while making a bed, the better. One chair is for fresh bedding and items that will be reused. The other chair, or laundry bag, is for bedding that will not be reused. The floor is the dirtiest part of a room; placing used bedding on a chair or in a laundry bag prevents needless soiling of it.

GENERAL HANDLING OF BEDDING

Whether making or changing a bed, do not flip, fling, or toss any bedding either off or onto it. Instead, fold the fresh bedding and articles to be reused and place them on the chair in proper sequence. Fold or carefully gather up the other bedding and place it on the soiled-bedding chair or in the laundry bag. Handle bedding gently to avoid the stirring up of dust, dirt, and germs that usually happens when large, billowy articles are flipped, flung, or tossed around.

Holding Bedding Handle bedding as little as possible, and hold it well away from yourself, to minimize transfer of germs or soil from used bedding to you and your clothing and from you to the fresh bedding.

When removing soiled linen from a bed, immediately place it in the laundry container or on the soiled-bedding chair. After making the bed, cleaning the room, and so forth, remove the soiled bedding.

Sequence of Bedding Simplify the work of bed making by placing linens, blankets, etc., on the chair in their order of use: bedspread on the seat, then the pillowcases, blankets, top sheet, draw sheet, waterproof sheet, bottom sheet, mattress pad, and mattress cover if any.

Fold Bedding To simplify work and lessen the spreading of soil, dust, and germs, fold all bedding except pillowcases. Fold fresh linen as you take it from the dryer, clothesline, or laundry bundle. Fold bedspreads, blankets, sheets (top, draw, waterproof, bottom), and mattress pads and covers while removing them from a bed unless they are to be changed; in that case simply pick them up and place them on the soiled-bedding chair or in the laundry container. Mattress pads and covers, however, usually are not removed when changing a bed unless they are to be laundered, or the mattress is to be turned or cleaned.

The two methods of folding bedding are the so-called *short* and *long*. Folding should be neat but need not be precise, as it is done to simplify the handling of bedding and does not affect the patient.

Short or Crosswise Fold. In short or crosswise folding, the bedding is first folded the short way of the width, or crosswise, as in Fig. 13–1*a*. The second fold, *b*, simply makes a smaller package. Except for draw and waterproof sheets (Chapter 8), the short fold is suitable only for making an unoccupied bed. However, other than for your convenience, it is not necessary to refold linen before putting it on an unoccupied bed.

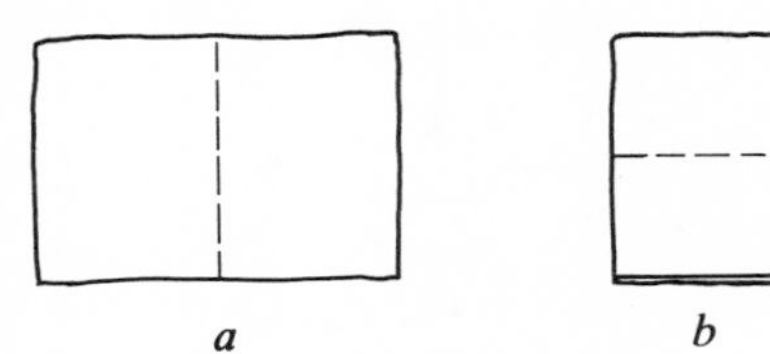

Fig. 13–1*a, b* *"Short" fold of bedding*

Long or Lengthwise Fold. For long or lengthwise folding, first fold the bedding the long way, as in Fig. 8–18. The second fold is to make a smaller package. The long fold must be used for making an occupied bed, and may be used for an unoccupied one.

Plan your folding so that the "right" side or surface of a sheet or bedspread, which is the smooth side of the hems at the ends, will be properly placed when you make the bed:

Bottom Sheet. Right side up, to prevent a patient's feet from rubbing on the rough side of the hem at the foot of the bed if the sheet comes loose. If you are reusing the top sheet as the bottom sheet when remaking a bed, it should be folded as it is removed from the bed.

Top Sheet. Right side down, so that when the top sheet is folded back near the head of the bed, the patient's hands and arms will not rub on the rough side of the hem.

Bedspreads. Right side up, usually for the sake of appearance.

MAKING THE UNOCCUPIED BED

You may of course make an unoccupied bed any way you want. However, most people find that the method given here saves steps, time, and work. If you are making up a hospital-type, adjustable bed, first set it flat and at a convenient height, usually at your waist.

Mattress Pad Except for the unfolding, *short* and *long* folded mattress pads and covers are handled basically the same way, the cover being installed first:

1. *Place the folded corner* at the middle of the bed, as in Fig. 13–2*a*. A folded package of bedding usually is first placed over an upper quarter of the mattress, since most people find it easier to work from the head toward the foot of a bed. When installing a boxed mattress pad (Chapter 8), tuck the boxing in place around the corner of the quarter being worked, and draw it tight and smooth along both sides of the corner.

2. *If using short-folded bedding*, draw it across the width of the bed or cover the other top quarter, as in Fig. 13–2*b*, then unfold it toward the foot, as in *d*. When installing a boxed mattress pad, after opening it across the width of a bed, tighten it smoothly along the head and tuck the boxing in place around the corner, drawing it tight and smooth along both sides. After completely unfolding the pad, tuck the boxing in place at the foot, and work it smooth throughout the surface of the mattress.

3. *If using long-folded bedding*, draw it down the length of the bed to cover that side from head to foot, as in Fig. 13–2*c*, then unfold it across the bed as

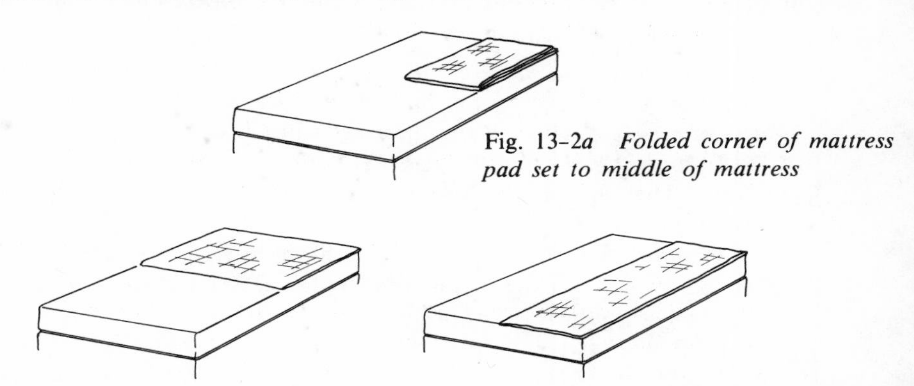

Fig. 13–2*a* *Folded corner of mattress pad set to middle of mattress*

Fig. 13–2*b* *"Short" fold pad opened across mattress*

Fig. 13–2*c* *"Long" fold pad opened to foot of mattress*

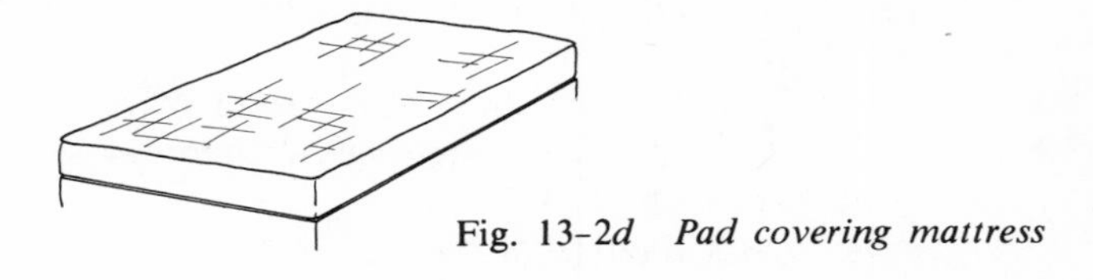

Fig. 13–2*d* *Pad covering mattress*

Fig. 13–2 *Basic plan for placing folded bedding*

in *d*. When using a boxed mattress pad, after opening it for the length of the bed, tuck the boxing under the mattress at both sides of the lower corner, working it tight and smooth on both sides. After completely opening the pad, tuck the boxing in place along the second side and at the head and foot, and work it smooth throughout the surface of the mattress.

4. *If using an unboxed mattress pad*, work as in Steps 1 and 2 or 3 above, but align the edges of the pad with those of the mattress throughout. If there are corner loops, tuck them under the corners of the mattress. The bottom sheet should hold an unboxed pad in place satisfactorily, although you may have to reposition the pad while installing the sheet.

Bottom Sheet The tighter a bottom sheet is installed, the smoother it will stay and the more comfortable your patient will be, especially if there is no draw sheet. Many experienced nurses prefer flat to fitted bottom sheets, provided the flat sheets are long enough and wide enough for ample tuck-in and tightening.

Fitted Bottom Sheet Install a fitted bottom sheet the same way as a boxed mattress pad. Since a fitted bottom sheet cannot be tightened as satisfactorily to the sides of a bed as a flat sheet, a draw sheet is advisable if your patient is confined to bed for more than about 8 hours a day.

Flat Bottom Sheet After a few times, you probably will make the bottom sheet smooth and tight enough while putting it on the bed so that going back over your work will not be necessary. Although the sheet may be folded either the short or the long way, folding it the long way (Fig. 8–18) gives you the convenience of doing all the work on one side of a bed before the other. The flat bottom sheet usually is installed with square corners:

1. *Place the folded sheet on the bed* with the fold corner at the middle, as in Fig. 13–2*a*. Depending on the sizes of the sheet and mattress, it may or may not overhang the sides of the mattress equally.

2. *Unfold the sheet package lengthwise* to cover the foot edge of the mattress. Then adjust the sheet between head and foot according to the type of bed:

Hospital Bed. For an adjustable hospital-type bed, allow at least 31 cm./12 in. of sheet for tucking under the mattress at the head of the bed. This is to keep the sheet from "crawling" as the head of the bed is raised and lowered, and as the patient moves about.

Nonhospital Bed. For a nonadjustable bed, distribute the amount of sheet at head and foot so that there is enough to tuck under the mattress at both ends. Equal amounts generally are best.

3. *Tuck the sheet under the mattress* at the head of the bed without pulling it away from the foot.

4. *Make a square corner* at the head of the bed, Fig. 13–3:

a *Hold the edge of the sheet* straight out to the side from the top edge of the head of the bed.

b *Draw the fold* of the extended sheet along the top edge of the side of the mattress.

c *Tuck the lower corner edge* of the hanging sheet, *b*, under the corner of the mattress just far enough to hold it securely in place.

d *Draw the fold of sheet* along the top of the side of the mattress down over the side.

e *Tuck the sheet hanging over the side* at the corner under the mattress as far as possible. Work the sheet smooth and tight in place on the side of the mattress without dislodging it on the top surface or at the head of the bed.

5. *On the same side of the bed*, tuck the sheet under the mattress at the foot. Without dislodging the sheet at the head, work it tight (see *Tightening a Sheet*, below) and as smooth as you can toward the foot when tucking it under the mattress. Then make a square corner as in 4 above.

6. *Tuck the side middle section* of the sheet under the mattress as far as possible, working it smooth.

7. *Go to opposite side of bed* and repeat steps 3–6 inclusive.

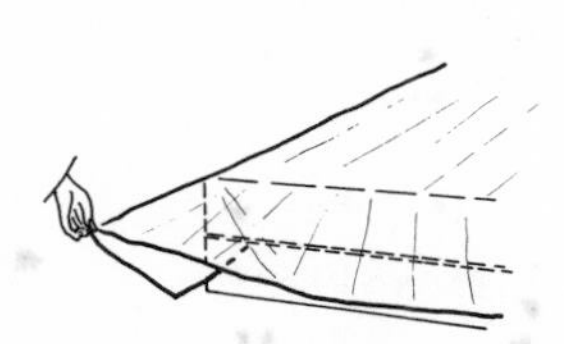

Fig. 13–3*a* *First step in making square corner*

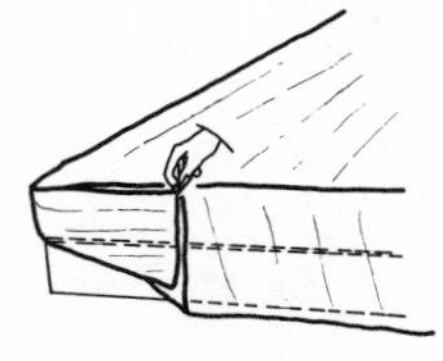

Fig. 13–3*b* *Second step*

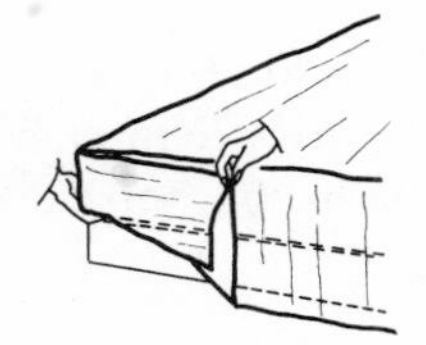

Fig. 13–3*c* *Third step*

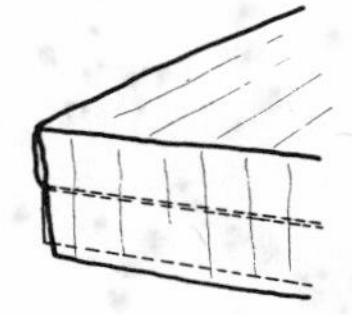

Fig. 13–3*d* *Fourth step*

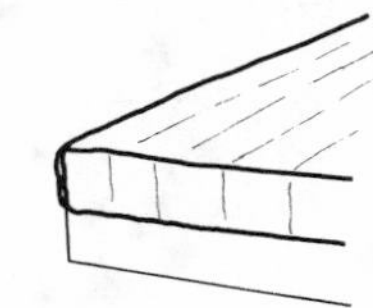

Fig. 13–3*e* *Completed corner*

Fig. 13–3 *The square bedding corner*

Tightening a Sheet Working a sheet so that it will stay tight in place for a reasonable length of time takes skill, not just strength. As in Fig. 13–4, with your hands any convenient distance apart, usually 31–45 cm./12–18 in., grasp the edge of the sheet, palms down, and loosely roll or crumple it up to about 10 cm./4 in. from the upper edge of the mattress, and pull it toward you. Pull hard enough to make the top surface smooth and tight, but not hard or far enough to dislodge the sheet between the corners of the bed; the warp or weft threads between corners should be straight. Then work the grasped sheet down and against the side of the mattress, shifting your grasp, without letting go of the sheet, to where you can lift the bottom of the mattress and push the sheet under it. Push the sheet in under the

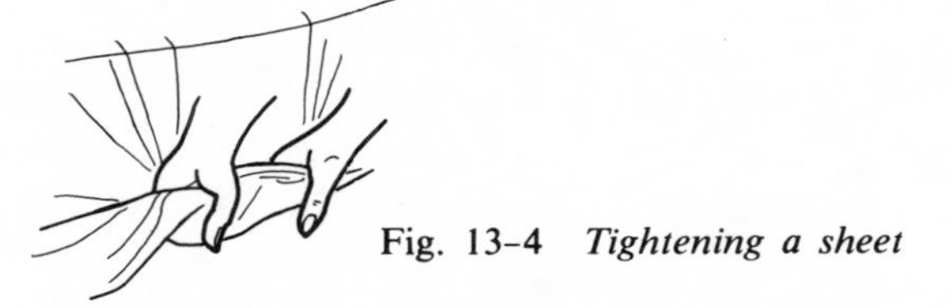

Fig. 13–4 *Tightening a sheet*

mattress as far as possible. The tighter you set the sheet against the side of the mattress, the better it will be held in place by the top edge of the mattress. While working the sheet in under the mattress, let it pull out of your grasp.

Waterproof Sheet A waterproof sheet (Chapter 8) covers the bed from side to side on top of the bottom sheet, as in Fig. 8–27. Installation is simple and fast:

1. *Fold the sheet in half the short way*, Fig. 13–1*a*, and place it on the bottom sheet with the folded edge midway between the sides of the bed. Move it toward the head or foot of the bed enough to lie within the area that will be covered by the draw sheet. Work the waterproof sheet smooth.
2. *Tuck an end of the waterproof sheet* under the mattress and push it as far as you can toward the far side of the bed without dislodging it on the top surface.
3. *Draw the waterproof sheet into place* on the other side of the bed and, keeping it smooth, tighten it the same as a bottom sheet.

Draw Sheet A draw sheet, installed the same as a waterproof sheet, completely covers the latter. A draw sheet may be used without a waterproof sheet, but the latter must always be covered by a draw sheet.

Top Sheet At the foot of a bed the top sheet must be tight enough to stay in place, yet loose enough for patient foot protection and comfort (Chapter 17). Depending on a patient's disability and probable length of time in bed, top sheets often are installed over a bedding frame (Chapter 8).

Fitted Top Sheet Fitted top sheets are not favored by most experienced nurses because they restrict a patient's feet, may cause bedsores (Chapter 15), and usually do not fit well over a bedding frame.

Flat Top Sheet Install the top sheet and other bedding across the foot of a bed before "locking" it in place by making the "corners." Before installing the top sheet, set the bedding frame, if any, securely in place. If a large bedding frame is used, it may be necessary to use two sheets for adequate coverage, staggering or overlapping them as necessary. To install a top sheet:

1. *Place the folded sheet on the bed* with the fold corner at the middle of it, as in Fig. 13–2*a*.
2. *Unfold the sheet package lengthwise*, passing it over the bedding frame, if any, to the foot of the bed. Align the other end of the sheet with the edge of the mattress at the head of the bed; as a rule this allows enough sheet for

adequate turndown over the blanket and bedspread. You may allow more sheet for turndown, but be sure to leave enough at the foot of the bed for satisfactory tuck-in under the mattress; the more tuck-in, the better the sheet will stay in place.

3. *Tuck the sheet in under the mattress* at the foot of the bed. Tuck it in as far as possible without dislodging it at the head of the bed or displacing or bending the bedding frame. At the same time, work the sheet smooth from side to side. There should be equal overhangs at the sides of the bed.

Blanket Install blankets the same way as flat top sheets except for placement at the head of the bed. There a blanket usually is set to cover a patient's shoulders, but of course may be set at whatever height your patient wants.

The "corners" may or may not be made after installing blankets. It depends on the bedspread.

Bedspread Install a bedspread or blanket cover the same way as a flat top sheet except:

1. *Placement at foot of bed.* Some bedspreads are made to hang down around a bed instead of being tucked under the mattress at the foot. Tucking under is generally considered the better way of installing a bedspread, but not enough better to make it worth spoiling a bedspread or its appearance.

2. *Placement at head of bed.* Ideally, the end of a bedspread aligns with the end of the blanket at the head of a bed, and the top sheet is turned down over them. However, many bedspreads are designed to cover the pillow at the head. These spreads really are too long for conventional sickbed use. But if it is a plain, lightweight bedspread it may be folded back smoothly at the end of the blanket.

Envelope Corner Envelope corners are made for the top bedding to hold it in place securely without pressing down on a patient's feet. All the top bedding—sheet, blanket, and bedspread if it is tucked under the mattress—are jointly made into the corner, as in Fig. 13–5:

a *Hold the edges of the top bedding* straight out from the top surface at the corner of the foot of the bed, X, and at Y, which is as far from X as X is from the corner of the mattress.

b *Draw the side edge of the bedding* at Y up and over the top of the bed, and lay it down on the top surface at a point that makes the edge of the bedding parallel with the end of the bed, as in *c*. While doing this, hold the covered bedding on the top surface in place along the edge of the bed. The bedding hanging over the side of the bed near the foot should reach to about 15 cm./6 in. below the bottom of the mattress.

NOTE: If making a bed with a bedding frame, you will have to experiment with the placement of Y to make the edge of the bedding parallel with the foot of the bed.

c *Tuck the corner of the bedding* hanging below the mattress under it. Tuck it as far under the mattress as possible without dislodging the bedding drawn up and over the top of the bed. While tucking it in place, slide it toward the head to tighten it. The tighter the bedding is under the mattress, the better the corner will hold.

d Draw the side edge of the bedding, Y, down over the side of the bed and let it hang free. While doing this hold the bedding above the tuck-in (as indicated by the dash lines) in place along the side of the mattress.

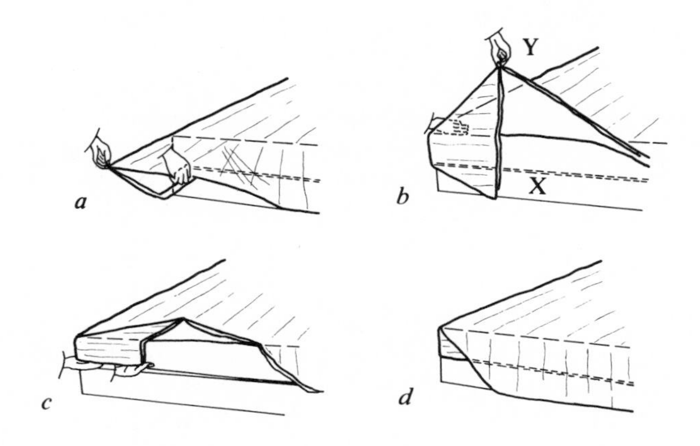

Fig. 13–5*a, b, c, d* *Envelope corner for bedding*

Loosening Bedding for the Feet If the top bedding is not installed over a bedding frame, it may not be loose enough to prevent pressure on the feet that can cause bedsores. To loosen bedding, grasp it—bedspread, blanket, sheet—midway between the sides of a bed and about 31 cm./12 in. from the foot. Pull the bedding straight up as much as is necessary to provide free movement for your patient's feet. Do not pull bedding up near the corners; they may come loose and let drafts of cold air into the bed.

Fan-Folding Bedding To make it easier for a patient to get into bed, the top bedding may be fan-folded toward the foot, as diagrammed in Fig. 13–6:

1. *To fan-fold*, pick up all top bedding—bedspread, blanket, sheet—at a point about one-third of the way from the sheet fold near the head of the bed to the foot. Draw the bedding down over itself to the foot.
2. *To replace fan-folded bedding*, grasp the top end at the sheet fold and draw it over your patient.

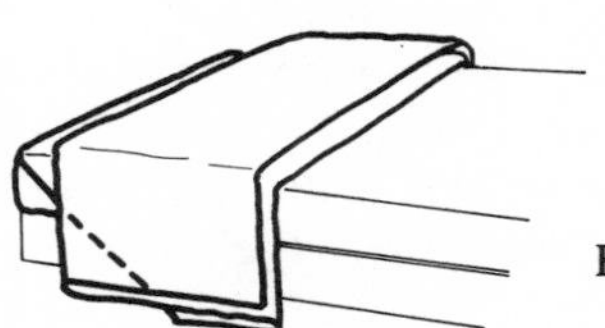

Fig. 13–6 *Fan-folded bedding*

Encasing Pillows There are several ways to cover a pillow with a pillowcase. A fast, simple method is:

1. *With the pillowcase right side out*, grasp the seam at the closed end with one hand.
2. *Turn the pillowcase inside out* over the hand grasping the closed end.
3. *Through the seam at the closed end* of the pillowcase firmly grasp an end of the pillow.
4. *Draw the pillowcase out over the pillow.*
5. *Work the corners of the pillow* into those of the case, and align the edges of the pillow with the side seam and crease in the case.
6. *If a pillow does not fill the case*, place the intended upper surface of the encased pillow down on the bed or other flat surface. Work a long side of the pillow against the corresponding side of the case. Draw the excess case out beyond the other long side of the pillow, and tuck it between the other casing and the pillow; tuck it in far enough to make the case fit tight around the pillow. Turn the encased pillow over carefully and place it as wanted on the bed. Although this method of fitting a too large case to a pillow does work, it is temporary at best. For long-term use, a case of the proper size should be obtained.
7. *Plumping up a pillow* after encasing it sometimes is needed to make it fill the pillowcase evenly. Point the open end of the pillowcase downward when plumping, to direct any blowout of dust or germs toward the floor and not at your patient or the freshly made bed.

MAKING THE OCCUPIED BED

Throughout making an occupied bed, your main consideration should be your patient's comfort and the prevention of exposure. Do the usual preparatory work. If your patient cannot leave the bed, assemble the necessary bathing materials (Chapter 23) and clean bed linen. Give the bath after removing the bedspread and blanket and replacing the top sheet with a Bath Blanket (Chapter 8). Keep your patient covered by the bath blanket as much as possible throughout bathing. In chilly weather or when bathing will be somewhat slow, another blanket on top of the bath blanket may be needed to keep from chilling your patient.

After the Bath After a bath, your patient should be dressed in a fresh bedgown or pajamas. Then assemble the bedding on a chair the usual way. Next, move or help your patient move from the middle of the bed toward the side that you plan to remake last.

To move a helpless patient for remaking a bed, stand at the side of the bed that you plan to remake last and, with a hand around the point of the patient's shoulder and the other hand on the hip, as in Fig. 13–7, gently roll the patient toward you to just your side of the middle of the bed.

Cover your patient, helpless or not, with a bath blanket to prevent possible chilling. If the bath blanket used during your patient's bath is dry, it may be used again.

If your patient is irrational or tends to move about carelessly, set the guardrail in place on the side of the bed nearer your patient if you have a hospital-type bed. For any other bed, set the back of a chair against the side to act as a temporary guardrail, or station someone there to hold the patient if necessary.

Remaking the Occupied Bed Except for the positioning of some of the bedding, and the fact that you should completely remake one side of the bed before starting the other, there is little difference between making occupied and unoccupied beds. The main advantage of remaking an occupied bed as given here is that it requires the least disturbance of or movement by your patient:

1. *Loosen* the draw, waterproof, and bottom sheets (and mattress pad and cover if they are to be changed) on the unoccupied side of the bed. Fold or roll each item separately, starting with the draw sheet, close to the patient. Since the old draw sheet will not be removed until remaking the other side of the occupied bed, it cannot be used as the new bottom sheet.
2. *Install the fresh* mattress cover and pad, if any, and the bottom, waterproof, and draw sheets basically the same way as on an unoccupied bed. If the old top sheet is to be used as the new bottom sheet, first cover your patient with the new top sheet. Then reach under it and pull the old top sheet to the foot of the bed and remove it. Fold it lengthwise and install it the usual way for a bottom sheet.
3. *Fold or roll each item* of fresh bedding separately—first the mattress cover and pad, if any, then the bottom, waterproof, and draw sheets—against your patient and press them as flat as possible.
4. *Move*, as in Fig. 13-7, or help your patient move over the folded bedding to the remade side of the bed. Keep your patient covered by the bath blanket. If needed, set the real or substitute guardrail in place on the side of the bed now nearer the patient.

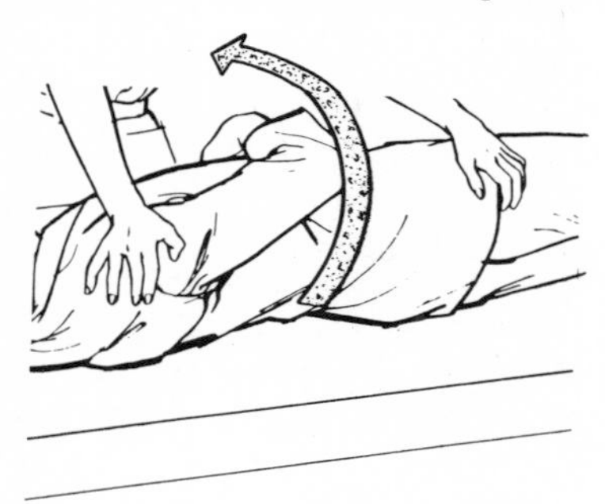

Fig. 13-7 *Moving a bed patient for remaking the bed*

5. *Remove all bedding* that will not be used.
6. *Complete installing* the mattress cover and pad, if any, and the bottom, waterproof, and draw sheets on the now unoccupied side of the bed. Tighten them the usual way from side to side to provide a smooth surface for your patient to lie on.

7. *Move* or help your patient move to the middle of the bed, then install the top bedding and pillows the usual way as for an unoccupied bed.

8. *Be sure to loosen* the top bedding to protect your patient's feet against bedsores.

AFTER MAKING A BED

After making a bed and helping your patient settle in it comfortably, remove all soiled linen for laundering. Then clean the room. To minimize the spread of dust, floors should be vacuum cleaned thoroughly, and furniture should be dusted with a damp cloth.

14 How to Move Your Patient Safely—for Both of You!

Patients who cannot move themselves must be moved or their positions changed at least every 2 hours. It is essential for their general well-being, and for the prevention of bedsores (Chapter 15).

The most important part of moving a patient is to do it safely for both of you. *Do not* jar or jolt your patient in any way. *Do not* drop your patient, even an inch or less, onto a bed, chair, or couch. *Do not* hold, press, or grasp your patient on a tender, sensitive, or painful area. *Do not* push your patient. When it is necessary to lift, pull, or slide your patient, do it with as little dragging or stretching of any part of the body as possible.

At the same time, take care not to strain yourself, especially your back—your patient needs you! With the use of easy-to-learn *body mechanics*, you should be able to move your patient safely for both of you. Doing it the correct way, you may move bed patients weighing up to twice as much as you. Most patients can and will cooperate in being moved; encourage it, provided it does not tax their strength.

You may or may not need assistance in moving your patient. When you do, be sure to show your assistant in advance exactly what to do and how to do it.

Although it need not be, *lifting* a patient often is hazardous for both the patient and the inexperienced nurse. This is due to lifting that should not be done, and to incorrect lifting. In both cases, the patient can suffer a serious fall, and the nurse can be permanently injured.

You can avoid the lifting that you should not do by being helped by an assistant or by a mechanical aid, as experienced nurses regularly are. Without an assistant or a mechanical aid, do not try to lift a patient who is heavier or taller than you . . . or one who is unable to help with being lifted . . . or a quadriplegic (one who has no use of arms and legs). For some paraplegics (patients with paralysis of a side of the body or of both legs), a mechanical lift can be most helpful, especially for those who do not have enough arm strength to move themselves. There are several kinds of mechanical lifts, below. Most are easy to operate, but should not be used without practice supervised by an experienced nurse. The doctor or your visiting nurse can advise you as to the type of mechanical lift best for your patient.

Most people who lift incorrectly do so simply because they do not know and apply *body mechanics.*

BODY MECHANICS

Body mechanics is the science or art of using your arms, legs, and back to lift, push, press, or pull objects without harmful stress or strain to yourself. There is a correct or safe way to perform every nursing care task. Sometimes there is more than one proper way; use whichever you find easier and more convenient. The methods of moving patients given in this chapter are based on good body mechanics; you probably will find them helpful for moving other objects.

Practice each of the following applications of body mechanics several times with a pillow before moving your patient. How you move and handle your patient is more important than the weight or size of your patient. You can sprain your back lifting a 10-pound sack of potatoes, or move a 200-pound patient safely—depending on your body mechanics. Applying the principles of body mechanics to moving your patient will give you confidence in your ability to do it safely, and the less chance there will be of harming your patient.

Lifting Most *lifting* injuries affect the muscles, nerves, and ligaments of the lower portion of the back, can be extremely painful, and usually are slow to heal. Recovery often takes several years and may never be truly complete. It is not difficult to injure your back by lifting. Keep your legs fairly straight and lean over until you can pick up an article, as in Fig. 14–1*a*, then force your back muscles to pull you up fairly straight, *b*; incidentally, the farther you hold a picked-up article away from your body, the greater the strain on your back. You can achieve the same result—an injured back—through putting down an article by bending over.

The safe way to lift an article, whether it is on the floor, Fig. 14–1*c*, or higher, is to squat down far enough to grasp it essentially without bending your back and, keeping your back straight and holding the article close to you, *d*, stand up. The work of lifting or putting down an article is done with your hips and knees, both of

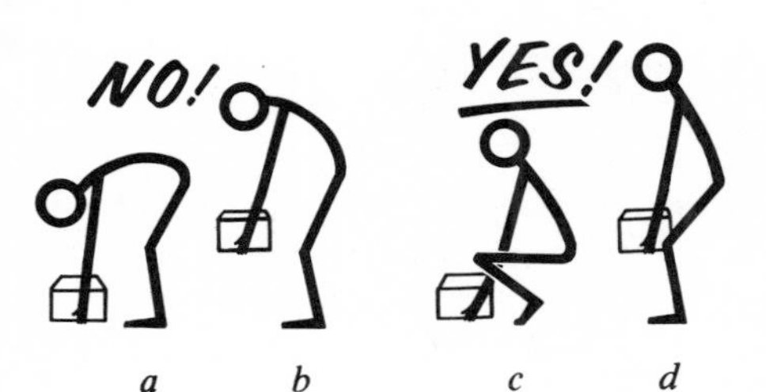

Fig. 14–1*a* *Bending over at small of back to lift article*

Fig. 14–1*b* *Straightening up from Fig. 14–1a*

Fig. 14–1*c* *Squatting to lift article*

Fig. 14–1*d* *Lifting with legs from Fig. 14–1c, keeping back straight*

Fig. 14–1 *Wrong and right ways of lifting*

which are continually used for lifting with every step you take. Of course, you will bend your back to some extent; but the straighter you keep it, the less chance there is of a lifting injury. Practice the proper way of lifting by squatting down and standing up several times without bending your back.

Whether your patient is down low or at chest height, always lift any part of the body other than a hand, foot, or the head by squatting down as far as necessary, setting your hands and arms in place to lift, then standing up by straightening your legs. Of course, in some cases the "squat" is only a slight bending of the knees. Regardless, keep your back as straight as you can at all times.

Pushing Never push a patient away from you. Always move or "pull" your patient toward you.

Pulling Pulling or moving a patient toward you is basically much the same as the method of lifting. Squat down to the proper height or level for moving your patient, and with your arms draw or pull the patient toward you. Keep your back as straight as possible throughout.

The so-called trick of the trade for safely pulling or moving a patient who cannot move without assistance is: do not try to move the whole body at once! First move one part, then an adjacent part; for example, first move the head and shoulders, next the trunk and hips, then the legs and feet.

Carrying Generally you should not try to carry a patient other than a child by yourself.

Children For mutual safety, you should not try to carry by yourself a child that you cannot readily lift from a bed, chair, or couch. Treat these children as adults. If a child is small, light, and passive enough for you to carry safely:

1. Squat down beside your patient to the proper height or level for lifting.
2. Slip an arm under the child's neck and opposite shoulder, and your other arm under the thighs about midway between the buttocks and knees.
3. Keeping your knees bent and back straight, pull or move the child close to your chest. Move your upper arm and shoulder to act as a rest for your patient's head, if possible; otherwise, temporarily remove your other arm from under the patient's thighs and position the head against your upper arm and shoulder.
4. Grasping the child firmly under the shoulders and thighs, stand up by straightening your legs, and walk to where you will deposit your patient. Depending on how heavy the child is, carrying may be more comfortable and easier for you if you lean backward slightly to put the weight on more or less a straight line of pressure down through your hips and knees.
5. To put a child down, simply reverse the process of lifting it. Squat or bend your knees as much as necessary to place your patient on the receiving bed, chair, or couch safely. Then withdraw your arms. Step to the other side of the bed, etc., and move or pull your patient safely back from the far edge to the desired position.

Adults For the safety of your patient and you, an adult should be carried by at least two people; more are often needed for very heavy patients. Since this procedure requires careful placements of the carriers' arms and good coordination or teamwork throughout, ask your visiting nurse for detailed instructions and, if possible, supervision before attempting it. Basically, the method of carrying adult patients is:

1. You and your assistants squat down beside the patient to the proper height or level for lifting.
2. You and your assistants slip your arms under the patient at enough places between the head and feet to give adequate and comfortable support. These places are usually at the patient's neck and shoulders, at the waist, the thighs about midway between buttocks and knees, and the ankles. However, if your patient's head must be supported, one carrier will have to support it and the shoulders, and the other the waist and between the buttocks and knees. If you have two assistants, one may be assigned to support the head.
3. Keeping your knees bent and backs straight, move or pull the patient close to your chests.
4. Hold your patient firmly, stand up by straightening your legs, and walk to where you will deposit your patient. Depending on the patient's weight, carrying may be easier and more comfortable if you and your assistants lean backward slightly to put the weight on a nearly straight line of pressure down through your hips and knees.
5. Put your patient down by reversing the lifting procedure. After withdrawing your arms, leave an assistant at the edge of the bed, chair, or couch to keep the patient from accidentally falling off. Step to the other side of the bed, etc., and pull or move your patient safely back from the far edge.

LET YOUR PATIENT HELP

Sick people who are physically able should be encouraged to help in being moved. Most of them want to help and feel better for doing so; also, the more they help, the safer and easier the moving usually is. Even those who are quite weak generally can help by pushing or pulling in time with their nurses' efforts to move them. Encourage your patient to help in being moved, but not to the extent where being helpful can be harmful.

Pushing Unless totally incapacitated, most patients can help in being moved, especially upward, in bed by pushing down with hands or feet while their nurses pull or slide their bodies toward the head. Patients should lie flat as in Fig. 14–2, or be in a semisitting position. Bend the knees upward, place the feet comfortably flat on the bed. As you move your patient toward the head of the bed, your patient pushes down on it with the feet. If your patient can push down hard enough to

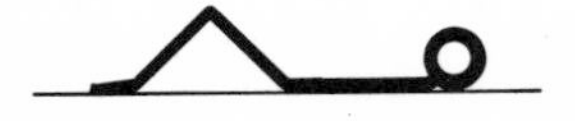

Fig. 14–2 *Patient flat on back, knees up, feet flat on bed*

arch the back and raise the hips, so much the better; it helps move the upper body toward the head of the bed.

Pushing with only one foot is not as effective as with two, but is a worthwhile help in moving. Even if both legs are paralyzed, or for any other reason cannot be moved by a patient, putting the feet in the pushing position will lessen the "drag" or resistance of the body to being moved.

A patient whose legs are immobilized, as in a cast, often may help being moved by pushing down on the bed with one or both hands.

Pulling Patients who can reach it should grasp the headboard and help pull themselves up in bed.

If your patient will be bedfast for much more than about a week and has at least moderate use of arms and hands, you should obtain a trapeze bar (Chapter 8). Ask your visiting nurse which type trapeze will be best for your patient.

MOVING YOUR PATIENT IN BED

Moving Upward The most difficult moving of a bedfast patient is upward or toward the head of a bed. It is done mainly for patient comfort and to incline the upper body so that a patient can read, watch television, look around the room, etc., with least effort; also, most people are not accustomed to lying flat on their backs for long periods of time while awake. With a hospital bed (Chapter 8), simply elevate the head to the slant your patient wants. With other beds, set the necessary pillows or bed wedge pillows (Chapter 8) in place after moving your patient.

If a headboard is low enough or it is an open frame, moving your patient up in bed is essentially a pulling task, helped when possible by the patient's pushing:

1. *Decide how far up in bed* to move your patient. It should be far enough for your patient's comfort.
2. *With the bed flat* and no pillows on it, set your patient's feet in place to help you by pushing, as in Fig. 14–2.
3. *Stand directly behind your patient* at the head of the bed. Reach under your patient's armpits and grasp the wrists, and lift and slide your patient toward the head. Your patient should push down on the bed with both feet while you pull.
4. *Elevate the head of the bed*, or place the pillows or bed wedge pillows to your patient's comfort.

Moving with Draw Sheet If your patient cannot help with being moved in bed, or you cannot get into a safe position for moving at the head, then use the draw sheet (Chapter 8). You will need an assistant to work with you:

1. *Station your assistant* on the opposite side of the bed.
2. *Loosen the draw sheet* on both sides of the bed, and roll it on both sides fairly close to your patient.
3. *Working together*, you and your assistant grasp the rolled draw sheet at

your patient's shoulders and hips, and lift and slide your patient up to the desired position in bed.

4. *Unroll the draw sheet*, tighten it to the sides of the bed, and tuck it under the mattress the usual way.

5. *Raise the head of the bed*, or arrange the pillows or bed wedge pillows for your patient's comfort.

Moving Downward Moving patients downward in bed usually is not very difficult, as most people tend to slide toward the foot of a bed. If it is necessary to move your patient down, first place the patient's feet flat on the bed, as in Fig. 14–2, with the knees raised enough to put the thighs and legs at an angle of about 90 degrees. Have your patient press down on the bed with both feet and strive to raise the hips as you move the upper part of the body downward in bed.

Moving Sidewise There are two easy ways to move a helpless patient sidewise or across a bed. The first method generally is for moving a patient a relatively short distance for a relatively short time, if the patient can be rolled over onto a side. The second method is satisfactory for all sidewise movement of all bed patients, although it may be somewhat difficult with a patient who is very obese (overweight) or much larger than you.

Method #1 This method of moving a bedfast patient across a bed often is used when making an occupied bed (Chapter 13). It may, however, be somewhat difficult for you if your patient is lying near the middle of a double or larger bed.

Stand at the side of the bed toward which you plan to move your patient. Reach across your patient, place one hand on the patient's shoulder and the other on the hip, as in Fig. 13–7, and gently roll your patient toward you.

Method #2 Stand at the side of the bed toward which you will move your patient.

Slip an arm under your patient's neck and far shoulder, and your other arm under your patient's back at the waist. Keeping your knees bent and your back straight, gently pull and slide the upper part of your patient's body toward you.

Release your patient and move down toward the middle of the bed. Put an arm under your patient's back at about the waist, and the other arm under the thighs about midway between the knees and hips. Keeping your knees bent and your back straight, pull and slide the lower portion of your patient's body toward you.

Release your patient and move the feet and legs into comfortable positions.

> NOTE I: If you cannot reach far enough across the bed to move your patient, loosen the draw sheet at the far side of the bed, return to the original side, and with the draw sheet pull your patient close enough to you for moving by hand. After completing movement of your patient, if the draw sheet is long enough tighten it on both sides of the bed and tuck it under the mattress the usual way. If the draw sheet is not long enough for handling this way, work enough of it back under your patient for tucking at the far side of the bed.
>
> NOTE II: Be careful throughout all this multiple moving not to jolt or jar your patient. Work in a steady, firm way with no abrupt motions.

MOVING PATIENT BETWEEN BED AND CHAIR

As a rule, it is best to move a patient from bed into an armchair. It may be a conventional chair or a wheelchair (Chapter 8); the arms are needed to help the patient get into as well as stay in it, especially if using a sliding board, below. To move your patient from bed to chair without a sliding board:

1. *Seat your patient on the edge of the bed* for a few minutes, feet dangling over the side. During this time help patient into robe and slippers.
2. Place a side of the chair close to the bed with the front of the chair a few inches from where your patient will stand while being helped into it. Whether the chair is to the right or left depends on how you will turn and lower your patient into it. If using a wheelchair, lock the wheels securely after placing it.
3. Stand facing the bed, help your patient to stand. For patients who can help being moved, it may only be necessary for them to place a hand on the arm of the chair farthest from the bed while the nurse holds them under the armpits and pivots or turns and backs them down into the chair. Patients who cannot help should keep their arms around the nurse's neck while being pivoted from the bed down into the chair; if their hands are free they may hold onto the bed, making it more difficult to move them.

NOTE: Throughout this work, which essentially is lifting and lowering a patient, keep your back straight and lift and lower only by bending and straightening your legs as necessary.

Moving a patient from chair to bed is a reversal of the above procedure, except of course that no foot dangling is necessary.

1. *Patients who can help* being moved should grasp the edge of the bed with the near hand while the nurse lifts them under the armpits and pivots or turns them around so they can back onto the bed.
2. *Patients who cannot help* being moved should keep their arms around the nurse's neck while being lifted and turned to back onto the bed.

Sliding Board Although in many cases a sliding board (Chapter 8) can simplify the moving of a patient between bed and chair, chair and toilet, etc., it should not be used until you and your patient have been thoroughly instructed by your visiting nurse or other qualified technician.

MECHANICAL LIFTS

There are many devices for lifting patients into and out of bed . . . transferring them to wheelchairs, commodes, automobiles . . . getting them into and out of bathtubs and shower stalls. Many of the lifts are much alike in design and purpose, but offer different conveniences that should be considered. Several lifts are available in mechanical and hydraulic models; some hydraulic lifts are self-contained and can be moved about freely, others are powered by water from the tub or shower bath. Ask the doctor or your visiting nurse which type of lift is best for your patient. If one will be needed for a fairly long period of time, try renting various models for trial before investing in one.

With the type of lift in Fig. 14–3*a*, a patient can be lifted out of bed, taken to other places, lowered into a chair, returned to bed—all with little effort by the nurse. The base is adjustable, opening to 86 cm./34 in., closing to 60 cm./24 in., and is low profile, enabling it to fit under fairly low articles, around fairly wide ones, and into somewhat narrow openings. This type lift is available in mechanical and self-contained hydraulic models. Accessories include sling seats, as in Fig. 14-3*b*, head and back supports, commode seats, and web straps for holding patients into seats.

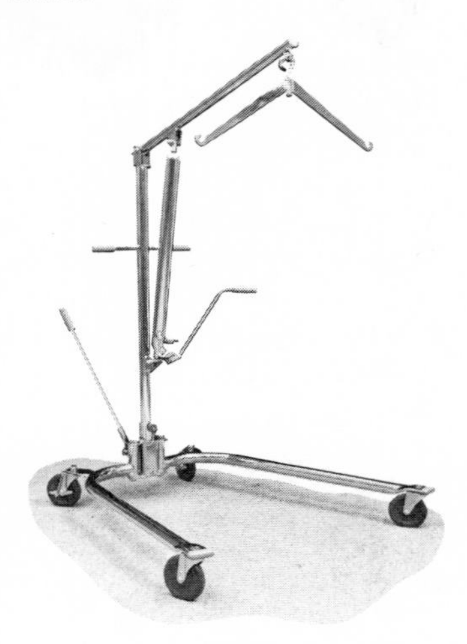

Fig. 14-3*a* *Standard lift*

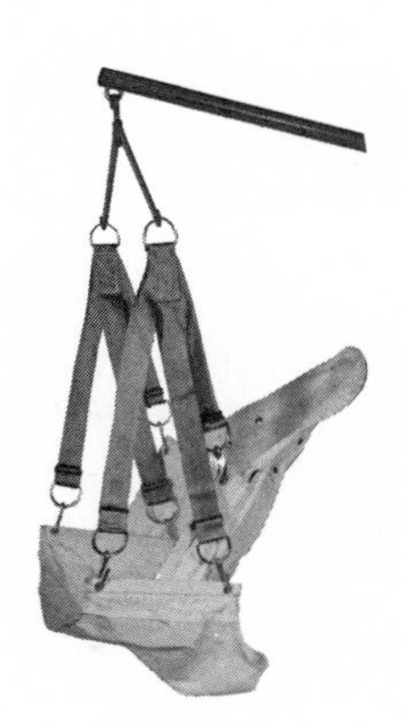

Fig. 14-3*b* *Sling seat*

Fig. 14-3 *Hoyer patient lift*

The completely portable Chec medical bath lift, Fig. 14–4, is easily installed in a bathtub or shower stall. The chair seat swings out for the patient and returns easily to position in tub or stall. Fingertip adjustment lets the seat slide gently downward and ascend smoothly. Hydraulic operation: connects to water faucet or spout.

The Hoyer bathlift, Fig. 14–5, is designed for patients who have some ability to help themselves and wish to bathe in privacy. Patients can have full control of operation, swinging themselves over the tub, lowering themselves to bottom of tub or some other level, lifting and swinging themselves out of the tub. Hydraulic jack system. Cannot be used on a rolled-rim or fiberglass tub.

The Invacare bath chair lifts, Fig. 14–6, can be operated by many patients witn either hand, unaided. The lifts may be positioned so that the ring seat height is the same as the transfer chair height, then raised so that the patient's feet will clear the edge of the tub. Chair then rotates and lowers into the water. The model in Fig. 14–6*a* is mounted on wood or cement floors and is secured to the side of the tub by a saddle (not shown). The model in Fig. 14–6*b* is easily mounted on and removed from the side of a tub.

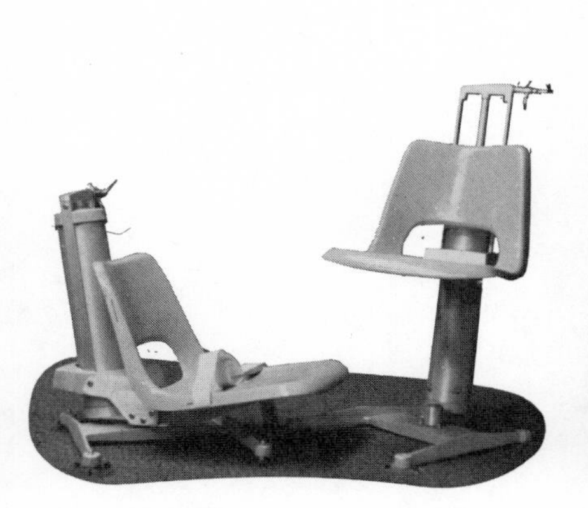

Fig. 14–4 *Chec medical bath lift*

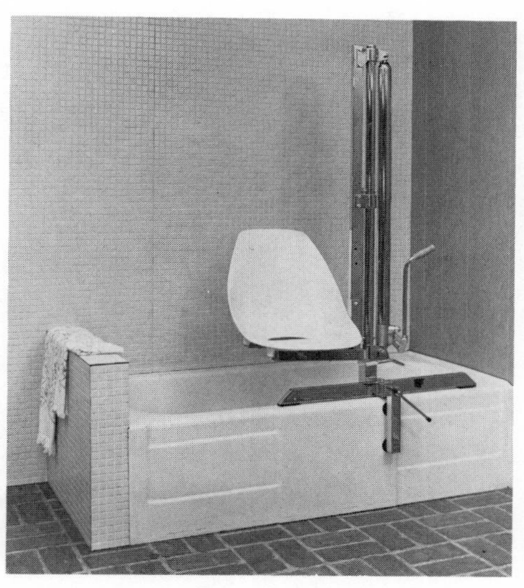

Fig. 14–5 *Hoyer bathlift*

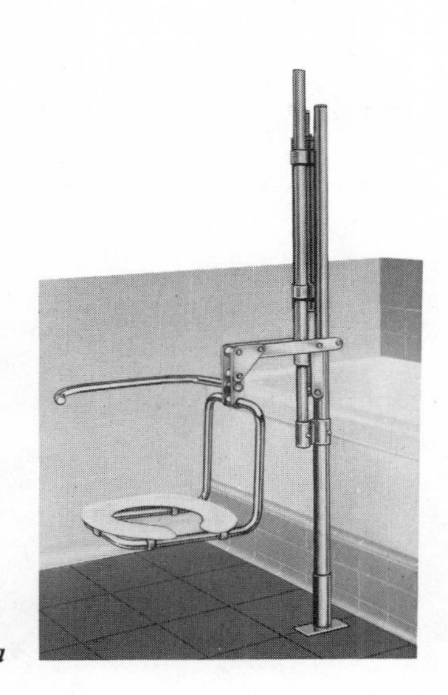

a

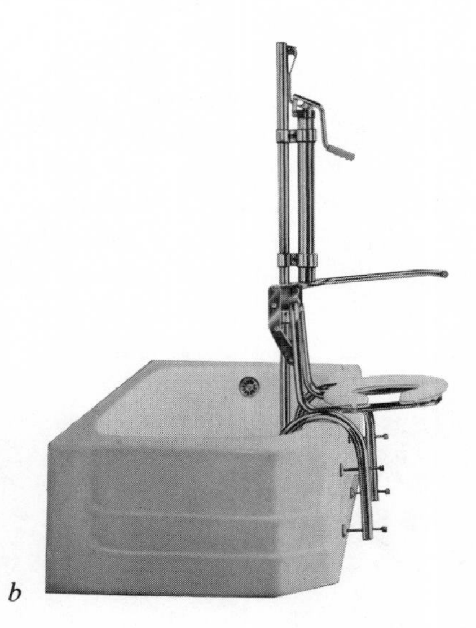

b

Fig. 14–6*a, b* *Invacare bath chair lifts*

15 Bedsores and What to Do About Them

If your patient is:

1. Elderly; or,
2. Very thin; or
3. Victim of a chronic disease; or,
4. Malnourished; or,
5. Confined to bed for longer than regular sleeping hours; or,
6. Unable to voluntarily move freely; or,
7. Receiving pain medication; or,
8. Overly active in bed; or,
9. In a cast,

one of the most serious nursing problems continually facing you is the prevention of *bedsores* (decubitus ulcers); they are also known as pressure sores.

NOTE: A high-protein diet (Chapter 40) can help prevent the development and speed the healing of bedsores. Ask the doctor about this kind of diet if your patient seems subject to bedsores.

Bedsores or *decubitus ulcers*, as in Fig. 15–1, result from pressure on various bony prominences or protuberances of the body such as heels (Fig. 15–1*b*), ankles, knees, hips, buttocks, the coccyx or "tailbone," elbows, shoulders and head, and toes and ears. Bedsores can develop in these areas if the blood supply is suppressed or cut off for 30 minutes, which is likely to occur when a person lies or sits in the same position for too long a time. Bedsores go through a definite disease cycle and, depending upon patient and treatment, commonly take several months to

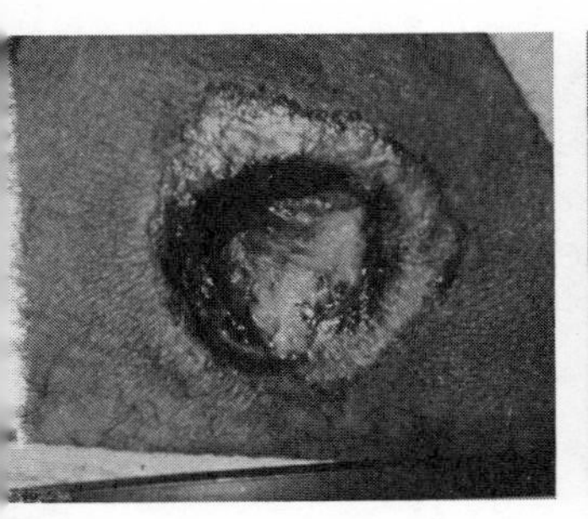

Fig. 15–1*a* *Relatively small bedsore*

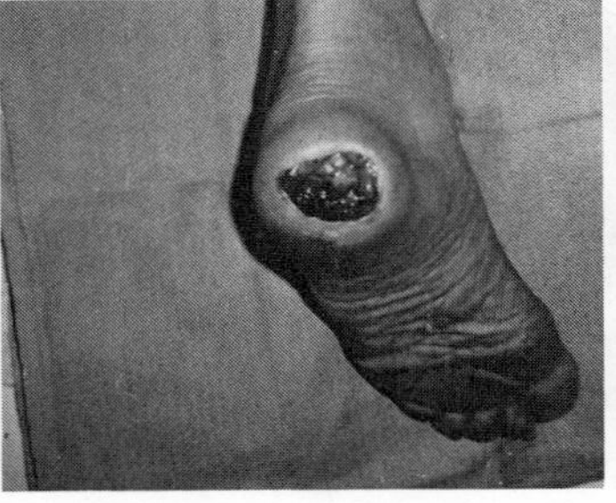

Fig. 15–1*b* *Bedsore on heel, exposes bone*

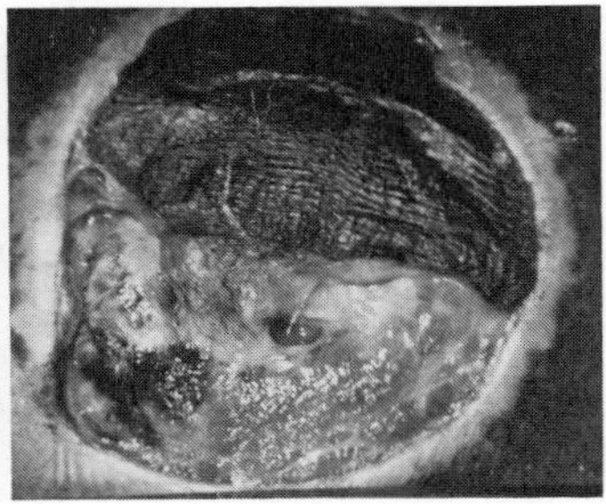

Fig. 15–1*c* *Bedsore with dead tissue (black area) sloughing off*

heal and may leave painful and disfiguring scars. Neglected or improperly treated bedsores may grow to 4 or more inches in diameter, and deep enough to expose the bone, as in Fig. 15–1*b*. Tissue around a bedsore can become so badly infected that it dies, as in Fig. 15–1*c*, in which case surgery, called debridement, and skin grafting may be necessary. In extreme cases, untreated bedsores can cut off the blood supply to a large area of the body, and may lead to extensive remedial surgery, even amputation. Certain types of bedsores may be fatal.

For patients, bedsores are debilitating, and sap energy, resistance, and morale. For even experienced nurses, bedsores are repellent and their persistence in the face of good treatment is frustrating. Fortunately, with relatively simple nursing care and procedures you can prevent bedsores.

EARLY DETECTION AND PREVENTIVE TREATMENT

If a potential bedsore is detected early enough, prompt treatment usually can keep it from developing.

A bedsore starts to develop after approximately 30 minutes of pressure (just the weight of the body or a limb) on a bony prominence that prevents blood getting into that area.

1. The first sign of a developing bedsore is a red area of skin that blanches or whitens when pressure is applied to it, such as pressing it firmly with your thumb or finger.
2. In the second stage, the red area turns a dusky blue-gray color that does not blanch when pressed. This indicates that the tiny capillaries (very small blood vessels) are blocked.
3. In the third stage, a blister develops. When it breaks, the dead tissue under the skin is exposed and there is immediate danger of a staph or strep infection developing to increase the basic seriousness of a bedsore.

Generally, development of a bedsore can be stopped if it is treated, below, in the first or red stage. When the second stage is reached, it is extremely difficult to arrest development of a bedsore, and it is nearly impossible when the blister begins to form.

Preventive Treatment The following treatment is quite effective in halting the development of bedsores, especially if it is given early in the first or "red" stage:

1. Wash the reddened area carefully with a mild solution of soap and warm water. Do not use a detergent.
2. Dry it thoroughly, but gently. Pat, do not rub.
3. Gently knead and massage the general area, *but not the reddened portion*, of the potential bedsore to stimulate local circulation of the blood. First coat the area lightly with a creamy hand lotion. Massage with the tips of your fingers, working in a circular, spiraling motion toward but not into the reddened area; massage of the reddened area might break the capillaries and contribute to development of the bedsore. Continue this treatment until the reddened area becomes approximately the color of the healthy tissue around it.

4. Many experienced nurses paint or coat a once reddened area with tincture of benzoin (a resin) to toughen the skin and increase its resistance to the development of another potential bedsore. If you do apply benzoin, when it is thoroughly dry sprinkle a little talcum powder over the area to keep it from sticking to the bedding or patient's clothing. Instead of benzoin, some nurses use alcohol on an area when massaging it, to toughen the skin and keep it dry.

WHY BEDSORES DEVELOP

Bedsores are caused by sharply suppressing or cutting off the supply of blood to flesh and skin for a period of about 30 minutes. Conditions favorable to the development of bedsores may be due to a patient's bed.

With most types of mattresses and bedding, a person's weight or downward pressure in bed is not distributed evenly. Soft parts of the body, such as calves, thighs, the belly, buttocks, etc., spread a person's weight fairly evenly over relatively large areas. But the bony prominences—heels, ankles, knees, hips, coccyx, shoulders, head, ears—push down sharply into the mattress or bedding and concentrate the patient's weight on fairly small areas. This creates enough pressure to slow down and eventually stop the circulation of blood through tissues covering a bony prominence. Also, when the upper bedding is too heavy or pulled too tight, its weight or pressure on a patient's toes can easily cause bedsores.

Whether a patient gets bedsores depends chiefly on the nursing care. However, there are several conditions that directly or indirectly affect the circulation of the blood and condition of the tissues, and make a person more likely to get bedsores:

1. *Age.* As a rule, the older a person is the poorer the circulation of the blood and the more easily it is blocked off from a fairly small area.
2. *Thinness.* The thinner a person is overall, the thinner the layers of flesh and skin over bony prominences and the more easily the flow of blood can be stopped.
3. *Chronic Disease.* The longer the onset of a disease and the longer it lasts, the greater the probability of bedsores due to loss of fat, wasted or atrophied muscles, and low hemoglobin (iron-containing pigment of the red blood cells).
4. *Malnutrition.* Persons suffering from malnutrition have a loss of fat, wasted or atrophied muscle tissue, and low hemoglobin. All these conditions help bedsores develop.
5. *Bedfastness.* The longer a person is confined to bed daily, and the greater the number of days of such confinement, the greater the effect of pressure on bony prominences is apt to be.
6. *Immobility.* The less a person can and will move about, the greater the likelihood of developing bedsores.
7. *Medication.* Patients receiving pain medication may not feel bedsore-producing pressures.

8. *Excessive Rubbing.* People often develop bedsores on heels and hips from moving or sliding up and down too much in bed and pressing themselves hard against it for long periods of time.

9. *Casts.* Patients may develop ulcers that are essentially the same as bedsores inside casts that are poorly padded or are too tight.

Important Contributing Factor A major factor that makes patients highly susceptible to developing bedsores is lack of bed cleanliness. It is primarily a matter of nursing neglect.

Incontinence. Persons who cannot control bladder or bowel excretions or emptyings are called incontinent. When they lie in their urine or feces for a long period of time, the contaminated skin and flesh become irritated and soften. The softer and weaker the tissues become, the less their resistance to pressure that can block the flow of blood and cause bedsores. Also, this macerated tissue is more open to staph (staphylococcus) and strep (streptococcus) infections (Chapter 11) that often are part of bedsores. These infections must be cured before bedsores can be treated successfully.

Perspiration. Patients who are feverish and perspire excessively must be watched closely for signs of skin irritation similar to those due to prolonged urine and feces contamination, above.

The only rule covering how often a bed must be cleaned or changed is—in each case—experience. If your patient cannot or will not ask for a urinal or a bedpan early enough, keep track of how often one is needed and give it to your patient 5 or 10 minutes before probable need. If your patient does not "go" regularly, you may be able to establish a routine by presenting the urinal or bedpan at regular intervals; often this will not work, but it is well worth the attempt. If a reasonably regular schedule of bladder or bowel evacuation cannot be established, or as sometimes happens there is a complete loss of control (see Chapter 28, Exercising Your Patient), consult your visiting nurse. If there is only loss of bladder control, ask the doctor or your visiting nurse about a catheter (see Urinals, Chapter 8). For loss of bowel control, there are special waterproof pants with disposable liners that are quite satisfactory for protecting a bed.

BASIC PREVENTION OF BEDSORES

There are three steps in a practical program to prevent bedsores:

1. Eliminate conditions that cause bedsores.
2. Take proper care of your patient; change body position frequently.
3. Always be on the alert for signs of possible or potential bedsores. Regardless of how successful the first two preventive steps appear to be, examine your patient frequently for signs of impending bedsores. Remember, a bedsore can develop after 30 minutes' absence of blood supply to an area.

Eliminate Conditions that Cause Bedsores Bedsores are caused by pressure on the bony prominences of the body. Pressure may be that of the body against a surface, such as a mattress, or it may be the pressure of some other object, such as bedding or a cast, against the body.

There are several ways by which you can sharply reduce, if not eliminate, the usual harmful pressures of the bony prominences against a mattress:

1. Instead of a conventional innerspring, or foam rubber or polyfoam mattress, use a waterbed or an air mattress.
2. Put a satisfactory flotation pad (Chapter 8) on top of a conventional mattress.
3. Place real or synthetic sheepskin (Chapter 8) on top of a conventional mattress.
4. Place special pads on your patient's feet. These bedsore pads (Chapter 8) commonly are small rubber or polyfoam "doughnuts" or sheepskin boots that absorb bed pressures commonly placed on toes and ankles. They often are used for elderly people, healthy or not, who do not move about much in bed while asleep and tend to develop bedsores on the sides of their ankles and knees.
5. Prevent downward pressure of bedding that can easily cause bedsores on a patient's toes by loosening the bedding at the foot of the bed after making it (Chapter 13). If your patient has injured, long, or very sensitive feet, a toe comfort board or foot support or guard (see Bedsore Prevention, Chapter 17, Foot Care) should be used.
6. The only way to prevent the pressure of a cast causing bedsores is the proper padding of the bony prominences before the cast is applied. If you suspect sores forming under the cast, notify your patient's doctor immediately.

Nursing Care One of the most important points of good nursing care for the prevention of bedsores is maintenance of a clean bed, see Important Contributing Factor, above. Another important point is the movement of your patient.

If your patient cannot or will not move about somewhat freely in bed, you must supply the movement needed to prevent bedsores. Moving is also done to keep the blood from settling in the overall lower parts of the body, such as the thighs and calves, when you lie on your back.

1. *Mattress.* If the mattress is conventional innerspring, foam rubber or polyfoam, at least once an hour throughout the day and night turn or make sure your patient turns over into a new position . . . onto the back, onto a side, onto the other side, onto the belly, onto the back, and so on. If using a waterbed or satisfactory flotation pad or sheeting (Chapter 8), turning a patient every two instead of one hour usually is sufficient.
2. *Position.* If your patient dislikes a position, use it less often or for shorter lengths of time. Also, ask your visiting nurse if a position may be harmful to your patient.
3. *Turning Your Patient.* See Moving Your Patient in Bed, Chapter 14. Hospitals have special equipment for turning patients to prevent bedsores and settling of the blood; these usually are impractical or too costly for home use unless they can be rented.

TREATMENT OF BEDSORES

Being open wounds, bedsores are extremely susceptible to staph and strep infections, which can be very serious (Chapter 11) and must be cured before the bedsores can be treated successfully. If for no reason other than to reduce the possibility of infection, treatment of bedsores should be started immediately upon discovery.

There are many proven successful treatments of bedsores. Some require prescription medicines, others use nonprescription or patent medicines that you can get from a pharmacist, and there are treatments with items common in the home. However, keep in mind that a treatment that works well for one person may not be effective for another. There also may be certain "medicines" that your patient should not be given. For these reasons, it is best to have the doctor prescribe a bedsore treatment. In general, bedsore treatments are similar to those for baby and diaper rashes.

An oldtime favorite and probably one of the most successful home treatments for severe bedsores is the same as a treatment for saddle sores on horses. Fill the bedsore cavity with ordinary granulated white sugar, cover with a piece of Saran or similar plastic wrap, tape it in place and leave it there for 3 or 4 days. Since sugar does not maintain life, bacteria do not grow in it; this prevents staph and strep infections. The mixture of sugar and body serum usually creates a substance that keeps a bedsore lubricated and encourages healthy tissue to grow back into the sore. This treatment generally is repeated every 3 or 4 days until the bedsore is healed.

> NOTE: The above treatment of bedsores is not recommended except in cases of emergency, since it lacks the antibiotics and other ingredients that may be essential for your patient. If you use this treatment, be sure to tell your patient's doctor exactly what you did and how your patient reacted to it. The doctor must have this information in order to prescribe future treatment.

Among the nonprescription ointments that have proved beneficial in treating bedsores are Vitamin A and D ointment, and chlorophyll ointment.

Daily exposure of a bedsore to sunshine is another generally accepted method of treatment. Heat lamp treatments for 15 minutes two or three times a day also are used. Be sure to keep a heat lamp 61 cm./2 ft. away from the sore; if it is closer, you may burn your patient. Examine your patient every 5 minutes for signs of redness that precede a burn.

16 Handicap Aids

In addition to equipment that is virtually essential for the basic good of a sick person (Chapter 8), there are many handicap aids that may do much for your patient's safety, comfort, and recovery. Unless the doctor orders complete rest, even if your patient is confined to bed you should encourage activity. Reasonable activity helps maintain a sick person's muscle tone and strength, and reduces the probability of blood clots and pneumonia.

Most of the handicap aids in this chapter encourage patient activity through self-service. Many of these aids may be practical suggestions for friends who ask what they can give your patient as a present. For best results, choose aids that fit the needs, interests, and personal likes of your patient, and encourage self-help. As a rule, it is best to avoid aids that are so difficult for your patient to use successfully that they are apt to discourage self-service activity.

There are many handicap aids of more specialized natures than those described in this chapter. Ask your visiting nurse for a catalog of aids or inquire at a hospital supply store (usually listed in the telephone or city directory under Hospital Equipment & Supplies). Most hospital supply stores stock a wide variety of handicap aids and will get the more specialized ones for you in a few days. In small communities, drugstores and hospitals often have a modest supply of handicap aids, and will gladly get others that your patient may need.

Many satisfactory versions of the simpler handicap aids may be made at home from commonplace materials. The more complicated aids, however, often cannot be made at home without the materials, tools, and mechanical experience needed for building the commercial models. Major problems with homemade handicap aids commonly are that they are too heavy or awkward for a patient to handle, or so light and delicate that they break easily.

TELEPHONE

An easy-to-reach telephone, either a special extension or an instrument with a long enough cord, should be regarded as essential for the safety of a patient who can be left alone at home for even a short time. A phone is, of course, ideal for patients who do not want or should not have visitors, as it enables them to pick and choose the people and times they want to "visit." For best results, get a phone that has a bell loudness control and cutoff switch. Ask the telephone office about other handicap aids that might help your patient, such as amplifier or volume-control phones for the hard-of-hearing.

EATING AIDS

The stainless steel eating utensils in Fig. 16–1 are cemented into resilient vinyl-plastic, bicycle-type handles with fingergrip knobs. When purchasing eating aids of this type, insist on those that will withstand normal dishwasher heat. In Fig. 16–1:

a The conventionally shaped utensils are designed for convenient use with either hand.

b The angled fork and large spoon are for persons with certain restrictions in the use of hands or arms. When ordering angle-handle utensils, specify that they are to be used with either the right or the left hand.

c The L-shaped spoon handle is mounted on a central swivel pin that permits the spoon bowl to remain level even though the handle is rotated through an arc of up to 60 degrees; double stops prevent excessive rotation or swing. A swivel fork and two sizes of spoons usually are available, all designed for use with either hand.

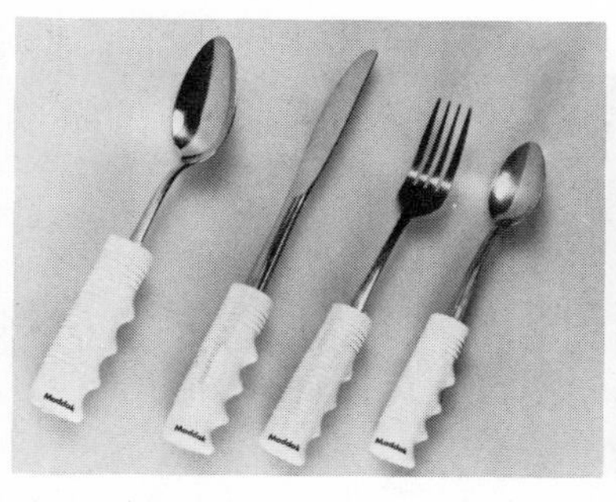

Fig. 16–1*a* *Conventional*

Fig. 16–1*b* *Angle-handle fork, spoon*

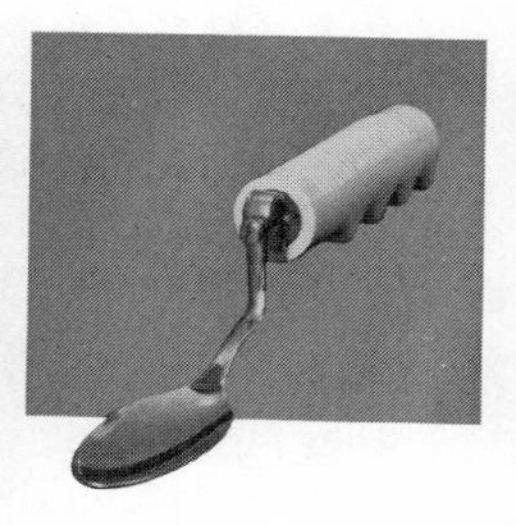

Fig. 16–1*c* *Self-levelling spoon*

Fig. 16–1 *Built-up handle utensils*

The exaggerated curves of the knife blades in Fig. 16–2 enable a person to cut meat and other foods with the use of only one hand. Cutting is done by a rocking action instead of the usual "sawing," which requires that the food be held in place. The simple rocker knife, *a*, is for cutting only. The combined rocker knife and four-tine fork, *b*, can be of great help to persons having only one hand available for self-feeding.

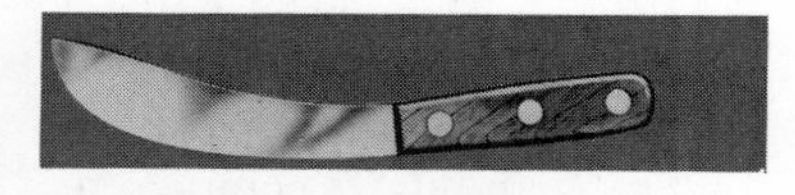

Fig. 16–2*a* *Rocker knife*

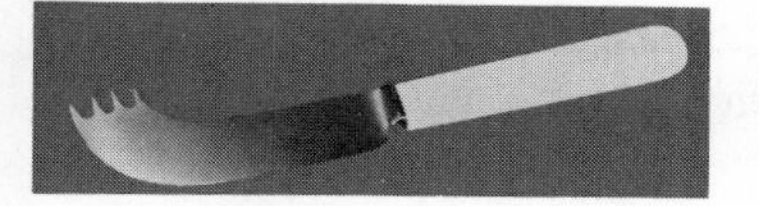

Fig. 16–2*b* *Rocker knife-with-fork*

Fig. 16–2 *Knives for one-hand cutting*

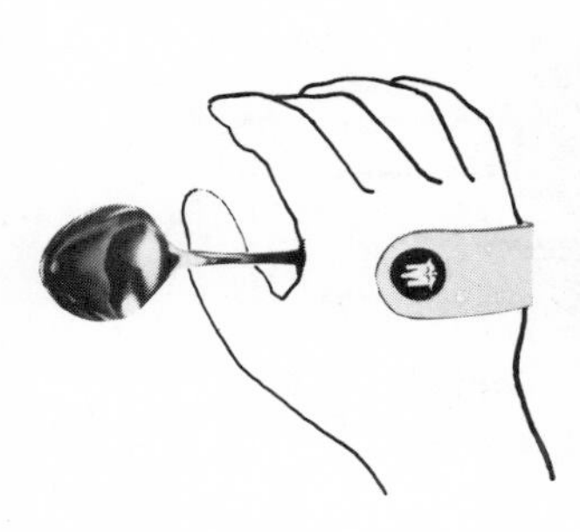

Fig. 16–3 *Utensil hand clip*

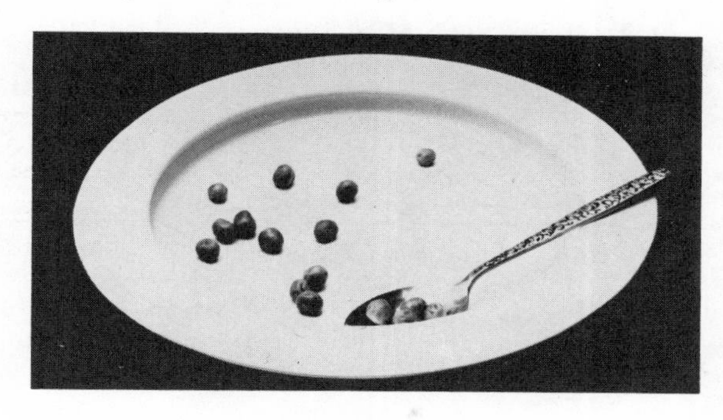

Fig. 16–4 *Inner-lip plate*

The spring-action plastic clip in Fig. 16–3 fits the hand ana holds a spoon or fork securely in place. This type eating aid may be excellent for persons who have difficulty in grasping and holding small utensils.

The inner-lip plate, Fig. 16–4, can prevent spills and make eating more enjoyable for elderly or handicapped persons who are feeding themselves. The inner lip holds food on the plate while the user brings the fork or spoon to the edge. This type of plate is molded of smooth, durable plastic and is lightweight, easy to clean, and dishwasher safe. There is also a nonskid plate that has a 15-cm./6-in. diameter rubber disc bottom support that helps keep it stationary on a smooth, slick surface.

Homemade Utensil Holders Simple versions of commercial utensil holders, Figs. 16–1 and 16–3, usually can be made at home in a few minutes. However, for long-term use the commercial aids may be more practical. In Fig. 16–5:

a The rubber-ball holder for a toothbrush, fork, or spoon is made by forcing the handle through the middle of a solid, soft rubber ball. First pierce the ball with a thin knife or other sharp object. A rubber-ball handle may not be practical for a knife. It depends on the shape of the knife handle, the sharpness of the blade, and the toughness of the food to be cut.

b The bicycle handgrip holder for eating utensils or a toothbrush is easily made by filling an ordinary bicycle handgrip with wet plaster of Paris and holding the handle in place until the plaster hardens. Work quickly—plaster of Paris sets in a very few minutes. This small amount of plaster will not weigh much.

c A rubber band may be used to hold the handle, if long enough, of a toothbrush, fork, or spoon against the palm of a person's hand. Fasten the rubber band at the end of the handle with adhesive tape to keep it from slipping off. This type of holder is seldom practical for a knife.

d The stitched holder is made from two strips of leather, cloth, or plastic, and a length of elastic tape. The lower strip should be about 1.25 cm./½ in. longer than the width of the user's hand, and at least 2.5 cm./1 in. wide. The upper strip should be at least 2.5 cm./1 in. shorter than the lower one, and

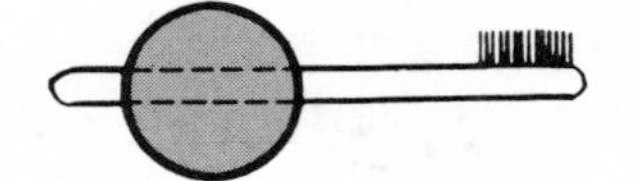
Fig. 16–5*a* *Rubber-ball holder*

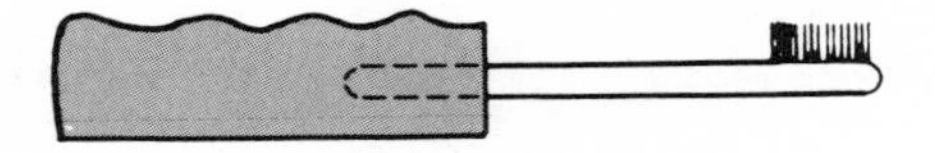
Fig. 16–5*b* *Bicycle handgrip holder*

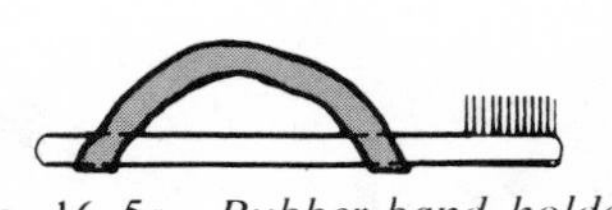
Fig. 16–5*c* *Rubber-band holder*

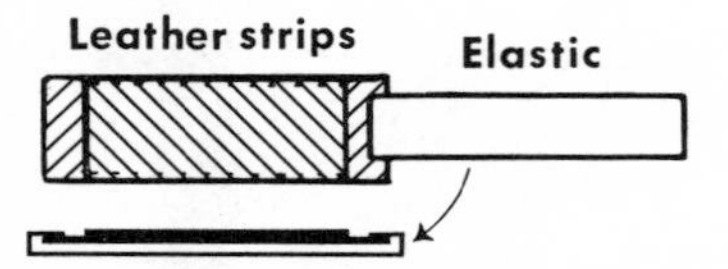

Fig. 16–5*d* *Stitched leather holder*

Fig. 16–5 *Homemade handicap aids*

wide enough to fit snugly over the handle of a toothbrush, fork, etc., when stitched to the sides and an end of the lower strip. Sew a length of elastic tape to the ends of the lower strip; it should be just tight enough to press the holder snugly against the palm or back of the user's hand.

WRITING AIDS

Writing aids for persons who have little or no ability to flex their fingers must be made to fit their hands and fingers. The holders shown in Fig. 16–6 are quite easy to make, but should be fitted to the user's hand step by step.

a The elastic-tape pen or pencil holder is made by sewing or stapling together the ends of a loop of 2.5-cm./1-in. wide elastic tape that is long enough to fit around the user's thumb and index or forefinger when held apart as in Fig. 16–6*a*. With a few stitches or staples, divide the loop into three slots or segments: one each for the thumb, finger, and pen or pencil. The elastic-tape holder is generally easier to make than the wooden block type, below, but may be more difficult for your patient to use since it offers less positive control of the pen or pencil point.

b To make a block pen or pencil holder, cut a piece of wood to the size and shape that the user can grasp firmly. Unless the user has very large or small hands, start with a piece of wood about 8 x 4 x 4 cm./3 x 1¾ x 1¾ in. Shape it gradually and carefully, with frequent testing, to a block that the user can grip firmly and comfortably. Drill a hole in the shaped block to hold the pen or pencil; it must be at an angle that is practical for writing or printing when the user grasps the block. It may be necessary to wrap an adhesive tape or paper around the sides of the pen or pencil to make it fit tightly in the hole.

As a rule, balsa wood is excellent for making a holder of this type. It is lightweight, easy to cut and drill, soft enough for most rough spots to be pressed into comfortable shape for a user's hand, and readily available in hobby and model shops. Instead of wood, a block of foam-type rigid lightweight plastic may be used; however, plastic holders often are not as durable as those made of balsa.

NOTE: The rubber-ball type of utensil holder, Fig. 16–5*a*, can be a satisfactory pen or pencil holder if it does not turn easily in the user's hand.

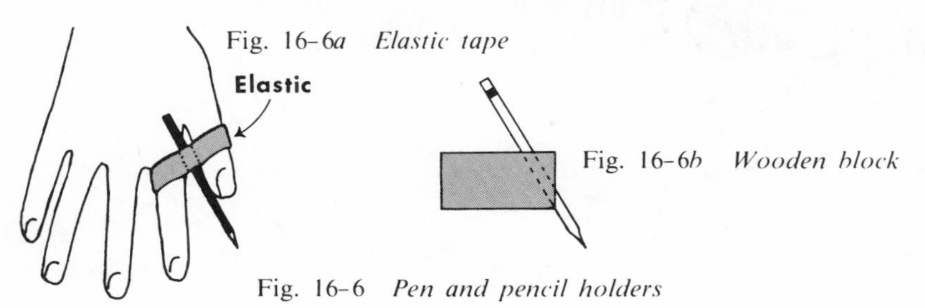

Fig. 16–6*a* *Elastic tape*

Fig. 16–6*b* *Wooden block*

Fig. 16–6 *Pen and pencil holders*

READING AIDS

The commercial page turner, Fig. 16–7, is excellent for persons having great difficulty turning pages of books and magazines. The 28-cm./11-in. long, curved, break-resistant plastic aid has a spring-action clip to hold it snugly on the hand. The rubber tip easily moves pages, even those of heavy coated paper. The wide, curved rubber-padded area is for turning very large sheets or pages.

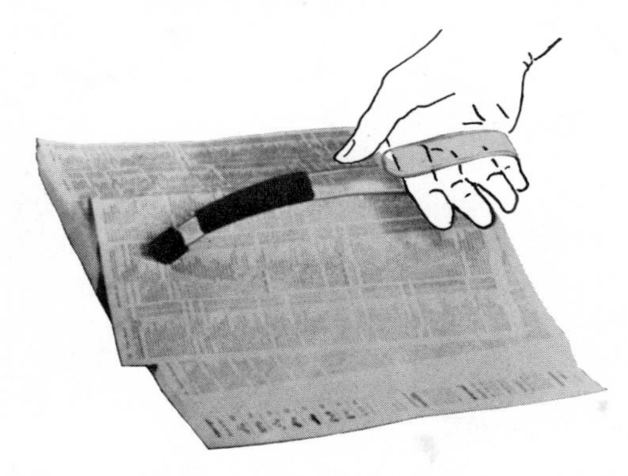

Fig. 16–7 *Page turner*

Homemade Reading Aids Instead of the commercial page turner, a rubber ball or cube may be used by persons who can hold it but have little or no use of their fingertips. Or a turner may be made by jabbing the pointed end of a rubber-eraser pencil into a solid rubber ball the same way as a toothbrush, Fig. 16–5*a*.

REACHING AIDS

Commercial reaching aids, such as the Matey Bantam in Fig. 16–8, usually have aluminum frames and plastic handles, triggers, and gripping jaws; a magnet on the tip of the jaw is to help in picking up small iron and steel items. Commercial aids come in lengths ranging from 67 cm./26½ in. to 82 cm./32½ in. There is a 56–cm./22–in. compact model that folds to 32 cm./12½ in. long for carrying in a

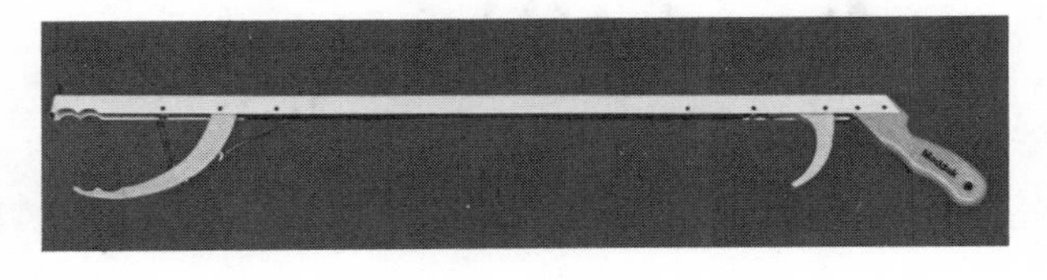

Fig. 16–8*a* *Matey Bantam holder*

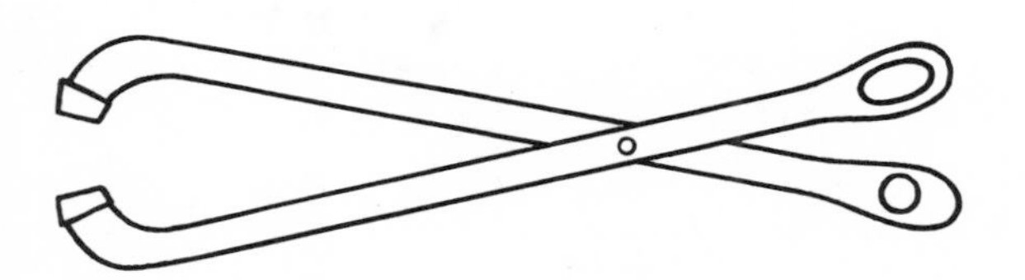

Fig. 16–8*b* *Homemade tongs*

Fig. 16–8 *Reaching aids*

pocket or a bag. There is also a reaching aid attachment for wood and aluminum canes. There are two basic types of commercial reaching aids—active and passive:

Active, in which a light spring keeps the jaw open. The trigger must be squeezed and pressure maintained on it to close and keep the jaw closed for picking up and holding an object.

NOTE: A special model of active reaching aid is made for persons who cannot operate the usual trigger type as in Fig. 16–8*a*. Instead of the trigger, on the side of the frame opposite the handle there is a lever to control the jaw. The user holds the handle with one hand and with the other hand or wrist moves the lever to close or open the jaw. Once the jaw is fastened onto an object, it is held until released by reversing the lever.

Passive, in which the gripping jaw is closed and kept closed by spring pressure. The hand lever is squeezed to open the jaw for picking up or releasing an object.

There are variations of both active and passive types of commercial reaching aids to fit the specialized needs of most handicapped persons.

Homemade Reaching Aids The homemade reach grabber or tongs, Fig. 16–8*b*, usually is made of 6-cm./¼-in. plywood. It can be any length convenient for the user; however, the longer it is, the heavier it will be and the more difficult it may be to handle. As a rule, the swivel or pivot pin is located about one-third of the distance from the top of the handle end to the pickup points, although it should, of course, be placed for the handle to fit and work with the size, mobility, and strength of the user's hand or hands. Small magnets may be fastened to the tong points to help in picking up iron and steel articles.

Instead of the scissors-type grabber in Fig. 16–8*b*, your patient may prefer the long-handle (about 48 cm./18 in.) commercial tongs sold by many houseware shops. Also, fairly long barbeque tongs may be satisfactory reaching aids, if the spring tension is not too great for your patient's hands or strength.

BED ASSISTS

As a rule, the more your patient moves about in bed without your assistance, the better. To encourage your patient to move independently, the bed should be equipped with a practical bed assist. The trapeze bar (Chapter 8) with a suspended triangular grab bar is an excellent assist, especially for most persons who are in body casts or have had strokes.

Homemade Bed Assists The board bed assist, Fig. 16–9, helps a patient to move from side to side and turn in bed, and move between the bed and a chair, but is not designed for raising or lowering oneself in bed. Fasten the board by C-clamps to the bedrail on your patient's so-called good side just above the hip level, or at any other point that is convenient for your patient to grasp for pulling or pushing.

Cut the board assist from 2-cm./¾-in. plywood, or 2.5-cm./1-in. solid wood. The board should be about 16.5 cm./6½ in. wide, and long enough, when stood on the floor, to reach a height suitable for your patient. Cut an 11.5-cm./4½-in. diameter hole centered between the sides of the board and at least 2.5 cm./1 in.

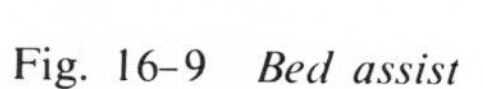

Fig. 16–9 *Bed assist*

down from the top. Cut the top of the board roughly parallel with the top of the large hole. Round off and sand smooth the edges of the handle area. For best results, varnish the complete board.

Instead of the board assist, an open-back kitchen or dining chair may be tied or clamped to the side of the bed. It is not as handy as the board assist, but generally is satisfactory for emergency or short-term use.

ENTERTAINMENT

Most people who are confined to bed or a wheelchair, or even just to the home, require some sort of entertainment. Helping to prevent boredom is important; but the more important effect of entertainment is taking their minds off minor problems, worries, and aches and pains that usually beset disabled persons. When arranging for entertainment of any kind, be sure it is something that your patient likes and wants, not merely what someone thinks your patient should have.

Television If the TV set controls cannot be within easy reach of your patient, get a set that has remote control. Nothing about television is quite as annoying as being unable to change channels, or turn it off and on.

Radio Disabled people often prefer radio to television simply because radio requires less effort to be "entertained." A small set with good sound that does not carry too far usually is best for both patient and family.

Record, Tape Players The major value of record and tape players is that they encourage a patient to create programs of music. A disadvantage of records is that a patient may worry and fret about the way they are handled.

Stereo The disadvantage of a portable or temporary stereo system is that unless the loudspeakers are balanced satisfactorily, the sound may irritate instead of soothe and entertain a person who is confined to bed or a chair. Stereo earphones may, however, overcome this problem.

Books and Magazines Do not borrow books or magazines from a lending library for a patient whose disease is in a communicable stage, or for one who must be protected against communicable diseases. If your patient has a highly communicable disease or sickness, it is advisable to burn books and magazines after use. Ask your visiting nurse.

Newspapers As a rule, there is no need to destroy newspapers that have been handled by sick persons, except those having the most virulent of communicable diseases. Few germs can tolerate the ingredients of printer's ink.

17 Foot Care

If your patient is confined to bed or a day couch and cannot be up and walk around for at least a few hours every day, an important part of your nursing duties is regular foot care. It is essential for any patient's well-being as well as comfort. It is of utmost importance if your patient has diabetes or any circulatory disturbance.

Foot care involves the soaking and washing of feet; the prevention of pressure or bedsores (Chapter 15); the trimming of toenails and prevention of ingrown nails; the exercises and equipment needed to maintain good muscle tone in the feet, ankles, and lower legs; and preventing foot drop and and foot rotation. Good foot care usually takes only a few minutes. For your patient's and your convenience, foot care usually is given while bathing a patient (Chapter 23).

The importance of proper foot care for persons with diabetes cannot be overemphasized. These patients have relatively poor blood circulation to their feet, making a cut or sore there very slow and difficult to heal. For this reason, extra care must be taken when trimming toenails not to cut or scratch the flesh. If you or your patient cannot be sure of trimming nails safely, have it done by a podiatrist or chiropodist. Also because of poor circulation to their extremities, diabetics tend to develop bedsores on their feet. They should always avoid tight footwear of any kind and too-short hose or socks.

SOAKING AND WASHING FEET

Before washing the feet as part of a bath (Chapter 23), soak them in a pan of warm water. A round or oblong plastic or other lightweight dishpan is excellent for this; if the pan is too small to hold both feet, soak one at a time. Soak feet for at least 5 minutes; 10 minutes or longer if you are trying to soften calluses, or soak off dead skin or encrusted dirt. Medicate the water only if the doctor prescribes it.

After soaking the feet, scrub them well; spread the toes and wash between them. Although the scrubbing feels good to most people, feet often are extremely sensitive to touching or tickling. In this case, since people cannot tickle themselves, hold the washcloth or sponge against the bottom or side of the washpan while your patient rubs the soles of the feet against it. Rinse feet thoroughly, especially between and around the toes; dry thoroughly, particularly between the toes. To dry the soles of ticklish feet, have your patient rub them hard against a towel.

Soak and wash feet daily unless the doctor orders a different schedule, as may happen when there are lesions or open sores on a foot.

FOOT BEDSORE PREVENTIVE TREATMENT

While washing feet, examine them closely for signs of pressure areas that could become bedsores (Chapter 15). The most likely areas are the tops and tips of toes, backs of heels, and both sides of the ankles. The first indication of a potential bedsore is a bright red inflammation of the skin at a pressure point. At the first hint of such redness, remove pressure on the area and lightly massage it, rubbing gently with a circular motion inward from the edges to stimulate circulation of the blood there. The more often you examine and treat it—once an hour is not too often!—the more likely you are to prevent development of a bedsore and the pain it will cause your patient. Continue treatment until the redness leaves and the skin takes on a healthy color.

| NOTE: Massage (Chapter 18) is not recommended as a regular part of foot care.

FOOT BEDSORE PREVENTIVE DEVICES

If your patient will be confined to bed for more than a few days, or tends to develop bedsores on the feet or ankles, special bedsore preventive equipment should be used. There are many good commercial devices; serviceable ones usually can be made at home.

Heel Protectors To guard heels against the effects of normal bed pressure there are commercial items, such as the Posey Ventilated Heel Protector, Fig. 17–1, that help prevent friction and skin breakdown while allowing free movement of the foot. The Posey device consists of a plastic shield with a washable, synthetic fur lining, and a special closure across the front to hold the protector securely yet comfortably in place on even a restless patient.

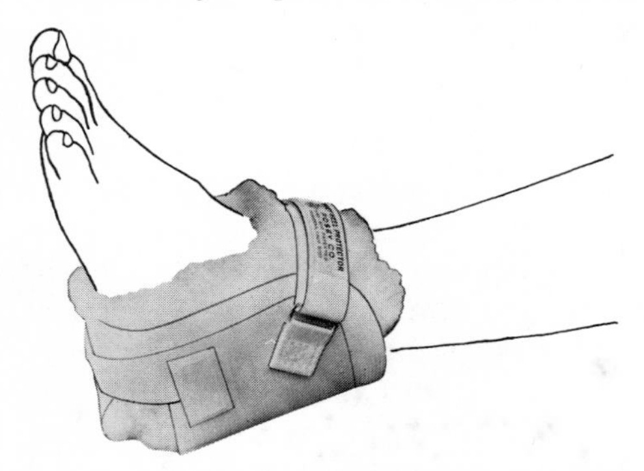

Fig. 17–1 *Posey ventilated heel protector*

Commercial heel protectors are sold in pairs. For short-term use, two pairs are usually sufficient. But if your patient's feet perspire heavily, and for long-term use, you should have three or more pairs. Change them at least once a day, more often if your patient's feet perspire heavily.

Homemade Heel Cups Sheepskin "cups," as in Fig. 17–2*a*, which protect your patient's heels against bed pressure, are not difficult to make. They may be genuine or artificial sheepskin, and machine or hand sewn. You need:

1. Sheepskin (which see, Chapter 8). Determine the amount needed after making the diagram. You need the same number of cups as you would heel protectors, above.

2. Sewing materials, including fairly heavy scissors or shears. Pinking shears usually are not practical for cutting genuine or artificial sheepskin.

3. A means of closing a cup and keeping it in place around your patient's ankle. "Touch and hold" tapes, such as Velcro®, are excellent for this. Twill tie-tapes are quite satisfactory.

4. A flexible tape measure.

5. Materials for making a full-size diagram of the cup. Use a paper, such as a fairly light wrapping or butcher paper, that you can wrap and fold around your patient's ankle and foot.

Make a full-size pattern of the planned heel cup (cups for both feet usually are made from the same pattern) based on actual measurements of your patient's foot, Fig. 17–2*b*:

NOTE: Throughout the making of the pattern and the cup be sure your patient's foot points straight up at an angle of 90 degrees directly to the front of the leg. If this is not done, the cup may encourage foot drop, below, which can be quite painful and difficult to cure.

1. Measure *length* of the pattern, A–B, Fig. 17–2*b-1*, the distance along the sole of the foot from about the middle of the arch, back under the heel and up the back of the ankle, to a point 2.5 cm./1 in. above the anklebone.

2. Measure *width* of the pattern, C–D, the distance from a point 2.5 cm./1 in. above the anklebone on one side of the foot, down under the heel and up the other side of the foot, to a point 2.5 cm./1 in. above the anklebone.

3. Cut a rectangular pattern based on the measured length and width, Fig. 17–2*b-1*.

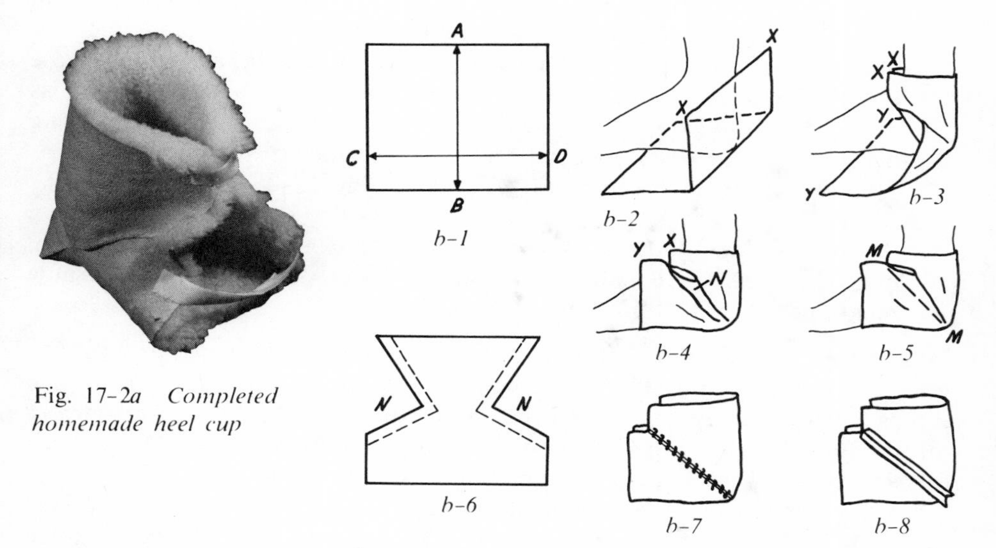

Fig. 17–2*a* *Completed homemade heel cup*

Fig. 17–2*b* *Homemade heel cup*

4. Place the front or A end of the rectangular pattern at the point on the sole of the foot from which you measured length, 1 above; center the foot between the sides of the paper pattern. Tape, or have someone hold, the front end of the pattern in place on the foot.

5. Set the B end of the pattern in place at the back of the ankle, at the point to which you measured length. Center the ankle between the corners of the pattern, X and X, to give you a basic shape of the pattern, as in Fig. 17–2*b-2*. Of course, the actual shape will depend on the size and shape of your patient's foot and ankle. Tape or have someone hold the B end of the pattern in place on your patient's ankle.

6. Wrap the upper corners of the pattern, X and X, Fig. 17–2*b-2, 3*, straight around the sides of the ankle. Keep the corners of the pattern at the same height as at the back of the ankle. While holding the corners of the pattern in place with one hand, rub downward with the other and press the sides of the pattern against the ankle and toward the front to a point just above the start of the bend between ankle and foot, as in *b-3*.

7. Wrap the front corners of the pattern, Y and Y, Fig. 17–2*b-3, 4*, up around the sides of the foot, keeping them the same distance from the back of the foot as the pattern is on the sole of the foot. While holding the corners in place with one hand, rub toward the back of the foot with the other and press the sides of the pattern upward and around the foot, working toward a point just in front of the start of the bend between foot and ankle, as in *b-4*.

8. While holding the foot portion of the pattern in place, 7 above, grasp the upper portion, 6, and work your hands toward one another until the paper pattern meets at about the middle of the bend between foot and ankle, as in Fig. 17–2*b-5*. The surplus or excess part of the pattern paper should fold outward, N, on both sides of the patient's foot. Draw a line along each crease of the pattern paper on the foot and ankle portions on both sides of the leg, as the dash line M–M in *b-5*. These lines represent the approximate lines along which the sheepskin will be cut and sewn together to form the heel cup.

9. Remove the paper pattern, spread it flat, Fig. 17–2*b-6*, and cut away the surplus on both sides, N and N. To prevent making these notches too large, thereby wasting a piece of sheepskin, cut the notches about 1.25 cm./½ in. outside the creases, as indicated by the dash lines. The paper pattern is now ready to use for making the heel cup.

Cut a piece of sheepskin the size and shape of the completed paper pattern. The notches, N and N Fig. 17–2*b-6*, probably will not be large enough for the sheepskin to fit snugly around your patient's foot and ankle, but it is easy to cut them to the proper size when the sheepskin is actually fitted in place. The fleece or fur side of the sheepskin is, of course, against the patient.

Sew tapes for closing and holding the heel cup to your patient's ankle and foot. The ends of the tapes should be about midway between the notches and the ankle and foot ends of the cup, as in Fig. 17–2*a*.

Set the cup in place on your patient, closing and holding it with the tapes, in order to enlarge the notches, N and N Fig. 17–2*b-6*, to make a smooth seam from about the bottom of the heel at the back to the middle of the bend between the top of the foot and the ankle. At this point, there are two ways of completing the heel cup; the first method generally is easier for persons who are not skilled in machine or hand sewing.

First Method. Press the foot portion of the heel cup snugly in place, and cut it to fit neatly along an imaginary line from the middle of the bend into the ankle at the top of the foot to the end of the notch at the back of the heel. Then cut the upper or ankle portion of the cup to make a smooth butt joint against the edge of the foot portion. Do this on both sides of the cup, then remove the cup and sew the edges of the notches together with a simple overhand or whip stitch, as in Fig. 17–2*b*-7.

Second Method. Instead of cutting the edges of the notches for a butt joint as above, cut each to leave a .6-cm./¼-in. seam allowance. Cut off the same amount of fleece or fur from the sheepskin on each side of the notch. Pin or hold the edges of the notches together and machine or hand sew them .6 cm./¼ in. from the edges.

Ankle Protector Ankle protectors are often advisable for people who are not confined to bed and need not wear heel protectors, but who at night tend to lie very still in bed and seldom turn over. This kind of bedsore prevention is especially important for elderly people who have poor blood circulation.

A practical and inexpensive type of ankle protector, commonly called doughnut, is shown in Fig. 17–3. It is often available at ski shops as well as drugstores and hospital supply stores. As a rule, four doughnuts are needed, one for each side of a patient's ankles.

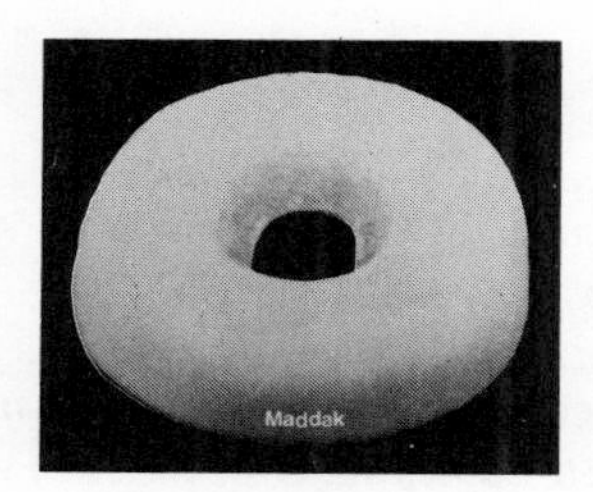

Fig. 17–3 *Polyfoam doughnut for anklebone*

Place a doughnut over each protruding bone of an ankle and fasten it securely in place. This may be done by putting a sock over the foot and ankle if the patient is not overly active. For active patients, doughnuts may be fastened in place with strips of 5-cm.-/2-in. gauze bandage or elastic bandage.

Homemade Ankle Doughnuts Suitable ankle doughnuts can be cut from 2.5-cm.-/1-in.-thick soft polyfoam plastic or a similar material. Polyfoam usually can be cut rather easily with a fairly large scissors or shears; a sharp kitchen knife or an electric carving knife may be used. You also should have a compass or dividers with at least a 4-cm./1½-in. span and a soft lead pencil tip. To make a doughnut:

1. Draw a circle with a 7.6-cm./3-in. span on a suitable piece of polyfoam. A slightly smaller circle may be drawn for a child's doughnut.

2. Cut the polyfoam neatly along the edge of the circle.

3. Working outward from the center of the round of polyfoam, cut out the area that will cover the anklebone itself. With this hole over the bone, pressure will not be on the bone but instead will be spread or distributed on the polyfoam surrounding it. Do not make the hole larger than necessary; the larger it is, the weaker the doughnut will be.

Toe Protection A toe comfort board, bedding frame, or foot cradle keeps bedding off a patient's feet for general comfort, improved air circulation, less foot perspiration and, most importantly, prevention of pressure on the toes that can easily cause bedsores (Chapter 15). There are several commercial products or devices for this, and practical homemade substitutes for short-term use.

For toe protection only, the bedding frame, Fig. 8–7*a*, is placed at the end of the bed. It adjusts for height, fits all beds, and is easily taken apart for small storage space. Two such supports, one on each side of a bed, can provide a complete bed cradle to hold upper bedding off a patient's body as well as the feet.

The foot cradle design in Fig. 8–7*b* fits across and clamps to the mattress at any point on standard hospital and twin-size beds. It easily converts to a foot support, Fig. 17–5.

The Posey foot guard, Fig. 17–4, also gives the patient's toes excellent protection against bedsores.

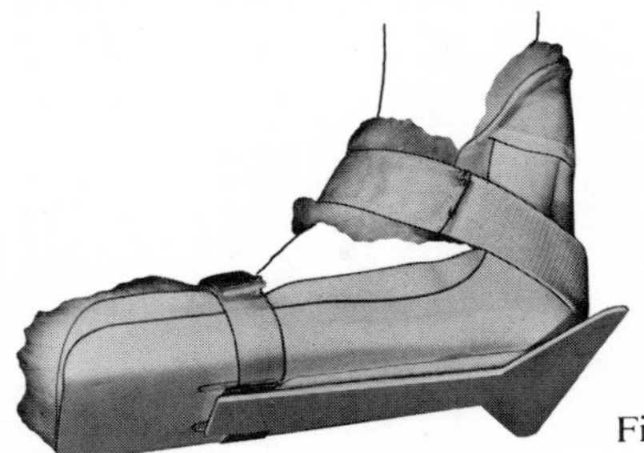

Fig. 17–4 *Foot guard*

Toe Protection Substitutes A satisfactory toe comfort board for short-term use can be cut from a sturdy cardboard box or carton, as in Fig. 8–7*c* and *d*. Select a box that is rigid and strong enough to support the bedding, and large enough to let your patient's feet move about freely.

For very short-term protection of the tips of the toes against bedding pressure, put slippers with stiff soles on your patient's feet. The slippers must be large enough to fit very loosely at the tips of the toes.

> NOTE: If you do not use toe comfort or foot support devices, be sure to loosen the upper bedding at the foot of the bed when making (Chapter 13).

FOOT DROP

Foot drop results from long confinement in bed with the foot extended from the ankle instead of being kept in the normal flexed or bent position, preferably at a right angle to the front of the leg, as in Fig. 17–5. Recovery from foot drop can be quite slow, and in severe cases may require surgery. Foot drop may be prevented by the use of foot support devices. A person who cannot walk around, even with aids, for at least 2 hours a day should have a foot support in bed regardless of how short confinement will be; without such support, a patient may also suffer foot rotation, below. There are several commercial support devices that function as toe comfort and foot support boards. Serviceable foot support boards can be made by the average person who is moderately handy with the simpler carpentry tools.

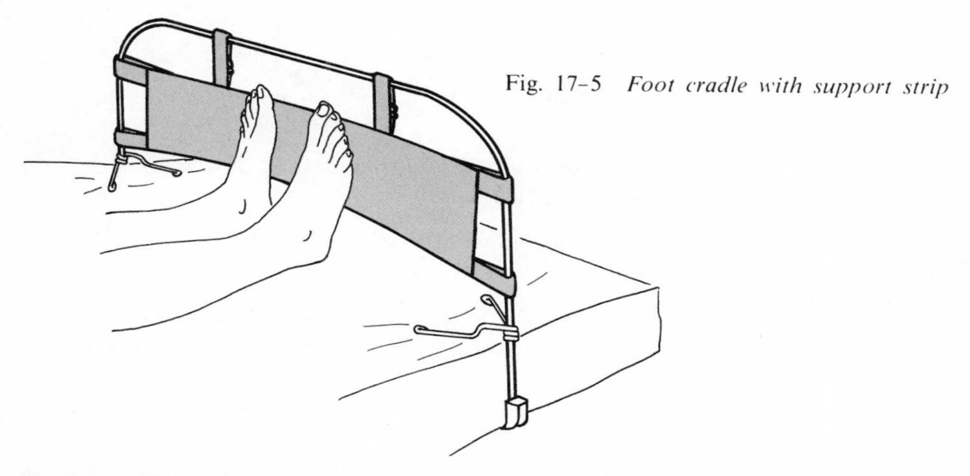

Fig. 17–5 *Foot cradle with support strip*

Commercial Foot Support Board The commercial-type foot support board in Fig. 17–5 is a bedding frame, Fig. 8–7*b*, with a support strip added. Since it clamps to the mattress at any convenient point on a standard hospital or twin-size bed, it is easy to set properly for your patient. Commercial support strips come in a choice of washable fabrics, and are simple to install.

For a foot support board to be beneficial, get your patient into a comfortable sitting or lying position in bed with both feet pointing straight up. Set the support board firmly against the soles of the feet or bottom of the heel protectors. Explain to your patient the real need of a foot support board, and why there should be no attempt to move away from it.

Foot Support Guard The Posey foot guard, Fig. 17–4, functions as a toe comfort board by holding the bedding up off the toes, prevents foot drop, and by means of its T-bar stabilizer helps prevent foot rotation, below.

Homemade Foot Support Boards Full-length foot support boards, as in Fig. 17–6*a*, are for persons whose feet reach the end of a mattress when they are sitting or lying down in bed. Short boards, *b*, are for persons whose feet do not reach the end of the mattress.

Support board frames may be made of 1.3- or 1.9-cm./½- or ¾-in. plywood, and three or four 12.7- or 15.2-cm./5- or 6-in. metal inside corner braces and

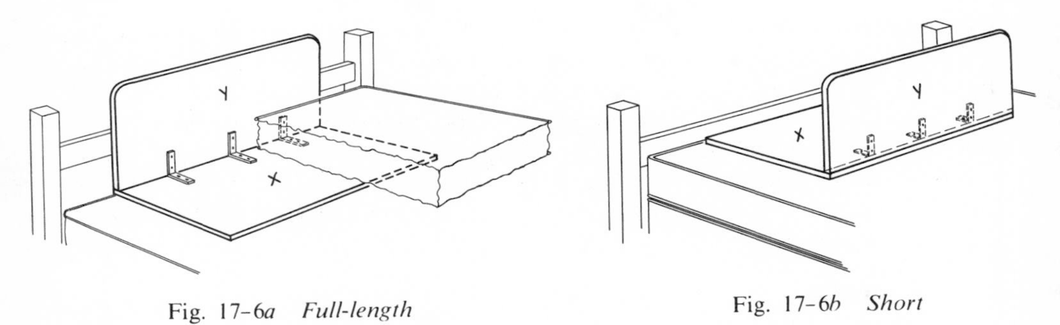

Fig. 17-6*a* *Full-length*

Fig. 17-6*b* *Short*

Fig. 17-6 *Homemade foot support boards*

screws. Tools needed are a screwdriver, medium sandpaper, and a saw if you do not buy the wood cut to size and shape.

Building Support Frames Foot support frames consist of a bottom or base, X in Fig. 17-6, to support the upright, Y, at a 90-degree angle:

1. *The base*, X, should be nearly as wide as the mattress it will be used with. The base for a full-length board, Fig 17-6*a*, should be about 61 cm./2 ft. long. For a short board, *b*, the base extends from where the soles of the patient's feet will be in bed to the end of the mattress.
2. *The upright*, Y, is as wide as the base, X. Measure height of an upright from a point at least 5 cm./2 in. above the patient's toes when the feet are in vertical position to the top of the base, which in use is:
   a. Directly under the mattress for a full-length board.
   b. On top of the bottom sheet or draw sheet, if any, for a short board.

NOTE: The top corners of an upright should be round-cut to let the bedding drape down better over the sides of the board and mattress. Also, round corners have less wear on the bedding.

Assemble the frame, setting the bottom edge of an upright on the top surface of the base, Fig. 17-6. Fasten them together with metal inside corner braces and screw them down tight. For twin and narrower beds, three corner braces usually are enough; place one at the center of the frame, the others about midway between the center and the sides of the frame. If using four braces, set each outer brace about 10 cm./4 in. from the sides of the frame; space the others equally between them. Round off the edges of a completed frame with sandpaper.

Padding Support Frames Foot support boards usually may be padded adequately with four or five layers of thick pile toweling or terrycloth covering the front of the frame (where the patient's feet go), plus a layer wrapped around the sides, top, and bottom of the upright and base, to hold the other layers in place. Fasten the holding layer to the frame with enough thumbtacks to keep it tight and free of wrinkles.

FOOT ROTATION

Foot rotation, which causes an unnatural and ultimately very painful position of the hip, occurs when instead of pointing almost straight ahead of the front of the leg, a patient's foot turns excessively outward. Some foot rotation is normal. But if allowed to continue too long, the damage caused by excessive foot rotation can become almost as serious and difficult to repair as that caused by foot drop, above. Foot rotation may be prevented by devices such as the Posey foot guard, sandbags, rolled blankets, and pillows.

Foot Guard The Posey foot guard, Fig 17–4, serves as a toe comfort board, prevents foot drop, and by means of the T-bar stabilizer helps prevent excessive foot rotation.

Sandbag Protection If your patient's foot turns outward excessively and continually, place a sandbag along the outer side of the ankle and foot, as in Fig. 17–7. Generally only one sandbag is needed. But if a foot resists being held upright, it may also be necessary to place a sandbag along the inner side of the foot and ankle. However, since some foot rotation is normal, as a rule you should not set sandbags so close that a patient cannot move the feet or foot comfortably.

Commercial sandbags are available at most hospital supply stores. One can be made by filling a cloth bag with dry sand or buckshot; dirt seldom is practical. Use cloth that will hold the filler. As a rule, the filled bag should reach from a point about 2.5 cm./1 in. beyond the bottom of a patient's foot to about 7.5 cm./3 in. above the anklebone, and from the back of the heel to about halfway to the tips of the toes. A filled bag should be firm enough to hold shape, yet soft enough to conform to the shape of the patient's foot and ankle.

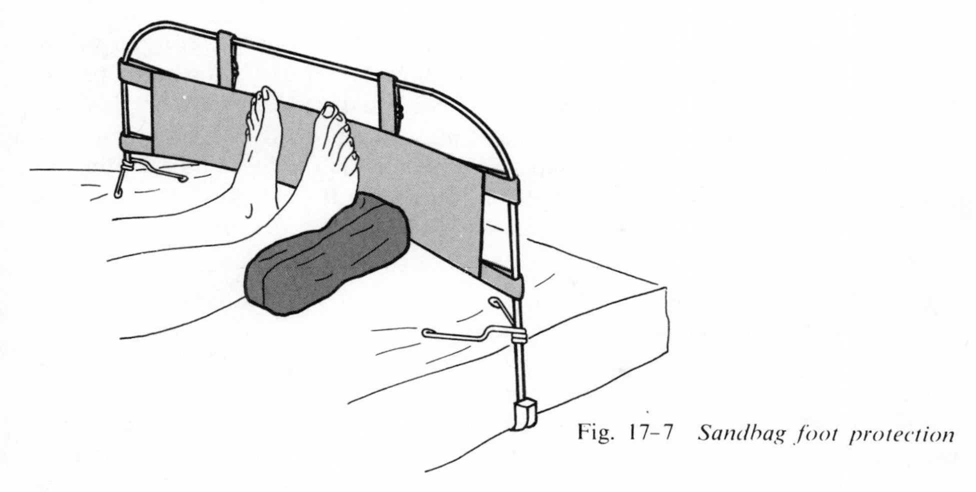

Fig. 17–7 *Sandbag foot protection*

Rolled-Blanket Protection A tight roll of blanket about 15 cm./6 in. in diameter extending from the hip to the sole of a foot may be used to prevent foot rotation.

Pillow Protection Instead of sandbags or rolled blankets, pillows may be used to prevent foot rotation, but because of their bulk and softness generally are not satisfactory except in an emergency.

CARE OF TOENAILS

After your patient's feet are washed and dried, trim the toenails and, if necessary, take steps to prevent ingrown nails. Toenails that are too long can scratch and even cut the feet, which may be a very serious matter for persons having diabetes or circulatory problems.

As a rule, toenails should be trimmed every 2 weeks or when they extend to the edges of the toes, whichever occurs first. Trim nails straight across from side to side, as in Fig. 17–8.

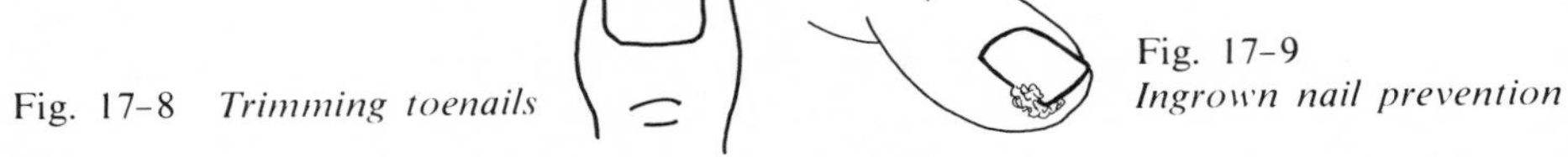

Fig. 17–8 *Trimming toenails*

Fig. 17–9 *Ingrown nail prevention*

The corners of toenails must be loose and free to keep them from growing into the flesh. Ingrown nails can cause intense pain just by pressing against the flesh; in severe cases they may cut the flesh and cause infection. At times surgical treatment may be necessary. Ingrown nails occur most often on the big or great toe, but can be on any toe. If there is a tendency toward an ingrown nail, pack a small ball of cotton under it at each side, as in Fig. 17–9; keep it there until the nail has grown safely out beyond the edge of the toe.

CALLUSES

Foot calluses, especially those that are hard and/or widespread, can cause severe discomfort after a person has been bedfast for more than a week or so. Then the calluses or thickened skin tends to become dry, brittle, and break away from the flesh. To soften hard calluses and make the process of losing them less uncomfortable, once or twice a day rub them with oil, a lanolin lotion, or Vaseline®; eventually they will slough off, leaving soft, normal skin.

EXERCISES

When patients are to be kept off their feet for more than a few days, exercise the feet regularly several times a day. Without this, foot and ankle muscles become weak and flabby, and the patient may suffer foot drop, above. If one foot is immobilized, as in a cast or when heavily bandaged, exercise the other.

Almost any strong movement of the foot, toes, and ankle can be good exercise. Wriggling the toes, alternately curling them tightly and stretching them outward, can exercise all the muscles of the foot and some of the ankle. Twisting feet from side to side and pressing hard against a foot board is excellent for toning foot and ankle muscles. Bending feet as far forward and backward as possible is another good exercise. Rotating feet in a circular motion, first one way then the other, helps keep ankle movement free.

FOOT LUBRICATION

Dry foot skin usually causes discomfort, and skin tends to become dry and itchy when people are off their feet for more than 2 or 3 days. For patient comfort, especially when the feet are callused, after giving all other daily foot care rub them with oil, a lanolin-base hand or body lotion, or Vaseline®. Use it to "grease" the skin, but not in a thick layer. Rub it in gently. If there is excessive lubricant after rubbing for a few minutes, wipe it off gently with your hands. Leave a thin coating of lubricant on the feet. It should not make them stick to the bedding; as a rule a lubricant allows feet to be moved more freely in bed.

18 The Body/Back Rub

Do not confuse the term *body rub*, as used here, with *massage*. A body rub is done to soothe and relax muscles and nerves; it calms and may help a patient go to sleep. Massage, on the other hand, is done primarily to stimulate and activate nerves, muscles, and blood circulation for the purposes of relieving pain, reducing swelling, and helping a person use and want to use certain parts of the body. Body rub and massage have their places in good care of a patient. But except as an aid to preventing bedsores (Chapter 15), massage should be done only when prescribed and, when possible, by a trained therapist. If massage is prescribed, ask the therapist or your visiting nurse if you can do it, and to show you how.

Trained therapists use many massage movements. Two of them, *stroking* or *effleurage* and gentle *kneading* or *petrissage*, are basically those used in the body rub. Other and more severe massage movements may include pressing, tapping with fingertips, and thrusting into the deeper parts of the body.

Any kind of "massage," even a back rub, may be inadvisable if a patient has or has had problems with blood clots (thrombophlebitis), since it can loosen blood clots and let them move through the veins to the heart or brain. This is a major reason why many doctors oppose massage and insist that it be done only by a skilled therapist. Do not, except on the doctor's specific order, massage or allow massage treatment on the abdomen or the front part of the body.

BACK RUB

The body rub is basically a gentle rubbing, stroking action combined with some firm but not hard kneading of the skin and flesh. In most home nursing it is done only on a patient's back, from the hairline or back of the skull downward almost to the buttocks; this type of body rub is called the *back rub*.

Although it may be done at any time, a back rub usually is given as part of preparing a patient for sleep. It is especially beneficial for a patient who is confined to bed or must lie down for most of the time. Lying for many hours on end, whether in bed or on a couch, taxes or tires the nerves and muscles of the back. The back rub is one of the best ways of inducing relaxation and helping a patient sleep naturally.

Another excellent time for a back rub is when you turn over your patient. If your patient cannot turn over or needs help doing it, finish the turn by giving a quick back rub. At the same time, examine the pressure areas on the shoulder bones, scapulae, or "wings" . . . back of the head . . . lower part of the back at the lumbar area . . . hips and buttocks . . . ankles, heels, and toes for redness that may be signs of potential bedsores. Treat these trouble spots with *light massage*, below.

Body Rub Lotion and Powder You may use a hand, body, or lanolin lotion when giving a back rub. It lets your hands move more easily. If the lotion is cold, warm it before application so as not to shock your patient's nervous system. Alcohol generally is not recommended for a rub because of its drying effect on the skin. Preparation of an oldtime body lotion that patients usually like because of its fragrance and lack of drying effect is given under Body Lotions in Chapter 9.

After completing a back rub, you may lightly rub a little talcum or body powder on the areas.

Cornstarch is a good substitute for commercial body powder or talcum. It is especially helpful in creases and between touching parts of the body to prevent moisture buildup and skin irritation.

Don't Keep in mind that the purpose of a back rub is to soothe and relax your patient. Often an inexperienced nurse is tempted to finish the back rub of a spouse-patient with a smart swat on the bottom as a sign of affection. It is best to refrain from such love pats, as they tend to undo all the good soothing effects of the back rub.

GIVING THE BACK RUB

For a good back rub, have your patient lie prone (face down, or on abdomen) with the head turned to a side. Remove the pillow from under your patient's head; if using a hospital bed, set it flat. Expose the patient's back down to the buttocks, Fig. 18–1.

As a general rule, there are four basic movements to a back rub and they are given in sequence. Within this, however, nurses tend to develop their own variations, such as the length of time for a movement, how close together the hands are, the speed of rubbing, and so forth. With experience and from observing the kind of movements that soothe and relax your patient best, you probably will develop your own system of giving a back rub.

In most cases, it takes at least 5 minutes to give a good, effective back rub. Spend more time if you can.

First Movement After smoothing lotion on your patient's back if desired, start the back rub at the hairline or the base of the skull, Fig. 18–1*a*. With two fingers of each hand, stroke on both sides of the spine from the base of the skull straight down to the tailbone or coccyx. Stroke slowly, smoothly, firmly without any circular motion. Do this at least six or seven times, more if you can. As a rule, after the first few strokes you will feel your patient begin to relax.

Second Movement Again starting at the base of the skull or hairline and using the same two fingers of each hand as in the first movement of a back rub, move your hands in a contracircular (one hand clockwise, the other counterclockwise) motion, Fig. 18–1*b*, while working down along both sides of the spine to the tailbone. Move slowly, at a soothing speed; avoid any jerky, irregular motion.

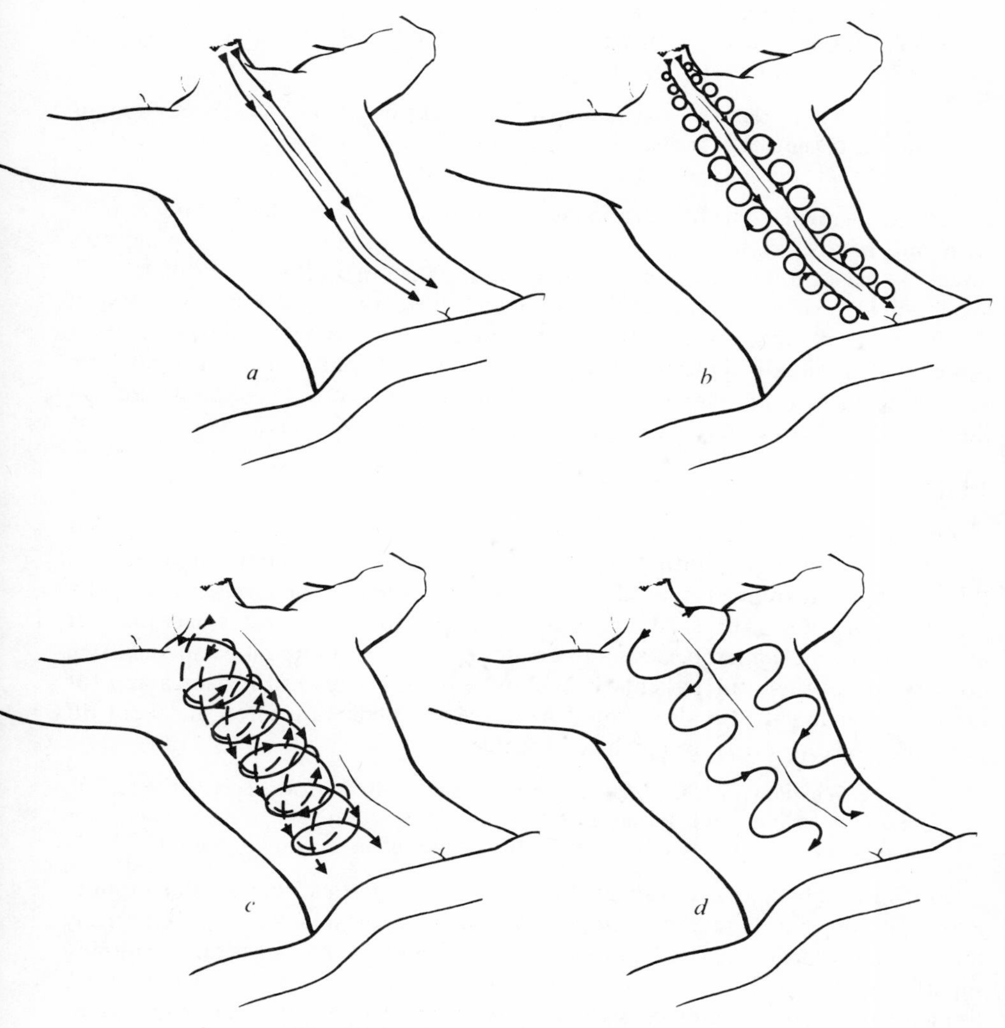

Fig. 18–1*a, b, c, d* *Back rub movements*

Press firmly while rubbing, but not hard. Do this five or six times, all the way from top to bottom; more often if you can.

> NOTE: Instead of working from top to bottom, some nurses get better results by working upward from the tailbone to the base of the skull.

Third Movement In the third movement of a back rub, work first on one side of the patient's back, fairly close to the spine, then the other. Start at the top of the shoulder. Work with your hands flat and fingers together. Rub your hands inward toward each other with a circular motion, Fig. 18–1*c*, that gently pushes the patient's skin up between your hands then smoothes it flat. Press firmly while rubbing, but not hard; do not press hard enough to "dig" into the flesh with your fingertips. Rub completely down one side of the back, then the other. Repeat this four or five times, more often if you can.

> NOTE: Again, the direction in which you work, from shoulders to buttocks or buttocks to shoulders, or one way one time and the other the next, is a matter of which is better for you and your patient.

Fourth Movement The fourth and last movement of a back rub generally is done with your hands flat, fingers close together, a hand on each side of the spine. Rub down the back outward away from the spine and then in up close to it, Fig. 18–1*d*. Work slowly, keep your motion smooth and even; the regular rhythm is very soothing and relaxing. Repeat the fourth movement at least six times, preferably more, while gradually lightening the pressure of your hands to just a soft touch on your patient's skin. If you wish, sprinkle body or talcum powder or cornstarch on the back just before making the last few complete movements.

LIGHT MASSAGE

The so-called light massage should be used only for treating pressure areas that appear to be developing into bedsores. The massage is to stimulate circulation of the blood. Do it frequently until the bright redness leaves the danger area and a healthy flesh color returns. As a rule, 2- to 3-minute massage periods once an hour are adequate. But longer periods and greater frequency can do no harm and often are highly advisable for patients who show a tendency toward bedsores and for diabetics. Such patients also should be turned in bed more often and kept off potential bedsore areas as much as possible.

> NOTE: When giving a light massage to a potential bedsore area, it is important not to press hard on the flesh. By pressing hard you may rupture some of the cells in the endangered area and thereby increase the chance of its developing into a bedsore.

To give a light massage, rub gently with your fingertips in a circular motion. Rub over the entire reddened area, from an inch or so outside it completely through it. Repeat this over and over again, changing the direction of rubbing slightly each time in order to stimulate the blood to move in all directions. Remember, the purpose of the light massage is to help the blood back into areas that it was forced out of by outside pressure on the body.

19 Temperature

Because temperature and its changes can be such accurate indications of a patient's condition, keep careful records and always take a reading the last thing before consulting the patient's doctor or your visiting nurse, especially in an emergency condition.

As used here, *temperature* means the heat balance of the body. Heat is always being produced in the body by muscles and glands and at the same time being lost or dissipated, primarily through the skin and lungs. The balance between production and loss of heat is body temperature; as a rule it stays fairly steady or constant, the condition called normal temperature.

Infections, diseases, and weather conditions cause changes in the production and loss of body heat. The body tries to eliminate or adjust for such causes; but when they are too strong for the body to control, there is a net increase of heat or a fever, or a net loss of heat or a chill.

Temperature is measured by *fever* or *clinical* thermometers. The greater the elevation of the temperature above normal, the more serious a patient's condition is.

> NOTE: The word *temperature* is often used loosely to denote fever or body heat above normal; for example, "has a temperature (fever)."

TEMPERATURE DEGREES

Body temperature is measured or graded in degrees and tenths of a degree Fahrenheit, such as 98.6° F, or Celsius (often called centigrade), such as 37° C. Celsius or centigrade is the metric system of measurements, and is gaining almost universal use. However, Fahrenheit readings are quite common, and in some institutions both Celsius and Fahrenheit degrees are used. Although you should know whether your thermometer is Fahrenheit or Celsius, there is such a great numerical difference between their readings that the doctor or visiting nurse will know which it is regardless of what you call it. A Celsius-Fahrenheit Table and methods of converting one temperature reading to the other are given at the end of this chapter.

TEMPERATURE-PULSE-RESPIRATION

Changes in body temperature usually accompany changes in a patient's pulse and respiration or breathing (Chapters 20, 21), as shown in Table 19–1. Since these related changes are the rule rather than the exception, you should expect, for example, higher rates of pulse and respiration when a patient's temperature is 40° C/104° F than when it is 37.8° C/100° F. However, keep in mind that a change in one factor does not cause a change in another, but that changes in all are due to the patient's condition.

TABLE 19–1
Related Temperature, Pulse, Respiration Readings

Temperature °C/°F	*Pulse* Beats/minute	*Respiration* Breaths/minute
37.2°C/ 99°F	80	18
37.8°C/100°F	88	19
38.3°C/101°F	96	21
38.9°C/102°F	104	23
39.4°C/103°F	112	25
40.0°C/104°F	120	27
40.6°C/105°F	128	28
41.1°C/106°F	136	30

NOTE: This table is only a guide; individuals may vary greatly from the pulse and respirations in relation to the degrees of temperature.

NORMAL TEMPERATURES

For most healthy people, normal body temperature is 37°C/98.6°F taken orally. However, normal temperature for many people may be slightly higher or lower than these figures. The difference seldom is more than about one-half a degree, and may be important only as a sort of starting point for determining how high a fever or deep a chill a patient may have.

It is also normal for body temperature to fluctuate slightly during a 24-hour period. When people sleep, temperature tends to drop. With most people it gradually rises to slightly above their normal temperature over a period of about 12 hours after waking from a normal night's sleep. These changes usually occur every day regardless of a person's state of health. Some efficiency studies suggest that there is a direct relationship between a person's peak of efficiency and highest normal temperature during a 24-hour period. And it is fairly common for graveyard-shift workers and other so-called night owls to reach their maximum efficiency and highest temperature sometime between two and five o'clock in the morning, and for day-shift workers to reach theirs at about the middle of the afternoon. Also, many people who dislike and are slow at housework during the daytime do it faster, better, and almost cheerfully at ten or eleven o'clock or later at night.

In feverish sick people, the lowest temperature usually occurs between about three and five o'clock in the morning, and the highest about 12 hours later. This is normal and no cause for concern, depending, of course, on the change in temperature in relation to the patient's established pattern of temperature.

Recorded temperature readings usually make a clear pattern or graph of a patient's general condition at a particular stage of a sickness or infection. Changes from this pattern are of primary importance, as they indicate improvement or worsening of the patient's state of health.

ABNORMAL TEMPERATURES

As mentioned above, there are a variety of normal body temperatures and normal changes in them. It is the abnormal or excessive changes, especially when they are sudden, that may indicate a grave condition in a patient. Ask the doctor or your visiting nurse what temperatures and changes to expect for your patient, and what to do when those conditions occur.

> NOTE: Aspirin is a common, generally safe drug for reducing fever. But ask the doctor in advance if and when it may be given to your patient and in what dosage.

Abnormal temperatures also may be caused by foods, beverages, and environment. Many people break out in a sweat after eating highly seasoned food, for example, or shiver and shake with chills after drinking ice water. But such spells usually last for only a few minutes and are of no real concern, although it may be advisable to avoid such food and drink until a patient's health is fully restored. Environment also can raise or lower body temperature abnormally. Unusually hot rooms, beds, heating pads, and baths increase body temperature; cold air, drafts, cold baths lower it. Except in severe cases, such as prolonged exposure to a blizzard, abnormally high or low temperatures seldom last more than a few minutes after a normal environment is restored. Environmental means often are used to combat abnormal temperatures due to sickness or infection. For example, patients running high fevers may be given cold baths or placed under thermal pads to help reduce temperature.

What to Expect with Changes in Temperature There is no set rule as to how much change in temperature may be serious. Some people get a higher temperature with less provocation or cause than others; of two adults having temperatures of 37.5° C/98.8° F, one may be in good health and the other seriously ill. It is common for children to run a higher temperature than an adult in less time and with less cause.

The possible seriousness of a change in temperature depends on the actual temperature and how much it differs from the previous reading. If over a period of 4 or 6 hours your patient's temperature goes from, say 37° C/98.6° F to 38.1° C/100.6° F, usually you need not be particularly worried. If the previous reading was, say, 37.7° C/100° F and the new one 38.9° C/102° F, you probably should not be worried. But if the temperature has gone from 38.9° C/102° F to 40° C/104° F, or has made a drastic jump from 37.2° C/99° F to 39.4° C/103° F, you should contact the doctor at once.

If temperature drops to more than about 2 degrees below normal, you can be fairly certain that your patient is going to have a chill. It will not be just on the surface of the body; instead, the cold completely penetrates the body and can be quite uncomfortable. The moment a possible chill is indicated, start increasing environmental heat by turning on an electric blanket, piling more blankets on the bed, applying hot water bags or heating pads to your patient. However, be ready to stop environmental heating as quickly as you start it, since chills usually are followed by fairly sudden rises in temperature.

Dangerous Temperature Extremes Body temperatures below 35°C/95°F and above 40.5°C/105°F always should be regarded as signs of grave danger to a patient. Unless you have been told otherwise, contact the doctor or your visiting nurse immediately if either of these extremes occurs.

TIMES OF TAKING TEMPERATURES

When your patient is in the acute stages of an illness or infection, take the temperature at least four times a day, preferably at 4-hour intervals as, for example, at 8 A.M., 12 Noon, 4 P.M., and 8 P.M. If possible, one reading should be taken between 3 P.M. and 5 P.M., the period in which most fevers reach their highest point. After the acute phase has passed and the patient is convalescing, temperature should be taken twice a day.

Even if your patient's temperature is not above normal, it should be taken at least twice daily for as long as the disability continues.

RECORDING TEMPERATURE

Whether you use Metric/Celsius or Fahrenheit readings, standard 5-lines-per-inch graph or drafting paper is excellent for recording a patient's temperature, Fig. 19–1:

1. Mark each heavy horizontal line a whole degree of temperature. Unless your patient is subject to extremes, temperature spans of 36–41°C/96–104°F should be adequate.

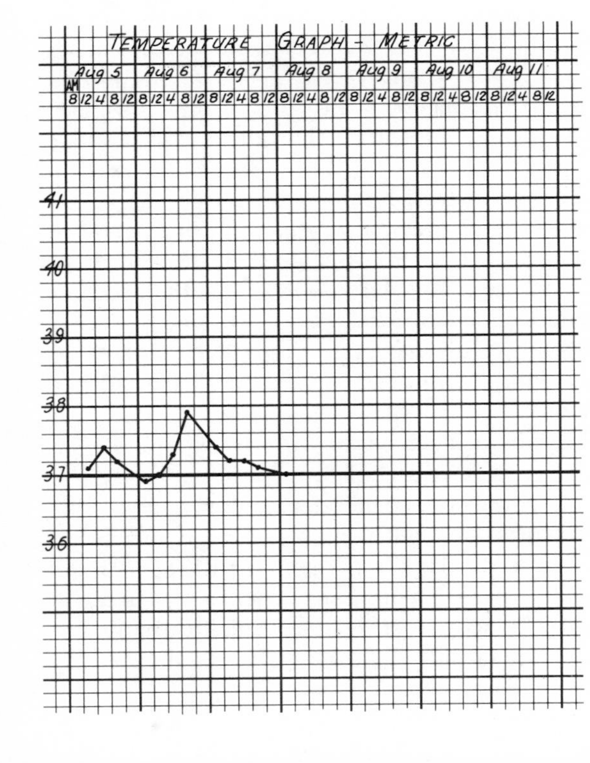

Fig. 19–1*a* *Temperature Graph—Metric/Celsius*

2. Light horizontal lines represent two-tenths of a degree of temperature. They usually are not marked, but you may if you wish.

3. Horizontal lines representing normal temperature, 37° C in Fig. 19–1*a*, and 98.6° F in *b*, may be made more noticeable by making them thicker or a different color from the other graph lines.

4. Vertical columns, not lines, represent the time in hours when you take temperature, such as at 8 A.M., 12 Noon, 4 P.M., 8 P.M., and 12 Midnight, or any other convenient but regular schedule. Readings usually are taken 4 hours apart at the same times each day. The doctor or your visiting nurse will tell you how many readings to take; it may or may not be necessary to take your patient's temperature at midnight and at 4 A.M. Time columns really need to be designated "A.M." or "P.M." only at the start of each cycle of temperature readings.

5. Heavy vertical lines usually divide the graph into dates, which should be clearly marked, Fig. 19–1. A week commonly is recorded on one graph. Of course, if more than five readings per day are required, you may have to draw extra-heavy or differently colored vertical lines to separate the dates.

6. Record each reading by placing a dot on the proper temperature line in the middle of the time column. As each reading is recorded, draw a straight line between it and the dot placed for the previous reading. This provides a

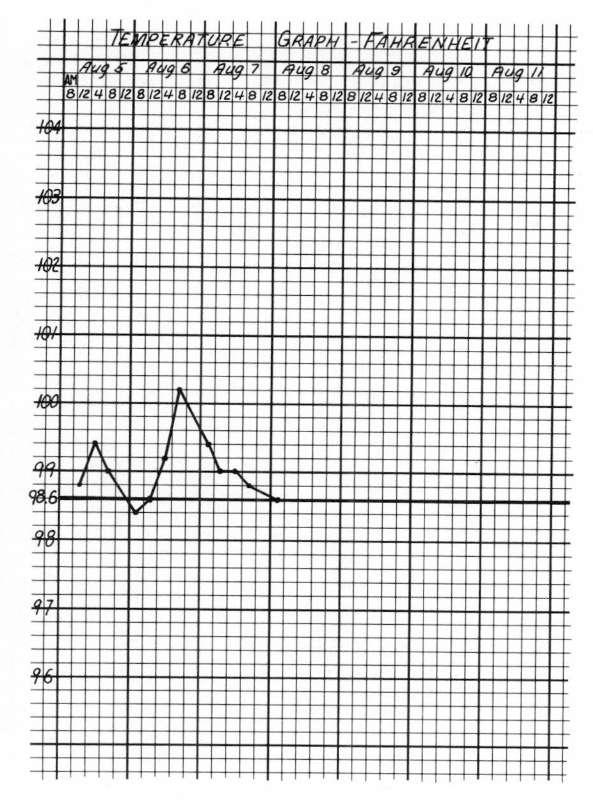

Fig. 19–1*b* *Temperature Graph—Fahrenheit*

pictorial outline or profile of the patient's temperature, and simplifies indications of changes in the patient's condition and the comparison of conditions day by day.

7. Show clearly on the temperature graph whether the readings are oral, axillary, or rectal, below. If axillary, place a capital *A* on the graph; if rectal, an *R*. For oral, no letter indication is needed.

THERMOMETERS

There are two types of *fever* or *clinical* thermometers: the mechanical or conventional, as in Fig. 19–2, and the electronic, as in Fig. 19–3. The mechanical thermometer is less expensive, and is complete in itself. Because of cost, an electronic thermometer may not be practical unless your patient has a long-term ailment and temperature readings must be taken daily. Electronic thermometers are much easier than the mechanical for the average person to read, but they need suitable batteries at all times.

Mechanical Thermometers The common mechanical or glass thermometers usually contain a column of mercury or alcohol that expands and rises in an enclosed tube as temperature rises, and theoretically contracts or drops as the temperature decreases. However, after a reading is taken, the column of mercury or alcohol usually remains at or near the high-temperature registration point in the tube until it is "shaken down," below, which always must be done immediately before using a mechanical thermometer.

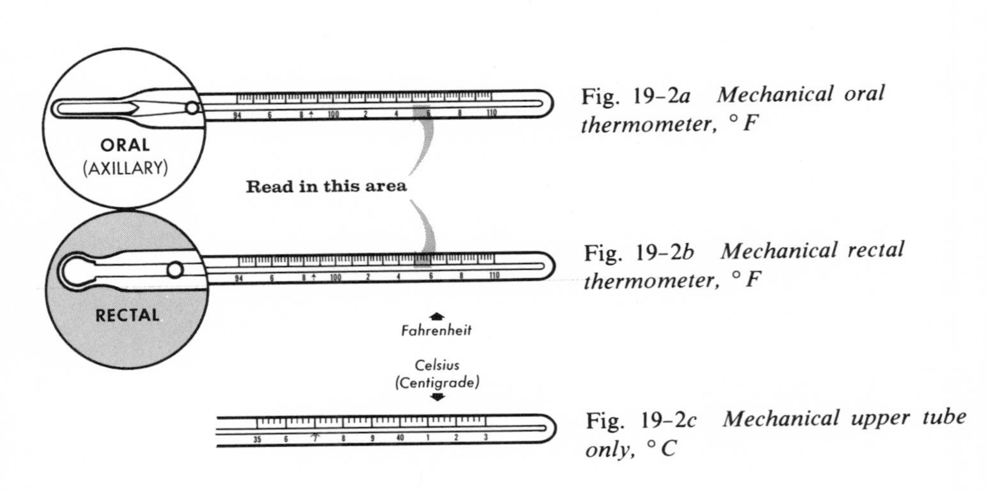

Fig. 19–2*a* *Mechanical oral thermometer, ° F*

Fig. 19–2*b* *Mechanical rectal thermometer, ° F*

Fig. 19–2*c* *Mechanical upper tube only, ° C*

The *oral* thermometer, Fig. 19–2*a*, usually has a thin, elongated tube at the bottom and is for measuring temperature in the mouth (orally), or in the armpit (axillary). The *rectal* thermometer, *b*, has a nearly round bulb at the bottom and is for measuring temperature in the rectum (rectally). Each method of measuring temperature has advantages and disadvantages, see Taking Temperature, below; ask the doctor or visiting nurse which method is best for your patient. When recording or reporting temperature, specify how it was taken, since the methods do not give identical readings.

> NOTE: Some manufacturers make both oral and rectal thermometers with round bulbs at the bottom. To distinguish it from the oral, the rectal thermometer may have a red top.

Thermometer Markings Most mechanical or glass clinical thermometers are graduated or marked in degrees and two-tenths of a degree, Fig. 19–2. There usually is a small arrow or arrowhead indicating normal oral temperature, 37° C/98.6° F. On many thermometers, the markings higher than oral normal are in red.

When reporting temperature, use the professional wording to avoid possible misunderstanding. If, for example, a temperature is 98.8° F, instead of saying "ninety-eight-and-eight-tenths degrees Fahrenheit," say "ninety-eight-point-eight degrees." It is not necessary to say Fahrenheit or Celsius (or centigrade). Report temperature accurately; if a reading is about midway between "point-six" and "point-eight," report it as "point-seven."

Shake Down Thermometer Just before taking your patient's temperature with a mechanical or glass thermometer, shake it as often as necessary to force the top of the column of mercury down below the 36° C or 96° F mark. To shake, hold the end of the thermometer opposite the bulb firmly with your thumb and fingers, swing your arm full downward, and end with a sharp snap of the wrist. Do not shake or snap a thermometer too violently; it may break. Before using a thermometer, read it to make sure that the mercury has been shaken down sufficiently.

Reading a Thermometer With your back to the light, hold a mechanical thermometer by the top end out in front of you and look for the mercury column, a shiny silver line, between the markings of the glass tube. Twist and turn the thermometer slowly between your fingers until the mercury line catches the light; take the reading at the exact top of the column. Many thermometers have a magnifying effect; that is, viewed from some angles the column of mercury is hairline thin while from other angles it is quite thick.

Cleaning Thermometers After taking temperature orally or rectally with a mechanical thermometer, wash it! (Before washing a rectal thermometer, wipe off all lubricant, see Taking Temperatures, below, with toilet or facial tissue or a cotton ball.) Wash a thermometer with a cotton ball that has been saturated with liquid soap. Start washing at the top end of the thermometer and wipe downward with a twisting motion to the botton of the bulb. Rinse it clean under cool running water (do not use hot water, it can break a thermometer), then wipe it dry with another cotton ball, again starting at the top and working downward. Store the clean thermometer in its case, or in a glass of water.

Electronic Thermometers Electronic or automatic thermometers are available with dial readings, as in Fig. 19–3, or with digital readouts. Dial-type thermometers usually give readings in both Fahrenheit and Celsius. Digital readout models generally read only in one or the other; however, there are units that you can control by a switch to read in either Celsius or Fahrenheit. In relation to mechanical or glass thermometers, above, here are advantages and disadvantages of the electronics in general:

1. *Easier to use.* No need to "shake down" the thermometer before use, no squinting at calibrations or readings.

2. *Safer.* No glass tube to break during oral or rectal measurement, or through careless handling; no mercury to accidentally get into a patient.

3. *Faster acting.* Electronic thermometers usually give a final reading in about 30 seconds.

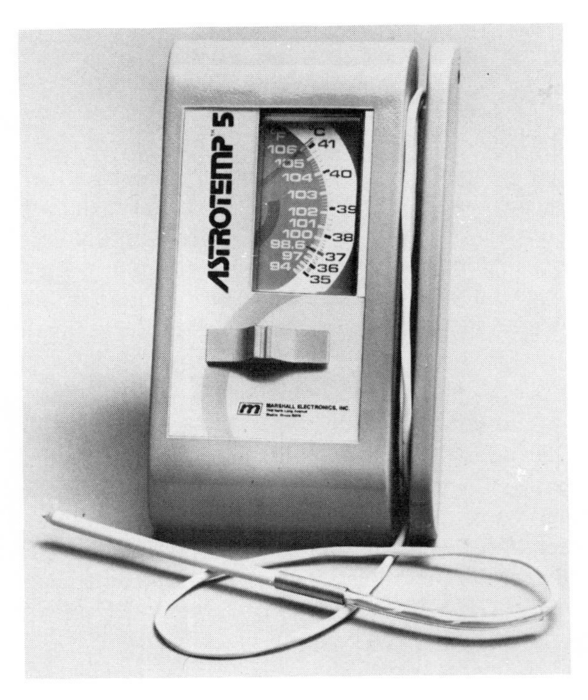

Fig. 19–3 *Electronic Fever Astrotemp 5*

4. *Versatile.* Electronic thermometers are suitable for taking temperature all three ways—orally, axillary, and rectally. The part inserted in the mouth, armpit, or rectum is commonly called the probe. Plastic probe covers usually come with or are readily available for electronic thermometers; their use eliminates the need for washing a probe after every use for the same patient (wash probes the same way as mechanical thermometers, above). You must,

of course, specify how your patient's temperature was measured—orally, axillary, rectally—when reporting or recording it, since the different methods give different readings regardless of the kind of thermometer used.

5. *Cost.* Electronic thermometers are usually much more costly than the mechanical or glass types, and may not be practical unless temperatures are to be measured frequently.

6. *Batteries.* Electronic thermometers are powered by small batteries, and for accurate measurements it is imperative that they are at proper strength. Under normal conditions, most batteries suitable for thermometers have a useful life of about 1 year; as a general rule they should be replaced at least once a year regardless of use. The better makes of electronic thermometers have indicators that show when a battery is too weak for reliable readings.

Testing Thermometers As a rule, there is no need to test a reliable make of mechanical or glass thermometer for accuracy. They are tested carefully by the manufacturer; they do not deteriorate with age or frequent use. The only thing that could spoil their accuracy is mistreatment resulting in breakage. Of course, you can test a glass or mechanical thermometer the same way as an electronic.

Electronic thermometers seldom need to be tested or checked for accuracy unless they have been dropped or severely shaken, or possibly subjected to temperatures 15 degrees or so higher than their normal maximum readings.

To test a thermometer, place it and one of known accuracy to the same depth in a glass of water that is no hotter than 37.8°C/100°F. If after proper time the readings are not identical, note the difference between them in tenths of a degree and whether the suspect thermometer's reading is higher or lower than the accurate one. Then reduce the water temperature to 35°C/95°F, and again compare readings. If the difference between readings is the same, and it is not more than about two-tenths of a degree, the suspect thermometer probably is safe to continue using. You must, of course, make the necessary correction by subtracting or adding the observed difference between readings when reporting or recording future readings; also, be sure to report this to the doctor and your visiting nurse. If the error between the suspect and accurate thermometers is not the same for the two test readings, or if it is more than about two-tenths of a degree, you should replace a mechanical or glass thermometer, and follow the manufacturer's instructions for the repair or adjustment of an electronic thermometer.

TAKING TEMPERATURE

Body temperature is measured by a mechanical clinical thermometer, or probe of an electronic one, placed in the mouth (oral temperature), in the armpit (axillary temperature), or in the rectum (rectal temperature). Always specify which temperature was taken. In writing, after the temperature reading put a capital *A* for axillary, *R* for rectal; the absence of a letter indicates that it was oral temperature.

Oral Temperature Normal body temperature of the average healthy adult, measured orally, is 37°C/98.6°F. Do not take oral temperature for:

Infants

Mouth-breathers

Unconscious or semiconscious patients

Irrational or paralyzed patients

Patients who are extremely ill

Patients who cannot hold still for 3 or 4 minutes if you are using a mechanical thermometer. Electronic thermometers usually give a final reading in less than 30 seconds.

Patients who have had recent mouth, nose, throat, or extensive head surgery.

Patients who have been, within the past 20 minutes, eating, drinking, smoking, or exercising vigorously.

Do not leave a patient unattended while taking oral temperature. Watch children very closely.

After shaking down a mechanical or glass thermometer, or covering the probe of an electronic one, insert the bulb or free end of the probe in your patient's mouth; it is usually placed a little to one side in the mouth back under the tongue. Keep a mechanical thermometer there for at least 3 minutes; an electronic probe only until the thermometer indicates a final reading; be sure your patient's mouth and lips are tightly closed all the time. Read temperature immediately after removing the temperature or probe, and record it on the graph. Then clean and put away the instrument.

Axillary Temperature Axillary temperature, measured in the armpit, usually is about .3°–.6°C/.5°–1°F *lower* than oral, above. Axillary temperature, generally taken with an oral thermometer, Fig. 19–2*a*, may be used when temperature should not be taken orally.

Except for placement of the thermometer or probe, axillary temperature is taken and treated essentially the same as oral temperature, above. After shaking down a mechanical thermometer, place the bulb or free end of a probe in the center of the patient's armpit, and press the arm down tightly against the body to hold it in place. Keep a mechanical thermometer there for at least 5 minutes, the probe only until the electronic thermometer indicates final reading; then remove the thermometer or probe, read and record the temperature, clean and put away the thermometer. Cleaning a mechanical thermometer after taking axillary temperature, and putting a cover on a probe before doing it, may not seem necessary, but it is good nursing practice and should be done.

Rectal Temperature Rectal temperature, taken in a patient's rectum, generally is from about .3°–.6°C/.5°–1°F *higher* than oral, above. Rectal is more accurate than oral and axillary temperatures, and may be used when temperature should not be taken orally. Do not take temperature rectally following rectal surgery or if the rectum is diseased; in most cases it is advisable to ask the doctor or your visiting nurse if your patient's temperature should be taken rectally. Rectal temperature should be taken only with a rectal mechanical thermometer, although any electronic thermometer, with the probe properly covered, may be used.

After shaking down a mechanical thermometer or covering the probe of an electronic one, lubricate the bulb or free end of the covered probe liberally with Vaseline® or a lubricating jelly.

Rectal temperature of a person more than about 4 years of age is most easily

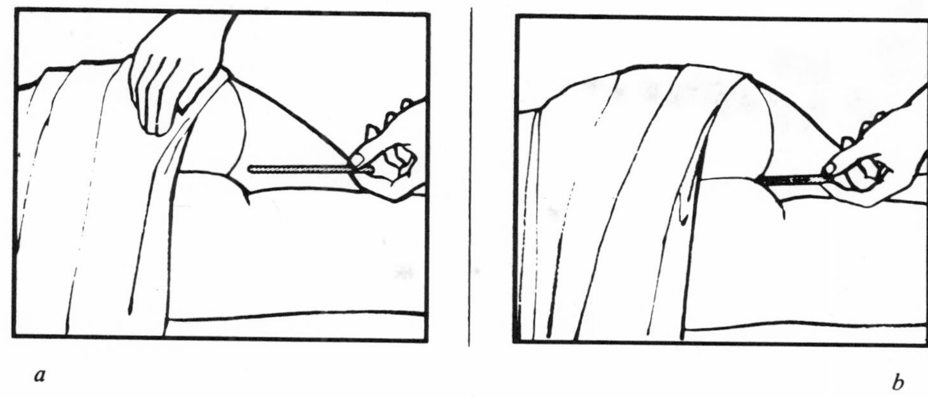

Fig. 19–4*a, b* *Taking rectal temperature*

taken with the patient lying on a side, as in Fig. 19–4. Turn back only enough covering to expose the rectum, *a*. Gently insert 1–1½ in. of the lubricated thermometer or probe in the rectum, *b*. Do not force the thermometer or probe; if well lubricated, it should slip in quite easily. Hold a thermometer in place for at least 3 minutes, a probe only until the final reading is indicated. Then remove the thermometer or probe; wipe a thermometer with a dry cotton ball or paper tissue; discard the probe cover. Then read and proceed as for Oral Temperature, above.

> NOTE: Rectal temperature of a child about 4 years old or younger is best taken with the patient lying face down across your lap. Always warn a child that taking temperature this way may be uncomfortable, but will not hurt. To help the patient relax and ease insertion of the thermometer or probe, have the child blow as if blowing up a balloon.

CELSIUS / CENTIGRADE—FAHRENHEIT CONVERSIONS

Originally temperature was measured in degrees Fahrenheit, based on the boiling point of water at sea level as 212° F and the freezing point as 32° F. With increasing use of the metric system of measurements, temperature is more commonly measured in degrees Celsius or centigrade, based on the boiling point of water at sea level as 100° C and the freezing point as 0° C. Below is a practical table of temperatures converted from one system to the other:

TABLE 19–2

Approximate Body Temperature Equivalents
Celsius to Fahrenheit

°C	°F	°C	°F	°C	°F
33.0	91.4	36.0	96.8	39.0	102.2
33.1	91.6	36.1	97.0	39.1	102.4
33.2	91.8	36.2	97.2	39.2	102.6
33.3	92.0	36.3	97.3	39.3	102.7
33.4	92.1	36.4	97.5	39.4	102.9
33.5	92.3	36.5	97.7	39.5	103.1
33.6	92.5	36.6	97.9	39.6	103.3
33.7	92.7	36.7	98.1	39.7	103.5
33.8	92.8	36.8	98.2	39.8	103.6
33.9	93.0	36.9	98.4	39.9	103.8
34.0	93.2	37.0	98.6	40.0	104.0
34.1	93.4	37.1	98.8	40.1	104.2
34.2	93.6	37.2	99.0	40.2	104.4
34.3	93.7	37.3	99.1	40.3	104.5
34.4	93.9	37.4	99.3	40.4	104.7
34.5	94.1	37.5	99.5	40.5	104.9
34.6	94.3	37.6	99.7	40.6	105.1
34.7	94.5	37.7	99.9	40.7	105.3
34.8	94.6	37.8	100.0	40.8	105.4
34.9	94.8	37.9	100.2	40.9	105.6
35.0	95.0	38.0	100.4	41.0	105.8
35.1	95.2	38.1	100.6	41.1	106.0
35.2	95.4	38.2	100.8	41.2	106.2
35.3	95.5	38.3	100.9	41.3	106.3
35.4	95.7	38.4	101.1	41.4	106.5
35.5	95.9	38.5	101.3	41.5	106.7
35.6	96.1	38.6	101.5	41.6	106.9
35.7	96.3	38.7	101.7	41.7	107.1
35.8	96.4	38.8	101.8	41.8	107.2
35.9	96.6	38.9	102.0	41.9	107.4

To change or convert degrees Celsius/centigrade to Fahrenheit, use this formula:

$$°F = (9 \div 5) \times °C + 32$$

To change or convert degrees Fahrenheit to Celsius/centigrade, use this formula:

$$°C = (°F - 32) \times 5 \div 9$$

20 Pulse

A patient's pulse usually is taken at the same time as temperature (Chapter 19) in most hospitals, clinics, and doctors' offices, and during house calls by a doctor or a visiting nurse. But as a rule taking pulse is not part of nursing at home unless ordered by the doctor. The main reason for this is that there is much more to taking a pulse than merely counting the number of beats per minute. It takes training and much experience to be able to identify and describe accurately the particular type of pulsebeat, such as bounding, thready, feeble, intermittent, rapid and the many other important characteristics based on the power and the rhythm of a heartbeat.

WHAT PULSE IS

Pulse is an extremely reliable indicator of the condition of a person's heart and how it is reacting to disease, infection, medication, and physical or emotional exercise, stress, fatigue, and stimulation. All such factors affect a heart's beating and the way it pumps blood through the arteries. As the blood flows and ebbs through the arteries, their walls expand and contract, or swell and shrink, in keeping with the rate (number of beats per minute), power (strong, feeble, etc.), and rhythm (steady, jerky, etc.) action of the heartbeat. Many so-called normal and abnormal factors affect or influence heartbeat.

Normal Factors For healthy men in the 18 to 60 age group, normal pulse rate is 70 to 74 beats per minute; for women the rate is about 8 to 10 beats higher, or 78 to 84 beats per minute. However, these are only common averages; some people are healthy with pulse rates as low as 50 or as high as 80. For healthy infants and children, normal pulse rate may range from 90 to 110.

Following exercise or excitement of any type, the pulse rate rises temporarily above normal. During periods of untroubled sleep or prolonged rest and relaxation the pulse rate usually drops to slightly below normal. Some medicines increase pulse rate, others decrease it. Healthy people usually have a strong, steady, regular pulsebeat. However, it is not uncommon for people who are for all practical purposes in a state of good health to have a heartbeat that may be quite different from the so-called normal one.

Abnormal Factors Any disease, infection, deterioration, or degeneration of the heart or any other organ or part of the body—and any physical or emotional shock, stress, abuse, or stimulation—can and usually does change the heartbeat and pulse. There is an important relationship between temperature, pulse, and respiration, Table 19–1, which must be considered in most fever conditions. One or more characteristics of a pulse may change; for example, a normal pulse may simply become faster, or faster and irregular, or faster, irregular, and weak.

Through education and experience doctors, professional nurses, and competent medical technicians know what type or kind of pulse should exist under certain conditions, and what to expect when there are variations. If it is necessary for you to take your patient's pulse, the doctor or your visiting nurse will describe exactly what characteristics to expect, what normal and abnormal differences may indicate, and when you should contact the doctor.

TAKING PULSE

Pulsebeat usually is counted over a 30-second period, and doubled to determine the minute rate. If the beat is irregular, count it for 60 seconds. A clock or watch with a sweep-second hand is recommended for taking pulse, but any timepiece with a second hand or a digital "seconds" readout may be used.

The power and rhythm of a pulse is a matter of the taker's identification of the characteristics of the beat. In case of doubt as to the proper medical term, describe as accurately as you can and in detail how your patient's pulse felt in relation to your own. Some of the more common terms for describing pulse are:

Alternating. Changing back and forth between weak and strong pulsations.

Bounding. The pulse reaches a higher than normal level, then quickly disappears.

Feeble, *Weak*. Difficult to feel, as opposed to a strong pulsebeat.

Intermittent. Occasional beats are missed.

Irregular. Appreciable changes in frequency and force.

Rapid. A pulse that is appreciably faster than normal, especially for an adult.

Regular. Very little variation in length, number, and strength of pulsebeats.

Thready. A fine, hardly noticeable pulse.

Taking Pulse Pulse usually is taken by pressing two fingers, the index or forefinger and the middle finger, lightly but firmly over an artery that readily can be felt through flesh and skin.

Do not take pulse with your thumb, because you may actually take your own instead of your patient's pulse.

Do not press on an artery hard enough to stop or hinder the flow of blood through it.

Unless the doctor or your visiting nurse specifies other points, pulse generally is taken at the:

Radial artery in the wrist.

Carotid artery in the neck.

Temporal artery at the temple.

Sometimes the pulsebeat may be visible in the neck or temple and can be counted without having to touch your patient, a great advantage when you do not wish to disturb a sleeping patient. However, observing the pulsebeat without feeling its quality gives you only the rate.

RECORDING PULSE

If you are required to take pulse readings on a regular basis, keep accurate record of them. Pulse usually is taken at the same time as temperature (Chapter 19), and is recorded essentially the same way on the same kind of chart or graph, Figs. 19–1 and 20–1:

1. Dates and times are indicated the same way on temperature and pulse graphs.
2. Heavy horizontal lines on a pulse graph represent tens of beats per minute. Each light horizontal line represents a change of two beats per minute. A span of 30 to 130 pulse rate is more than ample in most cases. Your visiting nurse will help you revise the graph if a greater span is needed.
3. Enter pulse rate on the graph in the same fashion as temperature on the temperature graph.
4. The power and rhythm of the pulsebeat may or may not be noted on the graph. If it is "normal" for your patient, you can jot down the date and time of the reading on a convenient part of the graph and write "normal"; or you can make no notation, thus implying that it is not abnormal—but you must do one or the other consistently! If the pulse is abnormal, such as alternating, feeble, thready, etc., write the most adequate descriptive term after the date and time notation. If no standard term seems adequate, write the date, time, and your description of the pulse on the back of the graph.

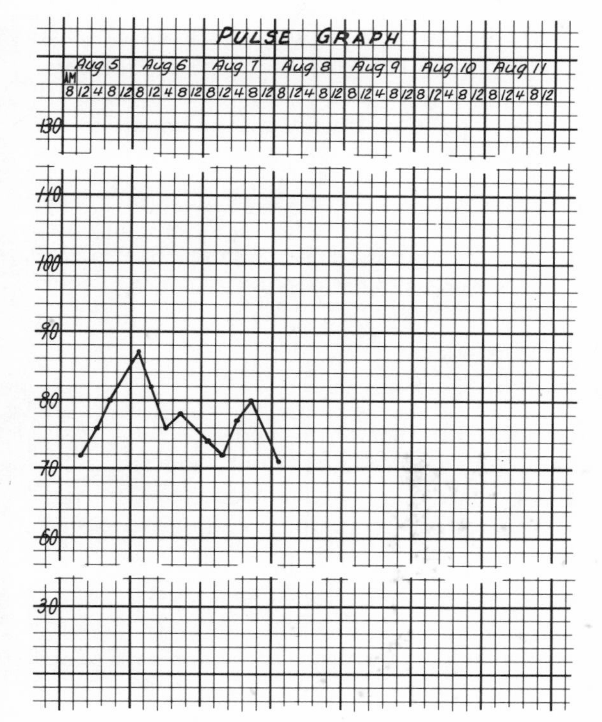

Fig. 20–1 *Pulse graph*

21 Respiration

Respiration, or the *rate and type* of breathing, can be a reliable indicator of a person's state of health. It can be a symptom of diseases, infections, and various bodily injuries; and it changes as a sick person's condition changes for better or for worse. However, changes in respiration also may be due to natural causes such as age, and changes in altitude and in a person's activity.

Rate of respiration is the number of complete breaths taken in one minute. A complete breath consists of one *inspiration*, or drawing of air into the lungs, and one *expiration*, or expelling of air from the lungs. In normal, healthy breathing, as a rule inspirations are noticeably longer than expirations. In feverish patients, the rate of respiration usually increases along with temperature and pulse, Table 19–1.

Type of respiration is a description based on the apparent ease or difficulty a person has in breathing, and the sound made by the air as it enters or leaves the lungs. Types of respiration are described medically as abdominal, thoracic, Cheyne-Stokes, costal, stertorous, labored, wheezing, etc. In taking a patient's respiration, it usually is as important to note the type as well as the rate.

Although it can be as important a state-of-health indicator as are temperature and pulse (Chapters 19, 20), a sick person's respiration usually is not taken in home nursing unless it is directly ordered by the doctor. This is due mainly to the average inexperienced nurse's being unable to correctly identify the many types of respiration. It takes several years to learn how to do this. When it is important for the doctor to know the type of a patient's respiration, usually it is too important to rely on a "guesstimate," no matter how well intentioned it is.

> NOTE: If you are required to take and report your patient's respiration, you will be given detailed information as to which changes in rate and type of breathing are important in this particular case. The doctor should explain the cause of the respiration and clearly describe, and possibly demonstrate, the type and rate of breathing to expect.

RATES OF RESPIRATION

Average normal rates of respiration for healthy persons are shown in Table 21–1 For an adult, a rate of less than 12/minute is considered "slow," and above 26, "rapid." However, rates usually vary to some extent with altitude, activity, and temperature. For descriptions of some rates and types of respiration, see Some Respirations, below.

> NOTE: With some diseases and infections, it is not unusual for the rate of respiration to rise to 60- or 80/minute, or fall to 10- or 8/minute. The doctor or your visiting nurse will tell you what rate to expect with your patient.

TABLE 21-1

Rates of Respiration

Premature infant	40–90/minute
Newborn	30–80/minute
1st year	20–40/minute
2nd year	20–30/minute
5th year	20–25/minute
15th year	15–20/minute
Adult	15–20/minute

NOTE: These rates are average; slight variations above and below are not uncommon.

Altitude On entering altitudes of 3,080 meters/10,000 feet or higher, a person's rate of respiration usually increases due to the air's containing less oxygen, or being "thinner," than at much lower elevations. However, most people soon adapt to living at a high altitude, and their respiration returns to near normal rates.

Activity Any physical, emotional, or mental activity, stress, excitement, or disturbance usually causes an increase in a person's rate of respiration as well as in heartbeat or pulse (Chapter 20). The ratio of respiration to pulse is fairly constant, approximately 1 to 5, or 21.5% of the pulse rate, as indicated in Table 19–1. As a general rule, respiration should be counted only when a patient is at rest and preferably does not know that it is being taken; people can control to a great extent both their rate and type of respiration.

Temperature The rate of respiration nearly always increases in keeping with an increase of temperature, as shown in Table 19–1. These are considered as being normal average temperature-respiration relationships. You should report differences in respiration, either slower or faster, to the doctor immediately unless you have been instructed otherwise.

TYPES OF RESPIRATION

Normal relaxed breathing is effortless, automatic, regular, even, and quiet. With illness, there can be a wide variety of breathing sounds—frictional, splashing, tinkling, bubbling, high pitched, whistling, rasping, forced, and so forth—and it may be done at regular or at irregular intervals, or at a mixture of regular and irregular intervals. Each sound and combination of sounds and frequencies is a symptom of known diseases, infections, and bodily injuries.

If you are required to take your patient's respiration, describe the sounds of inspiration and expiration as accurately as you can. Do not try to save words; it can be a great disservice to your patient and the doctor. Instead, describe a breathing sound in all the detail you need to tell exactly what you heard. For example, instead of merely "a bubbling sound," you may have heard "a bubbling sound like a pot of coffee perking quickly, or a pan of rapidly boiling water, but with sort of a weak splash as if you were pouring some out into the sink . . ." It is far better to give too much description than not enough. Do not be surprised if the doctor asks you to describe sounds several different ways or times; without meaning to, inexperienced nurses often leave an important point out of one description and add it to the next.

Some Respirations If taking your patient's respiration is part of your duties, the doctor probably will describe the sounds and frequencies of breathing that you should expect and report. Here are some of the more common types of respiration:

Abdominal. The abdomen rises and falls with each respiration, but the chest does not. See *Thoracic*, below.

Cheyne-Stokes. Respirations gradually increase in rapidity and depth until reaching a climax, then decrease until breathing may stop for 5 to 50 seconds, after which the cycle begins again. Cheyne-Stokes breathing is commonly a forerunner of death; however, it also may last for quite some time, a few days to several weeks, then disappear.

Dyspnea. Labored or difficult breathing.

Sigh. A very deep inspiration followed by prolonged expiration.

Stertorous. Breathing with rattling or bubbling sounds; "snoring"; noisy breathing. Usually caused by breathing with the mouth open.

Stridulous. A high-pitched crowing or barking sound made during inspiration. It is usually due to an upper airway obstruction such as laryngitis, croup, or a foreign body.

Thoracic. Breathing done entirely by expansion of the chest when the abdomen does not move. See *Abdominal*, above.

Wheeze. A high-pitched, often somewhat musical whistling or sighing sound. It commonly accompanies the difficult breathing that occurs with asthma, croup, and other respiratory disorders.

TAKING AND RECORDING RESPIRATION

Because breathing is controlled by a person's voluntary as well as involuntary muscles, when possible take respiration without your patient's knowing what you are doing. If your patient seems to be deliberately breathing a certain way, take respiration when your patient is asleep.

Count each inspiration and its expiration as one breath or complete cycle of respiration. With your hand in the same position as when taking pulse (Chapter 20), watch the rise and fall of your patient's chest or upper abdomen for one minute. If the movement cannot be clearly seen, place your hand gently on your patient's chest or back and count the respirations. Count several times, for the sake of accuracy, when respiration is fast and irregular. Try to identify the type of respiration in medical terms or by comparison with your own breathing. Also note any abnormal condition, such as pain, associated with your patient's breathing.

Recording Respiration Except in cases of serious illness, taking respiration is not a regular part of home nursing care. But if it is required of you, keep accurate record of the readings. Generally, unless a patient is obviously "putting on an act," respiration is taken at the same time as temperature and pulse (Chapters 19, 20), and is recorded on basically the same kind of chart, Figs. 19–1, 20–1, 21–1:

1. Dates and times are indicated the same way across the top.
2. Heavy horizontal lines represent tens of respirations per minute. A span of 10–40 respirations is adequate in most cases. The doctor or your visiting nurse will advise you if a greater span is needed.
3. Light horizontal lines indicate two respirations per minute.
4. Enter the rate of respiration on the chart the same way as for temperature and pulse, connecting the dots of successive entries to form a graph or profile of respiration.
5. The type of respiration and any abnormalities may be noted on the face of the chart, but inexperienced nurses usually do better by writing them on the back. Write the date and time of the respiration; identify it by accurate medical terms or by describing it in your own words; and add any abnormalities as to your patient's breathing or general condition.

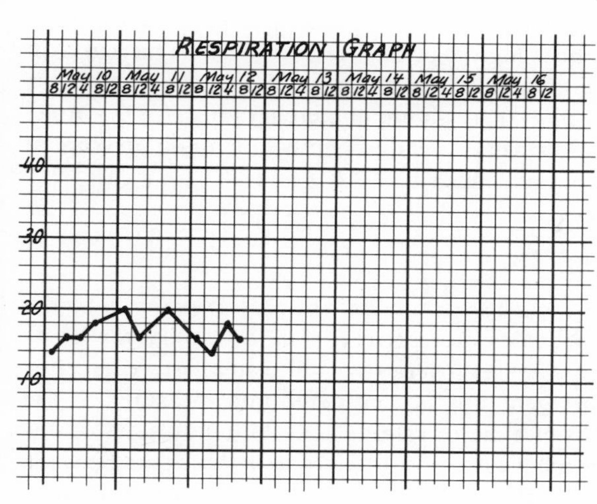

Fig. 21–1 *Respiration chart*

22 Blood Pressure

Instruments for measuring blood pressure are readily available. But whether you need one, or even if it is advisable to have one, depends on: (1) your patient's problem; (2) your ability to measure blood pressure accurately; and (3) the accuracy of your instrument.

Your Patient. Blood pressure is only one of the many vital signs, such as temperature, pulse, and respiration (Chapters 19, 20, 21) that a doctor takes into account when analyzing a patient's condition. However, many people believe that blood pressure is of utmost importance in all cases, and tend to worry unduly about it. So generally it is best not to mention blood pressure to your patient, let alone take it, without consulting the doctor. If it is necessary, the doctor will tell you.

Your Ability. To be of real help to your patient and the doctor, you must measure and record blood pressure accurately. Major errors in measuring or recording temperature, pulse, and respiration can as a rule readily be detected by the doctor or your visiting nurse. But with blood pressure, there often is no other vital sign to suggest that a reading is not accurate.

Your Instrument. The accuracy of your instrument (see Sphygmomanometers, below) is a prime factor in your ability to take blood pressure accurately. Have the doctor's nurse compare your instrument with the doctor's before you use it. After it has been dropped or severely jolted, or any time you think it may have become faulty, have it inspected and tested by a skilled repairman; hospital supply houses can direct you to competent technicians. In the original sphygmomanometers, blood pressure was measured by how high it pushed up a column of mercury. In modern units, pressure may be measured by other means, but it is expressed or given as the height in millimeters (mm) of a column of mercury (Hg); for example, 120 mm Hg, or, simply, 120 mm. However, instead of expressing blood pressure in "mm Hg," it may be given as "points," such as "120 points."

WHAT BLOOD PRESSURE IS

In a very general meaning, *blood pressure* is the force or pressure exerted by the blood in circulation on the walls or sides of an artery, vein, or capillary (such as the hairlike tubes connecting the smallest arteries with the smallest veins). For practical purposes, blood pressure generally is considered and measured as the pressure of blood against the walls of a major artery. Since blood pulsates as it is pumped through the arteries by the heart, and there is a slight pause between heartbeats, there are two basic types of blood pressure: *systolic* and *diastolic*. The difference between them is *pulse pressure*.

Systolic Pressure. This is the greater force or pressure, and is caused by the systole or contraction of the left ventricle (lower chamber) of the heart as it propels blood into the arteries. Systolic blood pressure rises during any kind of activity, stress, excitement, or worry, and falls during normal sleep and prolonged periods of rest. For a normal, healthy, relaxed, seated adult, systolic blood pressure may be as low as 100 and as high as 140 mm Hg. Systolic pressure persistently more than 140 is generally believed to be abnormal. However, with older persons, less resilience in the blood vessels and other physiological changes due to age must be taken into account when pressures above 140 are obtained. For healthy young persons, systolic pressures of 100 to 120 mm Hg are usually normal. In recording blood pressure, *systolic* is always placed at the left as in *120*/60.

NOTE: If you are instructed to take the blood pressure in both arms, as sometimes happens, be sure to indicate which reading is the right arm and which is the left.

Diastolic Pressure. This is the lower blood pressure that exists during the period of relaxation or the slight pause between heartbeats. It depends primarily upon the elasticity or resilience of the arteries and capillaries. Normal diastolic pressure usually ranges from about 60 to 90 mm Hg. A diastolic pressure persistently above 100 is considered abnormal and, as a rule, of greater danger to a person than a persistently high systolic pressure. In taking and recording diastolic pressure, some doctors prefer one reading, others want two (see Taking Blood Pressure, below). When recording blood pressure, the *diastolic* is always placed at the right, as in 120/*70*.

Pulse Pressure. This is the difference between systolic and diastolic pressures measured at the same time. Pulse pressure generally is considered normal when the systolic pressure is about 40 mm Hg greater than the diastolic. Pulse pressure of more than 50 mm Hg or less than 30 is generally considered abnormal and a sign of potential danger for the patient.

VARIATIONS OF BLOOD PRESSURE

Blood pressure normally varies with a person's age, sex, and muscular development; states of stress, worry, and fatigue; and the altitude. All these factors are taken into account by a doctor when evaluating a patient's blood pressure readings. Without the knowledge and expertise for proper evaluation, an untrained person who takes blood pressure and tries to interpret or analyze it for a patient can easily do more harm than good.

Patients have every right to know what their blood pressure is. But only competent doctors should try to explain what it means in a particular case. If you must take your patient's blood pressure, the doctor will tell you what certain readings may mean and whether you should tell your patient.

RECORDING BLOOD PRESSURE

Blood pressure readings usually are recorded on a very simple form, Fig. 22-1, which can be made at home with ordinary ruled binder paper. Enter the date, time, and systolic/diastolic pressures. If just an occasional reading is required, at

BLOOD PRESSURE RECORD

DATE	TIME-A.M.	READING	TIME-P.M.	READING
July 5	8:00	150/90	4:00	120/70
	12:00 Noon	130/80	8:00	130/85
July 6	8:00	120/70	4:00	140/90
	12:00 Noon	130/90	8:00	130/70

Fig. 22-1 *Blood pressure record*

any convenient place on a temperature chart (Fig. 19–1) you can make a date and time entry followed with "B.P." and the systolic/diastolic figures.

Blood pressure always should be taken at the same point on a patient's body. If at any time a different point is used, be sure to note it on the chart.

TAKING BLOOD PRESSURE

There are two basic methods of measuring blood pressure. In *direct measurement* (usually done only in a hospital or clinic) a sterile needle or small catheter is placed in an artery and through it the fluctuations of blood pressure are transmitted to a device for recording it graphically. *Indirect measurement*, the more common method, is done by measuring the pressure actually exerted by the blood on the walls of an artery, usually the brachial in the upper right arm. The patient should be seated or lying down, with the arm at the level of the heart. A mercury-gravity, aneroid-manometer, or an electronic blood pressure measuring device or sphygmomanometer, below, may be used.

Indirect measurement of blood pressure is done two ways:

Palpatory, which is done by feeling with a finger a change of pressure in an artery, can be used only for measuring systolic pressure. Accurate palpatory measuring is the result of much experience and skill; it should not be attempted by unqualified people.

Auscultatory (listening) blood pressure measurement, the more common method, is for systolic and diastolic pressures. A stethoscope is needed unless using certain electronic devices. If you must take your patient's blood pressure, the doctor is most likely to prescribe the auscultatory method.

> NOTE: Under certain conditions, a doctor may want two, instead of one, diastolic readings taken at the same time. This requires a slightly different technique from the usual one, and you will be given adequate instruction.

Taking blood pressure accurately is not always easy for inexperienced nurses, but it is not necessarily difficult. For best results, ask the doctor or your visiting nurse to show you several times exactly what to do; if possible, you should take your patient's blood pressure and compare your readings with those made by the doctor or the visiting nurse.

Always measure blood pressure at the same point on your patient's body, as different points usually will have different pressures. Blood pressure usually is measured on the upper right arm, but several other points are satisfactory. The doctor or your visiting nurse will advise you where to take blood pressure when the upper right arm is not suitable.

Sphygmomanometers There are three basic types of sphygmomanometers or devices for auscultatory (above) blood pressure measurement: the *mercurial*, the *aneroid*, and the *electronic*. Mercurial and aneroid instruments, both of which require stethoscopes, are truly auscultatory in operation; with certain electronic instruments, changes in flashing lights as well as, or instead of, sound indicate a change from systolic to diastolic blood pressure.

Mercurial, also known as mercury-gravity, sphygmomanometers are an enclosed column of mercury attached to an upright scale, as in Fig. 22–2*a*. In operation, the pressure of the blood against an inflated cuff wrapped tightly around the measuring point on the body forces mercury up in the column for the systolic reading; a valve releasing air from the cuff allows the mercury to fall in the column for the diastolic reading. Mercurial sphygmomanometers usually are the least costly and the least likely to get out of adjustment. However, they do require the use of a stethoscope, Fig. 22–2*b*, and are the most difficult for many people to learn to use properly.

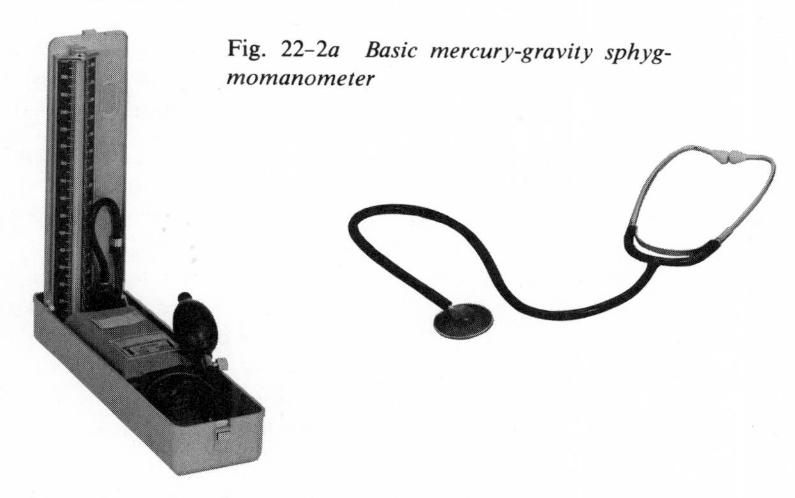

Fig. 22–2*a* *Basic mercury-gravity sphygmomanometer*

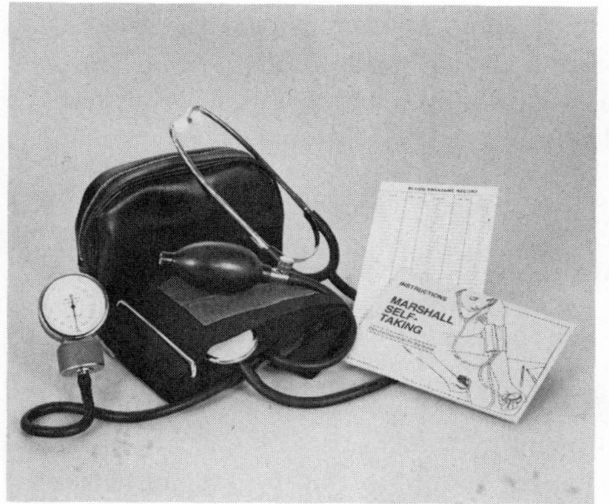

Fig. 22–3*a* *Aneroid sphygmomanometer*

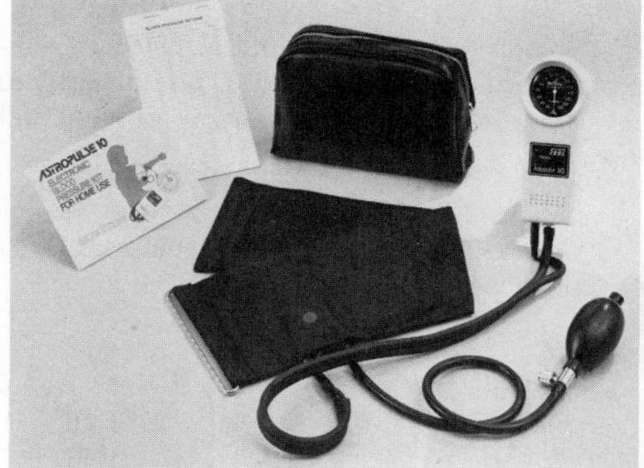

Fig. 22–3*b* *Electronic sphygmomanometer*

Aneroid, or aneroid-manometer, sphygmomanometers function much the same way as the mercurial type, but operate on air pressure instead of a column of mercury. Two other important differences are that the pressure readings of aneroid instruments are on a dial, as in Fig. 22–3*a*, and that the stethoscope often is built into the cuff. Aneroid instruments generally cost more than the mercurial of similar quality and efficiency, but weigh less and are easier to use and carry around.

Electronic sphygmomanometers, as in Fig. 22–3*b*, are the easiest to learn to use. No stethoscope is needed. In the type shown here, a microphone imbedded in the cuff "interprets" the systolic and diastolic pressure points and reports them to the user with a flashing light and sound signal as well as needle readings on the pressure gauge. Electronic sphygmomanometers are the most costly, and may not be practical unless you have long-term need of almost daily blood pressure readings. Electronic units also require batteries. Normally the batteries should last for a year or longer; however, they should be replaced once a year regardless of use to guard against possible corrosion. The better electronic sphygmomanometers contain battery testers that indicate when batteries are too weak for reliable use.

Repair and Testing Sphygmomanometers are precision instruments and, to be of genuine help, must be kept in good condition. Repairs seldom are needed, and should be made only by an authorized repair service, or returned to the factory according to the manufacturer's instructions.

Like any other precision instrument, a sphygmomanometer should be tested for accuracy from time to time, particularly if it has been dropped or received a severe jolt. Testing is easily done. Take readings at the same place on a person with an instrument of known accuracy and the suspect one within a minute of each other. There may be a very slight difference between readings, and if it is the same for the systolic and diastolic pressure, as a rule the suspect instrument is satisfactory for continued use. The difference in points of pressure and whether the suspect instrument "reads high" or "reads low" should be written, dated, and kept with the instrument. If, however, the differences between systolic and diastolic pressure readings is not the same, or there are more than about 5 points' difference between the accurate and suspect instruments, the latter should be repaired or adjusted according to the manufacturer's instructions.

Stethoscope A stethoscope, as in Fig. 22–2*b*, is needed with mercurial and aneroid sphygmomanometers for you to hear the loss of sound of heartbeat that marks the difference between systolic and diastolic blood pressures. There are many good types of mechanical and electronic stethoscopes in a fairly wide range of prices.

Cuff Blood pressure cuffs, as in Figs. 22–2 and 22–3, are a vital part of mercurial, aneroid, and electronic sphygmomanometers. Except in some electronic units, the cuff is wrapped around the point of measuring blood pressures, then inflated by a small hand squeeze-bulb air pump until the systolic pressure is measured. Releasing air from the cuff provides for measuring diastolic pressure.

Blood pressure cuffs for adults should be approximately 13 cm./5 in. wide; for infants and children, 2.5–6 cm./1–2.5 in. wide.

There are various types of cuff fasteners. The old-fashioned kind is an extension of the cuff that becomes narrower until the end is approximately 5 cm./2 in. wide. This strip is wrapped several times around the patient's arm or other point of measuring pressure and the end is tucked under a layer to hold it. There are also cuffs with hook-and-eye fasteners. Many nurses prefer the cuff with so-called touch-and-hold or Velcro® fasteners; it easily adjusts to fit any size arm.

Auscultatory Blood Pressure Measurement Regardless of the kind of sphygmomanometer used, auscultatory blood pressure measurement is done essentially the same way. A deflated cuff is wrapped around the patient's arm with the lower edge of the cuff about 2.5 cm./1 in. above the inner crease of the elbow, as in Fig. 22–4.

NOTE: If the doctor or your visiting nurse wants blood pressure to be measured at a point other than the brachial artery in the patient's right arm, it will be shown you.

If using a mercurial or an aneroid sphygmomanometer, place the stethoscope over the brachial artery on the body side of the elbow, Fig. 22–4. Hold the stethoscope firmly in place, but do not press it hard against the arm. The stethoscope is not needed with an electronic sphygmomanometer.

With the air pump, inflate the cuff until the reading in the sphygmomanometer is about 30 points (mm Hg) above the anticipated reading. It may be necessary to inflate the cuff to 150 or 200 points to reach above the systolic reading for your patient. To obtain the systolic reading, slowly release the air from the cuff until, with the stethoscope, you hear the first clear sound of your patient's heartbeat; note the numeral on the sphygmomanometer at the top of the column of mercury or on the dial of an aneroid unit scale—it is the systolic pressure reading. With many electronic instruments, a light will begin to flash when you have released enough air from the cuff for the systolic reading; some instruments also emit a sound at this point.

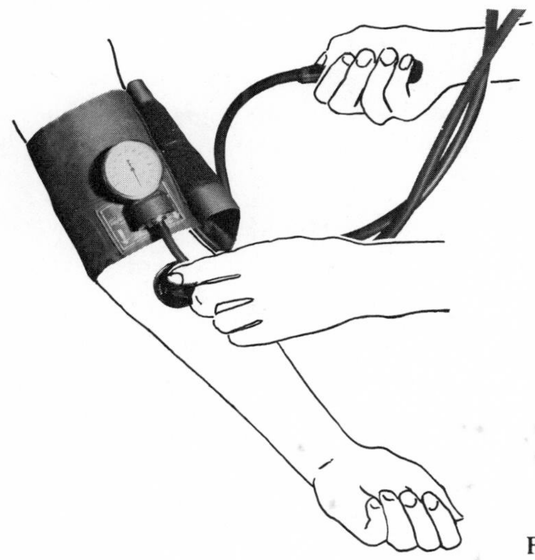

Fig. 22–4 *Measuring blood pressure*

After noting the systolic pressure reading, continue to release air from the cuff at the rate of 2–3 points per heartbeat, and note the reading at which you no longer hear the heartbeat—this is the diastolic pressure reading. With many electronic units, the flashing light and sound stop when diastolic pressure is reached.

Record the systolic and diastolic readings, such as 120/70 as in Fig. 22–1; systolic, the larger figure is always written to the left of the slantbar, and diastolic to the right. In reporting verbally, you would give systolic pressure as "over" the diastolic; for example, "120 over 70."

Practice taking blood pressure several times with your visiting nurse watching and guiding you. It is not difficult to take blood pressure readings accurately, but it does require some practice.

23 Wash and Bath Times

Except in very rare cases, patients should have a full bath every day for the physical and emotional uplift it generally gives, as well as the cleansing. A "full" bath may be a more or less conventional tub or shower bath, a sponge bath, or a bed bath. In addition to the full bath:

1. Your patient's face and hands should be washed before breakfast. Hands also should be washed before any other meal or snack.
2. After urination and bowel movements, whether in the toilet or in bed with a urinal or bedpan, the hands of the patient or whoever administers to a patient should be thoroughly washed. This is of major importance when the patient has a disease or sickness in the communicable or contagious stage (Chapter 12).

Towels, Washcloths, and Sponges Make it a strict rule in your home or wherever you are nursing that no one ever uses anybody else's towel, washcloth, or sponge.

Soap Unless the doctor prescribes a particular soap for your patient, as a rule any kind is satisfactory for good, protective washing and bathing. The amount of soap used and the thoroughness of the cleansing action is more important than the type of soap.

> NOTE: Scented soaps, bath oils, and salts may be used if a patient has no skin problems that could be aggravated by them. To be safe, first ask the doctor or your visiting nurse if such articles may be used.

WASHING FACE AND HANDS

As a rule, the wash water should be as warm as you or your patient can stand comfortably.

Washing Face You may wash your patient's face with a washcloth, sponge, or disposable paper tissues. Use the latter, and dispose of them immediately, if there are rashes or open sores or wounds on your patient's face; also, do not wash more than one area, or from one area into another, of rashes or sores.

Liberally soap the washcloth, sponge, or tissue. Scrub the entire facial area from neck to hairline and ear to ear. While scrubbing, press against the flesh; press firmly enough to rub the skin briskly, but not hard enough to cause pain. Usually it takes only 2 or 3 minutes to wash a face satisfactorily. After washing, rinse the face with (preferably) a fresh washcloth, sponge, or tissues, and clean water. Instead of a fresh washcloth or sponge, the one used for washing may be rinsed free of soap in clean water.

Dry the face with a towel or disposable paper tissues. Dry the skin with a patting motion instead of rubbing, unless your patient prefers the latter. If there are rashes or open sores or wounds on your patient's face, drying should be done with disposable paper tissues, and they should be used as carefully as when washing the face.

Washing Hands Wet the hands well, and work up a good, thick lather of soap. Work it briskly between the fingers, on the backs, fronts, and sides of the hands, and up the arms to a few inches above the wrists. Wash for at least 1 minute. Normally hands may be washed with or without a washcloth, sponge, or disposable paper tissue; some people like to wash their hands with a nailbrush. However, hands with rashes or open sores or wounds should be washed with disposable paper tissues with the same care as used for washing faces in a similar condition.

After washing hands for at least 1 minute, rinse off the lather and dry hands with a towel or paper tissues. Treat hands with rashes or open sores or wounds with the same care used for drying a face in like condition.

This method of washing and drying hands, if done regularly by all members of a family or household, will do much to prevent the spread of a communicable disease or sickness.

Washing and Trimming Nails As a rule, it is not necessary to wash your or your patient's fingernails with a nailbrush, except as part of the first hand washing of the day and after urination or a bowel movement. Of course, some people like to wash their fingernails every time they wash their hands, and there certainly is no harm to it.

Fingernails usually should be trimmed when needed after washing and drying the hands; the nails are less brittle then. How short the nails should be cut is a matter of personal choice. Short nails usually do not collect soil as readily as longer ones, but the latter often are easier to wash clean.

A complete manicure may be a welcome treat for your patient.

BATHS

In addition to the various kinds of full baths, there are two *types* of bath: cleansing and therapeutic. Often they are essentially the same, the difference being that in simple therapeutic baths special ingredients such as salt, baking soda, herbs, oil, etc., are added to the water. The doctor or your visiting nurse will tell you exactly how much additive to use, how to mix it with the water and apply them, how hot the bath should be (see Tables 23–1, 23–2, bath water temperatures), and how long it should last. More complicated therapeutic baths, such as blanket, earth, paraffin, etc., should not be given except by experienced nurses and technicians.

Of course, every bath is therapeutic in that it has healing properties. Warm baths tend to soothe people mentally and emotionally as well as physically, thus relaxing and calming nervous, uneasy, or agitated patients. Warm baths also may help to relieve pain. Cold baths take heat away from the surface of the body, and when followed by a brisk rubbing of the skin stimulate circulation of the blood. However, excessively hot or cold baths should not be given except upon direct orders by the doctor. Excessively hot baths can weaken a sick person, and if prolonged they may have a bad effect on the heart. Also, due to excessive sweating, it may be difficult to thoroughly dry and keep dry someone who has been given too hot a shower or tub bath for more than a very few minutes. An excessively cold bath can give a sick person a severe and painful chill; if given suddenly, such as by abruptly changing shower water from hot to maximum cold, cold water can cause serious shock.

You may merely have to supervise your patient's bath, whether it is a shower, tub, or sponge bath, and do little more than keep yourself ready for a quick assist if needed. In other cases, particularly when a bed bath is involved, you may have to do nearly all the washing and drying of your patient. However, in all cases you should encourage your patient to help with the bath in any and every way possible. Every bit of work your patient does, no matter how small and unimportant it may seem, will help you both, emotionally as well as physically.

Bathtime The time of day for bathing your patient usually is a compromise of what is most convenient for you, especially if you are employed outside the home, and what your patient likes. But if your working hours are of no importance and your patient has no special preferences, here are some points to consider. A bath about midway between breakfast and the noon meal, or noon meal and supper, can be a very welcome break in the day for both of you. A bath shortly before "bedtime" may be a great help in preparing your patient for sleep (Chapter 27). A bath before an expected house call by the doctor or your visiting nurse often puts a patient in a good mood for this important event. But no matter what time is selected for bathing, it should be when the bath will not be rushed. A major purpose of bathing is to refresh and relax a disabled person—which cannot be done when you rush through bathing the fastest possible way.

Bathing Equipment Whether it is a shower, tub, sponge, or bed bath, once started it should be completed without interruption, such as leaving your patient in order to fetch forgotten items. The first step in any bathing procedure is to get all the equipment and materials that will be needed and put them in a convenient location. There are basic bath items, and those that are needed only for certain kinds of baths.

Collect all bedding (Chapter 13) that you will need and place it on a chair or chairs close by the bed. If your patient will have a bed bath, remake the bed as part of the bathing process. If your patient will have a shower, tub, or sponge bath, and if an immediate return to bed is not necessary, bathtime and for a while afterward is excellent for airing bedding; this depends, of course, on how much attention your patient needs while bathing.

Basic Bath Items Approved soap. Washcloth, sponge, or disposable paper tissues. Fingernail brush if necessary. Shampoo if hair will be washed. Therapeutic additives that are prescribed. Towels or disposable paper tissues. Medicinals (ointment, lotion, powder, etc.) ordered for application after the bath. Body lotion wanted by patient and allowed by doctor.

Items for Shower and Tub Baths Patient's bathrobe, slippers. Cane, crutches, walker, or wheelchair if needed. Backbrush. Shower cap if wanted. Safety strips, guardrails, bath seat, below, if needed for stall shower or bathtub. Mechanical lift (Chapter 14) for getting patient in and out of bathtub if necessary. A portable or hand-held shower head may be used for rinsing a tub-bath patient.

Items for Sponge Bath Same items as for shower and tub baths if the sponge bath will be in a stall shower or bathtub. If elsewhere, the safety mat is not needed. The patient may or may not sit on a bath bench or any other chair or bench seat placed conveniently for the bath.

Items for Bed Bath In addition to the basic bath items, above, you need a bath basin, bath blanket, and shampoo tray (Chapter 8) if the hair is to be washed. Put all bath items on one or more tables convenient to the side of the bed; TV tables or trays are excellent for this. To protect bedside furniture against possible water damage, cover them with newspapers or plastic (a house painter's plastic drop cloth is very good for this); protect the bed headboard the same way. Close or block off all windows, doors, or other openings that might allow a draft of air on your patient.

Bath Water Temperatures Bath water temperature usually is specified by name, as in Table 23–1, instead of by degrees of heat.

TABLE 23–1

Bath Water May Be Called

Cold	7.2–18.3°C/ 45– 65°F
Cool	18.3–23.9°C/ 65– 75°F
Tepid	23.9–29.4°C/ 75– 85°F
Warm	29.4–35° C/ 85– 95°F
Hot	35–40.6°C/ 95–105°F
Very hot	40.6–43.3°C/105–110°F

NOTE 1: *Lukewarm* generally means tepid to mildly warm. A lukewarm bath, however, usually is one in which a patient is, from the head down, kept in water 34.4–35.6°C/94–96°F for 15 to 60 minutes.

TABLE 23-2

Bath Temperatures

Room Temperature	*Recommended Water Temperature*
Below 24.4° C/76° F	34.4–35.6° C/94–96° F
Above 24.4° C/76° F	33.3–34.4° C/92–94° F
Hot summer days	32.2° C/ 90° F

NOTE II: The above bath water temperatures are general recommendations. A few degrees warmer or cooler as your patient wishes usually is all right.

NOTE III: In certain cases, your patient's doctor or therapist may prescribe specific water temperatures and lengths of time for baths, generally based on your patient's body temperature.

Strictly speaking, bath water temperature should be measured by a reliable bath thermometer; these usually are sold by pharmacies, and shops or departments that specialize in infants' wear. But unless bath temperature is of major importance, as a rule you can estimate it satisfactorily by dipping your elbow into the water. If you are in good health and have normal body temperature (37° C/98.6° F), water that is noticeably warm to you should be about 37.7° C/100° F; water that feels only body warm probably is about 35° C/95° F.

SHAMPOOING AND CARE OF HAIR

Hair may be shampooed and braided, if necessary, as a separate procedure (below), but usually it is done as part of the bath. If long enough, it should be combed and braided daily regardless of shampooing.

SHAVING

Although shaving often is part of a bath, if practical it should be done according to your patient's wishes. Shaving is very much a matter of habit. The man who shaves in the morning, or at noon, after work, just before going to bed, or at any other time, usually does it then chiefly because he likes to and has the habit of doing it then. To many men, shaving is almost an "omen" of getting the day off to a good start, or a "thanks" that the day's work is done.

If your patient will shave himself, let him use whatever method he likes and can handle. If you must do the shaving, both of you may be happier if you use an electric or a windup shaver instead of a blade.

WHAT TO DO FIRST

If possible, before ever attempting to give a bath have your visiting nurse show you and your patient step by step how it should be done. The visiting nurse undoubtedly has had practical experience bathing patients such as yours, and knows some "tricks of the trade" that will help you and your patient. Also, having been bathed by you and an experienced nurse, your patient will have more confidence in you when you must do it alone. Last but not least, your patient can jog your memory if you forget some phase of the procedure.

Patient Bandaged or in Cast As long as it can be kept dry, a bandage or cast may not, in itself, be sufficient reason to keep a patient from having a shower or tub bath.

Shower bath. If part or all of an arm or leg is injured, enclose it in a large plastic or other waterproof bag; make the top of the bag watertight by taping it to the skin about 2.5 cm./ 1 in. above the bandage or cast. Shoulder and body bandages and casts also may be kept dry in a shower bath by wrapping those areas with plastic and taping it to the skin for waterproofing, but seldom is worth the time and work.

Tub bath. As long as it can be kept out of the water, any area of the body that is bandaged or in a cast need not be given waterproof covering for a tub bath. Areas that cannot be kept out of the water should be protected the same as for a shower bath, above.

THE SHOWER BATH

Except for making sure that the bottom of the stall shower or bathtub is safe for your patient, the guardrail is installed, and the bath seat is in place . . . possibly helping your patient in and out of the stall shower or tub . . . and turning on the water to the proper temperature and pressure, as a rule there is little you need to do for a patient who will have a shower bath. Of course, you must stay close by in case of a fall or other accident.

> NOTE: Most patients who can leave their beds can have shower baths. Whether it is practical is another matter. See Giving the Shower Bath, below.

Safety Strips and Tub Mat The bottom of a stall shower or bathtub should have permanent-type antislip safety strips, as in Fig. 23–1, set 2.5–5 cm./ 1–2 in. apart. Safety strip material is available in most hospital supply stores and other places that carry basic home care materials. Safety strips usually are plastic tape with a strong adhesive backing and a rough top surface, and are easily cut with a scissors or knife. Safety stripping is not expensive.

If the bottom of a stall shower or bathtub cannot be equipped with safety strips, install a rubber or plastic safety tub mat on it to help keep your patient from

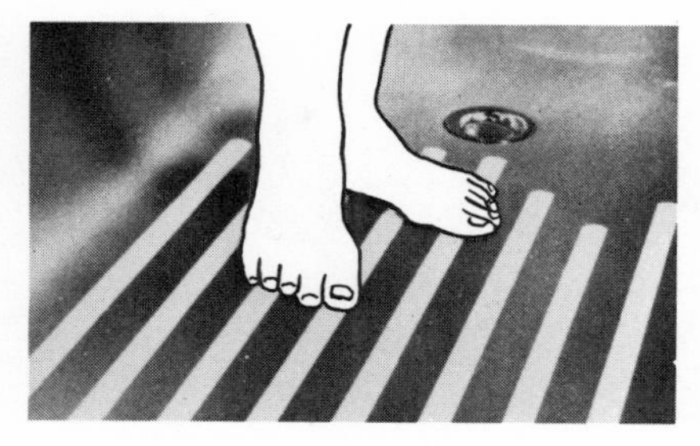

Fig. 23–1 *Safety strips for shower / tub*

slipping. For best protection, the bottom surface of the mat should be studded with small suction cups. Run about 1.5 cm./ ½ in. of water onto the bottom of the stall shower or bathtub, and press down hard on the mat at several points to make the suction cups stick. Do this at enough places to set the mat firmly, so you cannot readily move it in any direction. Be sure that the mat does not block the outlet drain, or cut a large enough hole in it over the drain.

> NOTE: Remove a safety tub mat and clean the bottom surface thoroughly once a week. Without regular cleaning, deposits of soap, body oils, and water pollutants may form a slime that in time will let a mat slide despite its suction cups.

Bath Seats If your patient cannot stand while taking a shower bath, install a bath seat. Usually there are several models to choose from at hospital supply stores. In Fig. 23-2:

a *Bathtub Transfer Seat* fits over the side of a standard bathtub, allowing the patient to sit with feet outside the tub, and turn around while lifting feet

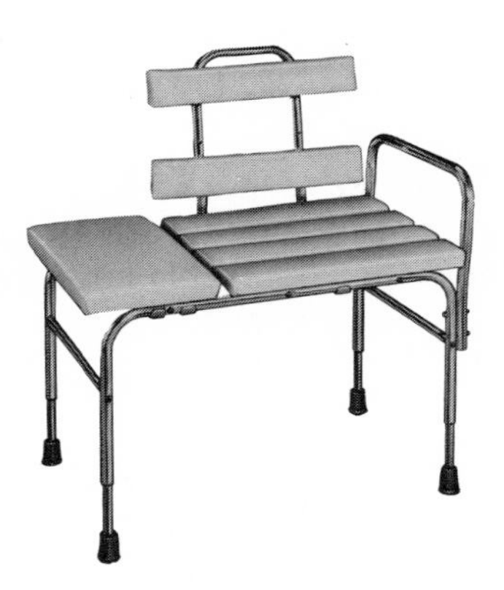

Fig. 23-2*a* *Bathtub transfer seat*

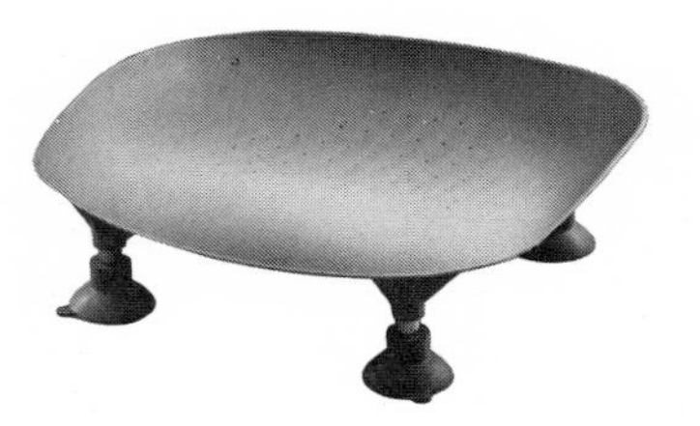

Fig. 23-2*b* *Bath seat*

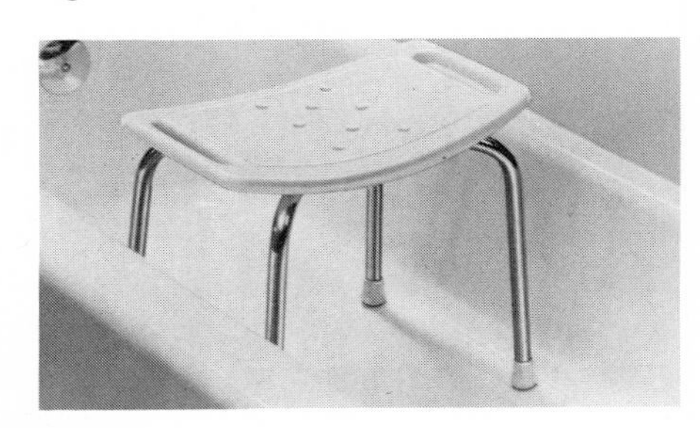

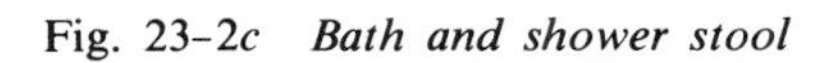

Fig. 23-2*c* *Bath and shower stool*

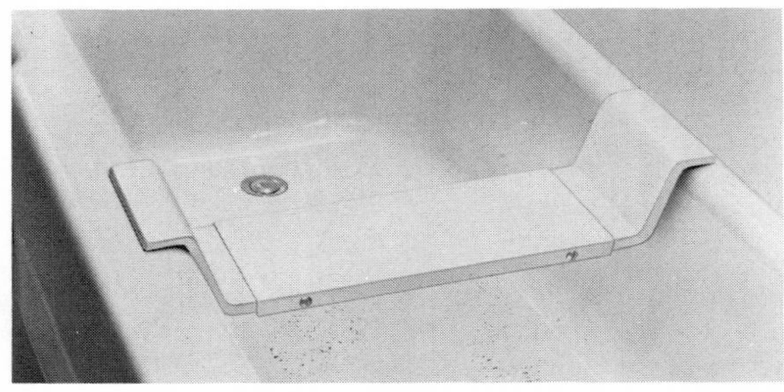

Fig. 23-2*d* *Bath-Ease safety seat*

Fig. 23-2 *Bath seats*

into the tub. The legs outside the tub usually are adjusted to raise the seat slightly higher than it is inside the tub, so that any water will run off into the tub. Some models have adjustable-height backrests.

b *Bath Seat* for general use by convalescents in bathtub or stall shower. The molded plastic flow-through seat allows water to circulate more freely around a patient's buttocks and in the perineal area. Extension legs allow the seat to be raised or lowered.

c *Bath and Shower Stool,* available with backrest, fits completely inside a stall shower or bathtub. It may be had with high legs for the shower bath patient, with low legs for bathtub use.

d *Bath-Ease Safety Seat* often is recommended for children, expectant mothers, elderly, and handicapped persons. Width adjusts to fit all tubs.

Instead of a commercial bath seat, a wooden or metal chair that does not have an upholstered seat or back may be used. An open-weave cane seat is not advisable because of the effects of the seat on the patient and of the water on the cane. For safety, the legs must have nonskid tips or caps. If conventional chair leg or crutch tips are not available, wrap a piece of automobile tire innertube or similar rubber around the end of each leg, and tack or tie it securely to the sides.

Guardrails Bath safety guard- or grabrails may be used for either shower or tub baths. For shower baths, a rail is chiefly to help support a patient who does not

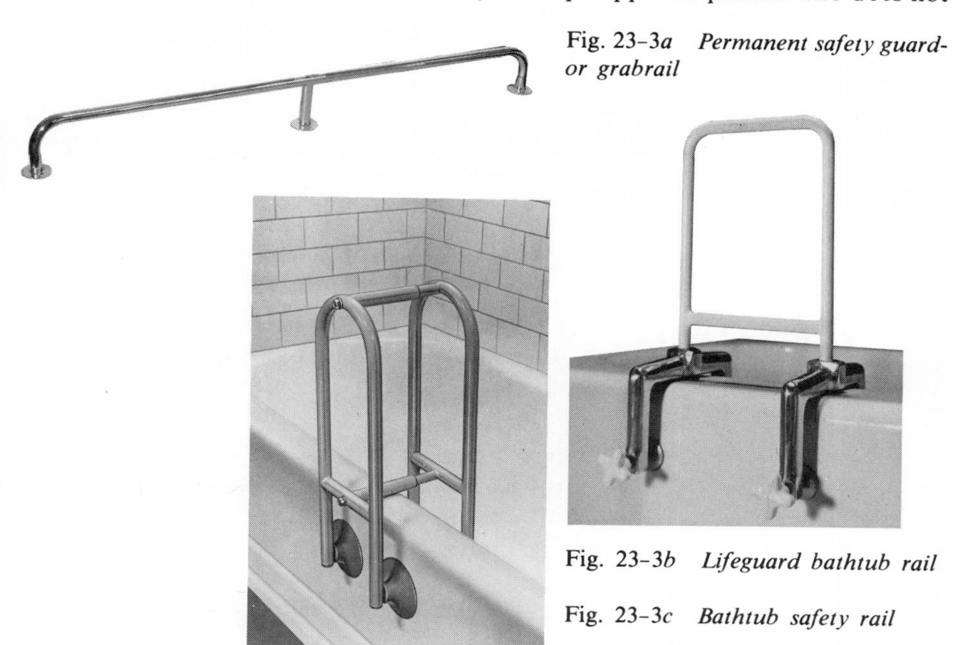

Fig. 23-3*a* *Permanent safety guard- or grabrail*

Fig. 23-3*b* *Lifeguard bathtub rail*

Fig. 23-3*c* *Bathtub safety rail*

Fig. 23-3 *Guardrails*

wish to sit, but is unable to stand safely alone. For tub baths, rails are used mainly by patients who, given something to grasp, can get in and out of the tub with little or no help from the nurse. Several models of rails, for permanent and for temporary installation, are usually available at hospital supply shops. In Fig. 23–3:

a Permanent Safety Guard- or Grabrail must be screwed to the studs of the shower stall or bathtub wall. Mount vertically, at a slant, or horizontally, whichever is most convenient for your patient.

b Lifeguard Bathtub Rail enables many bathers to stand erect while entering or leaving a bathtub. Models are available to fit all roll-rim or leg-type tubs, square or built-in tubs 5 inches or less across the top edge of the rim, and for built-in tubs with the top edge of the rim greater than 5 inches.

c Bathtub Safety Rail features a double handhold for double support of patients getting into and out of a bathtub. An adapter block is available for using this rail with roll-rim tubs.

Water Temperature Many people like shower baths to be somewhat warmer than the basic recommendations, Table 23–2. As a rule, this is all right unless a patient is very debilitated, below, or the doctor forbids it.

Ending a shower bath by abruptly turning the water from hot to cool or cold is fairly common. But first ask the doctor or your visiting nurse if it is allowed, because the change in water temperature might give your patient a severe shock. If allowed, it generally is advisable to make the change somewhat slowly in order to minimize possible shock.

Water Pressure and Massage Usually the shower bath water flow or pressure that your patient likes is all right. Shower baths have a massaging effect that in most cases is soothing and refreshing. Some shower heads can be adjusted to give soft to hard "massage"; do not direct too hard a massage on sensitive or tender parts of the body.

> NOTE: If your patient is bandaged or in a cast, above, make sure the shower water is not directed so it will dislodge or leak through the waterproof protection.

Duration of Shower Bath Except for very debilitated persons, below, as a rule if a patient wants a fairly long instead of a short or quick shower bath, it is all right. But keep in mind that it is more difficult for a person to get and stay dry after a long hot shower than a short one.

Very Debilitated Persons Patients who are especially weak or feeble should not be exposed to the possible additional weakening that may be caused by excessively hot water during a long shower bath. Their baths should last just long enough for satisfactory cleansing, and as a rule the water should not be warmer than recommended in Table 23–2.

Giving the Shower Bath Run the shower bath water long enough to reach the desired temperature and pressure, memorize the settings of the water controls, and turn them off before your patient enters the shower stall or bathtub. Help your patient in and out of the stall or tub only if necessary. Supervise or actually assist in the bathing according to the methods you and your patient have agreed to.

Getting Your Patient in and out of a Stall Shower Patients who can walk, even in only a very limited way, seldom need much extra assistance getting in and out of a stall shower. Often you need only help them keep their balance while stepping over the sill, reaching for a guardrail, or sitting down on or getting up from a bath seat.

Since they must be lifted and carried, it seldom is practical to bathe patients who cannot walk in a stall shower. Mechanical lifts (Chapter 14) are not designed for use with regular stall showers. Patients who are small and light enough to be lifted and carried safely by their nurses may be seated in a stall shower; but as a rule it will be a tight fit for both and not be really practical.

Getting a Shower Bath Patient in and out of a Bathtub As a rule, shower bath patients who can walk at all do not need much special aid in getting in and out of a bathtub. Generally it is just a matter of helping them keep their balance while stepping over the side of the tub, reaching for a guardrail, sitting, or getting up from a bath seat. Of course, many patients need no help at all, nor do they need a guardrail or a bath seat.

> NOTE: If instead of a shower curtain a bathtub has sliding doors, there may not be enough space for you to safely help your patient into and out of the tub. Remove the doors. If your patient must sit on the rim of the tub, pad the door rails with toweling.

How much you must aid a shower bath patient who cannot walk get into and out of a bathtub depends on the patient's condition and the assists, such as guardrails, bath seats, and mechanical lifts (Chapter 14) available:

1. If your patient can, even though needing assistance, stand and step over the side of the bathtub and it is equipped with a bath seat (Fig. 23–2) and a temporary guardrail (Fig. 23–3*b*, *c*), place the rail so that your patient can step over the tubside between it and the seat, and grasp the rail as an aid to sitting down and getting up.
2. If your patient cannot step over the side of the bathtub and it is equipped with a bathtub transfer seat (Fig. 23–2*a*), help your patient onto the seat as much inside the bathtub as possible. Move your patient's legs one at a time to inside the tub and to the front. Help your patient move along the seat to any convenient point about midway between the sides of the tub.
3. If your patient cannot step over the side of the bathtub and it is equipped with a bath seat, stool, or safety seat (Fig. 23–2*b*, *c*, *d*), or a substitute chair, seat your patient in a safely balanced position on the rim of the tub about midway between the front and rear edges of the back seat. Move your patient's legs one at a time to inside the tub and to a comfortable position in front of the bath seat. Then assist your patient from the sitting position on the rim of the tub to one on the bath seat; often it is necessary first to get a patient partway but safely onto the seat near the edge of it, then move to a more comfortable position.
4. There are several models of mechanical lifts (Chapter 14) for getting patients into and out of bathtubs. Each model features various safe and efficient ways of handling patients; adequate instructions should come with a

unit, whether it is bought, borrowed, or rented. Follow the instructions exactly. But even if you and your patient are completely satisfied with the instructions, ask your visiting nurse to assist the first time you attempt to move your patient with a mechanical lift.

Getting a patient out of a bathtub is essentially the opposite of the method used for getting one into it. However, as a rule it is best first for a patient to dry or be dried upward completely from the lowest part of the buttocks and thighs that can be reached while the patient is sitting on the bath seat. Then:

1. A patient who can stand and step out of the tub should do so. The backs of the thighs and between the buttocks, or if possible the complete perineal area and crotch, should be dried before the patient sits on the rim of the tub and the legs and feet are dried.
2. Assist a patient who cannot step out of the tub to a seat on the rim, or to the end of an elevated bath chair, and move the feet one at a time out of the tub. Help the patient stand so that drying of the backs of the thighs and between the buttocks or preferably the entire perineal area including the crotch can be done. Then seat the patient on the rim of the tub, or end of the elevated bath chair, for drying of the legs and feet.

Giving Shower Baths Aside from soaping or completely washing their backs and other places that they cannot reach, there is little you need to do for patients who can wash themselves. First soap or wash their out-of-reach places the usual way, then turn on the shower water and let them finish the bathing. Hair may be shampooed during the shower bath or later, below.

You may, of course, completely soap or wash, as above, shower patients who cannot wash themselves. After thoroughly soaping or washing them, turn on the shower water for rinsing and for the refreshing massage effect. However, reaching into a stall shower to wash a person may be too difficult to be practical; generally it is much easier to do such soaping or washing in a bathtub. Space permitting, you can get into the stall shower or bathtub, close the door or curtain, turn on the water, and wash your patient. This has, of course, been done time and time again; the main disadvantage is having to get out and dry yourself quickly enough to attend to your patient before the shower lasts too long or a chill sets in.

Drying As a rule, it is more practical for stall shower patients to dry themselves or be dried after getting out of the stall. This also applies to bathtub patients who can stand with little or no assistance.

A bathtub patient who cannot stand safely usually dries or is dried while getting out of the tub, above.

THE TUB BATH

Recommended water temperatures, duration of bath, precautions for very debilitated persons . . . safety strips, guardrails, bath seats, mechanical lifts . . .

and methods of getting patients in and out of a bathtub are the same for tub as for shower baths, above. There is, of course, no problem of water pressure; instead, there is one of depth. A portable or hand-held shower head may be used for rinsing a patient.

Water Depth Except for very debilitated patients, the depth of water for a tub bath generally is a matter of personal choice. Tub baths usually are about 10–30 cm./4–12 in. deep for patients who sit on the bottom of a tub. Shallow depths, provided the water reaches at least above the patient's anklebones, usually are satisfactory for those who use a bath seat. Depth of water may be specified by the doctor for a patient who requires special treatment of the buttocks or the perineal area.

> NOTE: Very debilitated patients should not be subjected to the possible weakening effect of excessively hot water or a long or a deep tub bath. The water should not exceed the temperatures recommended in Table 23–2 and be no more than 15 cm./6 in. deep, and the bath should last just long enough for satisfactory cleansing.

Getting Patient in and out of Bathtub Patients who require a bath seat or a mechanical lift are gotten in and out of a bathtub for a tub bath the same ways as for a shower bath, above.

Most people who can sit on the bottom of a bathtub, even if only by difficult means, will wish to. Fortunately, few of them need much help for entering or leaving the tub, lowering themselves to the bottom, or getting up from it; often all they want is the nurse's hand or arm to hold for balance while stepping over the side of a tub. For those who need help, as a rule the most difficult tasks are lowering them to sit on the bottom of a tub and lifting them up after the bath.

Getting in:

1. Get your patient into the tub and safely seated on the rim, back toward you. A patient who cannot step over the side of a tub is first seated on the rim, back to the tub. Then one at a time the legs are moved to inside the tub, the patient turning with them.
2. Reach under your patient's shoulders from the back, grasp each wrist firmly, and gently lower your patient down onto the bottom of the tub (see Chapter 14).
3. Turn your patient to sit lengthwise in the tub.

Getting Out:

1. Turn your patient sidewise in the tub, back toward you.
2. Reach under your patient's shoulders from the back, grasp each wrist firmly, and lift your patient up to sit on the rim of the tub. If possible, have your patient press down with both feet on the bottom of the tub while you are lifting.
3. Help your patient out of the tub. If your patient cannot step over the side, move the legs one at a time out of the tub, the patient turning with them while still sitting on the rim.

Portable Shower Head A portable or hand-held shower head or sprayer, Fig. 23–4, may be used for rinsing a tub bath patient. It adds a "massage" effect that usually soothes and refreshes a patient. Some such heads can be adjusted for soft to hard massage, which is further controlled by the water force. Do not use too hard a massage on tender or sensitive parts of the body, or direct the spray so that it can dislodge or leak through the waterproof protection of a bandaged area or a cast.

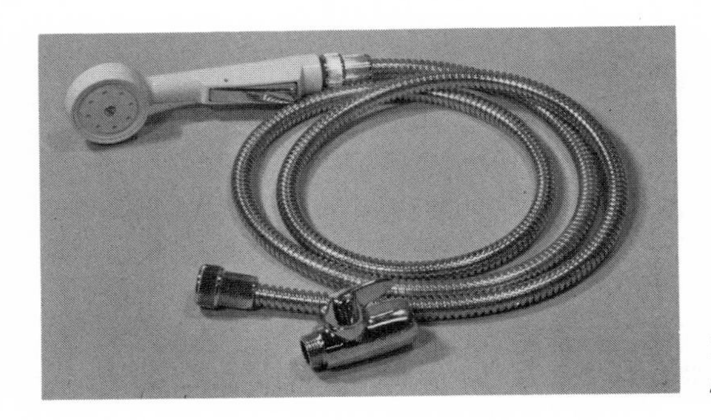

Fig. 23–4 *Hand-held or portable shower head*

Giving the Tub Bath Most patients who can sit on the bottom of a bathtub are able to bathe themselves completely, although help often is needed for washing the back of the neck, shoulders, and torso. Although your patient may be able to bathe without assistance, often it is necessary to help with the drying.

Most patients who need a bath seat also need help for bathing. Water in the tub should be at least ankle deep to provide a comfortable foot bath (Chapter 17). For the rest of the bath, a washcloth or large sponge may be used to take water where needed for washing and rinsing the body; or water may be dipped up in a pan or cup and poured over the patient; or it may be sprayed with a hand-held sprayer or portable shower head. The major washing "problem" places for these patients usually are between the buttocks and in the perineal area (between the vulva and the anus of a female, between the scrotum and the anus of a male). Most patients prefer and should be encouraged to wash these areas themselves; it may be advisable to assist by helping them lean over far enough to right or left to allow satisfactory washing and rinsing. As a rule, quite a bit of help must be given in drying patients whose condition requires use of a bath seat of any type, including a mechanical lift (Chapter 14).

THE SPONGE BATH

There may be occasions when a sponge bath is more appropriate or convenient for your patient than a shower, tub, or bed bath. It can be given in the bedroom or the bathroom; the latter usually is better if your patient can move or easily be moved into it. A sponge bath may be given in a shower stall or a bathtub, but probably will be easier for your patient and you if done beside the wash basin or lavatory. A bedroom sponge bath can be given with your patient sitting on the side of the bed; but as a rule it is more convenient for both of you, and a welcome change for your patient, if it is given beside an appropriate table in the room. The average person being given a sponge bath sits on a stool or chair because of being too weak, or otherwise unable to stand long enough. If your patient can and wishes to stand for a sponge bath, there should be no real reason not to. To give a sponge bath:

1. Bring all necessary equipment, such as towels, clean gown or pajamas, washcloth or sponge, etc. (see Items for Sponge Bath, above), to where the bath will be given. In addition to the usual bathing equipment, you need a bath blanket (Chapter 8) to cover your patient and protect against chills, a stool or chair for the patient to sit on, and a bath basin (Chapter 8) unless the sponge bath will be given beside the bathroom wash-basin or lavatory.
2. Seat your patient on a stool or chair convenient for the bath. If your patient will instead sit on the side of the bed, first cover that part of the bed with a protective sheet of plastic or other waterproof material and a large terrycloth towel.
3. Disrobe or help your patient disrobe, and immediately cover with the bath blanket. Fit it around your patient in such a way that it can be partially removed or opened, as need be, for washing an arm, leg, the chest, etc.
4. Fill the bath basin or lavatory bowl with water warm enough to satisfy your patient.
5. Sponge bathing usually consists of washing, rinsing off the soap, and drying one part of the body at a time, generally in this order: the face and neck ... an arm, including the hand, then the other ... the chest and abdomen ... (change the water) ... then one leg, including the foot, and the other ... the back, including the buttocks and between them ... and finish with the patient washing, rinsing, and drying the genital area if able to. Of course, in most cases the patient should be encouraged to do all the work possible.
6. When the bath is finished, help your patient dress, then put away all equipment, collect the laundry, etc.

THE BED BATH

In many respects, the bed bath is a combined procedure of remaking an occupied bed (Chapter 13) and bathing a patient. It is particularly important for most bedfast patients to help with the bathing as much as they can.

> NOTE: You must take every precaution to keep an unreliable, irrational, or comatose patient from falling out of bed during a bath. The surest way is to lower the bedrail only on the side of the bed where you are working and only when actually attending to your patient or making the bed. If you must turn away from your patient or move more than a very few steps from the bed, first raise the bedrail to its protective position.

You should study and memorize the following routine for giving a bed bath. It will save you much time and work:

1. Remove bedspread and blankets, fold and place them on a chair. Before removing the upper or top bed sheet, spread a bath blanket (Chapter 8) over it and your patient. Then remove the upper sheet by sliding it out from under the bath blanket; this way you avoid exposing or chilling your patient. Instead of a regular bath blanket, you may use a large beach towel. If you will use the upper sheet on the bottom or for a draw sheet when remaking the bed, fold and put it on the chair with the fresh bedding.

2. Put a towel under the patient's head. Wash the face and neck, rinse and dry them.

3. Remove the towel from under the patient's head, or use a second towel, and lay it under a shoulder and arm. Wash, rinse, and dry the arm from fingertips to shoulder, including the armpit. Then remove the towel and place it under the other arm and shoulder, and wash, rinse, and dry that arm. While washing an arm, raise it as high as possible to exercise the shoulder joint.

4. Fold the upper part of the bath blanket down to the patient's pubic area. Cover the upper part of the body with a towel to prevent exposure and possible chilling. Working underneath the towel, wash, rinse, and dry the front and sides of the torso from the neck and shoulders down to the pubic area and hips. Replace the bath blanket up to the top of the patient's shoulders.

5. Change the bath water, and rinse out the washcloth or sponge in clean running water.

6. Uncover a leg, and bend the knee upward so that the sole of the foot is flat on the bed. Place a towel crosswise under the leg. Wash, rinse, and dry it, all sides, from ankle to hip. Remove the towel and do the other leg.

7. Place a towel under both feet, lift them, set the bath basin on the towel, as in Fig. 23–5, and put both feet in it. If the basin is too small to hold both feet, bathe one at a time. Soak feet in the bath water for several minutes before washing them. Scrub the feet well, spreading the toes and washing between them. The scrubbing action feels pleasant to most people. However,

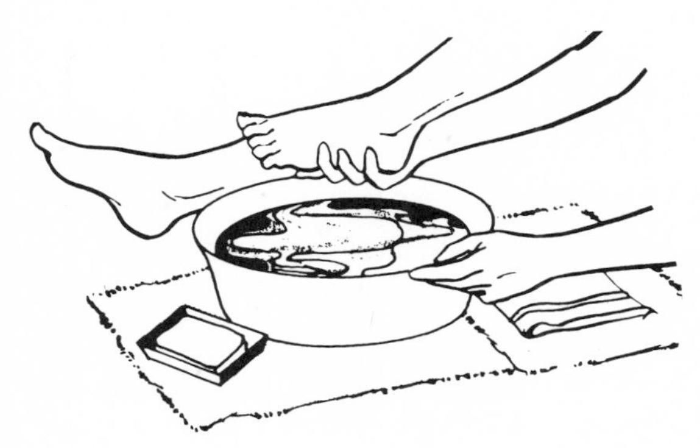

Fig. 23–5 *Washing feet in bed*

many feet are extremely sensitive to touching or tickling. In this case, since people cannot tickle themselves, hold the washcloth or sponge against the side or bottom of the basin while your patient rubs the soles of the feet against it. To dry ticklish feet, have your patient rub them hard against a towel. Be sure to dry thoroughly between the toes.

8. Change bath water again, 5 above.

9. Turn or assist your patient to turn over onto the abdomen if possible; if not, turn patient over onto a side. Lay a towel close against your patient and wash, rinse, and dry the back all the way down from the neck, including the buttocks and the anal area.

10. Then have or help your patient turn over onto the back. Wash, rinse, and dry the perineal area and between the buttocks. Most patients prefer and should be encouraged to do this bathing themselves. If they cannot, then you must do it, as it is most important for these areas to be kept as clean as possible at all times. With a male patient be particularly careful about drying the perineal area; unless the penis, scrotum, and groins are dried thoroughly, a rash often develops.

11. Comb your patient's hair; braid it, if shoulder length or longer, to prevent tangles and snarls, see Shampooing and Care of Hair, below. Shampooing may be done at this time.

The bed bath having been completed, remove all bathing equipment, dress your patient in a fresh gown or pajamas, and remake the bed. Move your patient as far as possible to the side of the bed away from you. Loosen the draw sheet, if any, and the bottom sheet on the side of the bed near you, and roll each one separately up against your patient. Then fold the fresh bottom sheet in half lengthwise, install it and the fresh draw sheet, if any, on the bed, and proceed as in Remaking the Occupied Bed, Chapter 13.

NOTE: How much work of a bed bath you must do, and how much your patient does, depends on your patient's condition. Most bedfast people cannot wash their backs and buttocks satisfactorily; but everything else that a patient can do, a patient should do. The more you do that your patient could have done, the slower your patient's recovery generally will be.

SHAMPOOING AND CARE OF HAIR

How often hair should be shampooed depends to a great extent on your patient. Some people like their hair washed daily, others may want it done once a week or even less often. However, sickness and being indoors most of the time can cause changes in a person's hair and scalp. The best rule of thumb for shampooing is—as often as your patient wants and your time permits. But it should be done as soon as possible if your patient's head starts to itch.

NOTE: Shoulder-length and longer hair generally should be braided daily regardless of shampooing, below.

Whether a shampoo should be wet or dry depends chiefly on your patient's condition. Unless the head, hair, or scalp requires special treatment because of sickness, injury, or surgery, as a rule a wet shampoo with its scrubbing, massaging, and rinsing is the more refreshing. But for bedfast patients a dry shampoo may be more practical; it can be quite refreshing.

Use the shampoo material your patient prefers unless there is a skin problem that demands special treatment. Sometimes a change in the hair or scalp due to sickness or confinement indoors may change the effectiveness or pleasing qualities of a shampoo as far as your patient is concerned. Explain the problem to your visiting nurse and ask about preparations that may be more suitable.

Follow the manufacturer's directions for preparing and applying a shampoo, plus any special instructions by the doctor or your visiting nurse.

Shampoo Equipment In addition to shampoo material, you need a comb, hairbrush, and a hand-held electric hair dryer with, preferably, a choice of heats and blower speeds. Blow hair drying after a wet shampoo always is advisable no matter how thoroughly the hair has been towel dried. Blow-drying after a dry shampoo blows away particles of shampoo that may have clung to the scalp, and usually makes the scalp feel fresher, cleaner:

1. *For a wet shampoo*, you also need at least three medium-size bath towels, or two large ones. For a wet shampoo in bed, you need a bed rinse/shampoo tray, Fig. 8–5; a hairbrush; two buckets or basins, one for clean water, the other for collecting used water; a small pitcher or pan for dipping water onto your patient's head; and a sq. m./yd. of waterproof material, or eight or ten sheets of newspaper, to protect the bedding.
2. *For a dry shampoo*, you need a plentiful supply of cotton balls or pledgets for applying the shampoo solution, and a stiff-bristle hairbrush for working it out of the hair.

Wet Shampoo out of Bed Nearly any practical way of washing a patient's head and hair during a shower, tub, or sponge bath, or at any other time outside of bed, is satisfactory. You should, however, first describe the method you use to the doctor or your visiting nurse. After rinsing and towel drying, for best results blow-dry your patient's head and hair with an electric hair dryer. When thoroughly dry, braid it if at all possible; see Care of Long Hair, below.

Wet Shampoo in Bed A wet shampoo in bed usually is given as part of the bed bath. Of course, it may be given at any other time you and your patient want. To give a wet shampoo in bed:

1. Remove the pillow from under your patient's head.
2. Brush hair thoroughly, preferably with a stiff-bristle brush.
3. Lower the head of the bed to the flat position.
4. Place the protective waterproof material or sheets of newspaper under your patient's head and shoulders. Set the shampoo tray in place, and work a towel snugly around the back of your patient's neck and tight against the collar of the shampoo tray to keep water from leaking out of it.
5. Set the bucket or basin in place to collect used water.
6. Wet patient's hair and pour a small amount of shampoo solution on it.

Work up a lather with your hands and fingertips. Scrub all areas of the head, then rinse. Apply a second amount of shampoo; work up a lather and again scrub, firmly but not hard enough to hurt, for several minutes.

7. Rinse out all shampoo. Apply a hair rinse preparation if your patient wants it; be sure to follow the manufacturer's instructions.
8. After completing a shampoo, remove the tray and wrap your patient's head with a large towel. Towel-dry the head and hair, finishing with an electric hair dryer for best results.
9. Braid hair; see Care of Long Hair, below.
10. Make your patient comfortable.
11. Remove, clean, and store the shampoo equipment.

Dry Shampoo out of Bed and in Bed Since each dry shampoo preparation has its own instructions, follow those on the container. When shampooing in bed, first spread a large towel under your patient's head to collect spilled and used shampoo material. After completing the shampoo, braid your patient's hair, see Care of Long Hair, below.

Care of Long Hair If your patient's hair reaches to the shoulders, braid it daily to keep it from matting; this is particularly important if your patient spends more than half the time in bed. Human hair mats, similar to the fur balls on cats and dogs, are caused by movement of the head against a pillow or pad. Badly matted hair must be cut out. Braiding prevents matting and keeps long hair out of a patient's eyes.

Simple braiding is easy to do and is satisfactory in nearly all cases. After brushing the hair thoroughly, part it at the middle of the head. Separate each side into three fairly equal strands, and braid them together the usual way; more and smaller braids may, of course, be made. Fasten the end of a braid with a rubber band or length of ribbon.

24 The Sitz Bath

Sitz baths are often given following surgery or to treat infection in the rectal, genital, or perineal areas, to soothe and clean them, and to reduce hemorrhoids (piles). The sitz bath also loosens and frequently washes away dried blood and feces, and helps prevent stitches from becoming tight and uncomfortable, which tends to occur a few days after surgery.

At home, sitz baths are commonly given in a special basin, as in Fig. 24–1, or in the bathtub, and normally are not difficult to give unless you must help your patient in and out of the tub (see Getting Patient in and out of Bathtub, Chapter 23). But ask your visiting nurse to supervise the first sitz bath you give your patient.

EQUIPMENT

The simplest special sitz bath equipment is a plastic basin, Fig. 24–1*a,* that fits into a standard toilet seat. As shown, it is used primarily for soaking the affected parts of a patient; if a flow of water is desired, it is poured over the patient from a small pitcher. A more advanced unit, Fig. 24–1*b*, consists of the basin, a plastic water reservoir or container, and tube from it to the basin; a pinch clamp on the tube may be operated with one hand to start, stop, and control the flow from the reservoir. The end of the tube may be positioned in the basin to direct the flow of water as needed against the patient. Basins normally do not require as much water as bathtub sitz baths. But unless your patient will have long-term sitz bath treatment, a special basin may not be a practical purchase.

Patients being given bathtub sitz baths usually should sit on rubber or plastic rings, as in Fig. 8–17*b*, placed on the bottom of the tub. There are several types of rings; ask the doctor or your visiting nurse which will be best for your patient.

For drying your patient after a sitz bath you should have very soft—the softer the better!—terrycloth toweling. If your patient is extremely sensitive, dry with sterile cotton squares or pads; discard each after making one drying stroke.

Rubber or plastic gloves (Chapter 8) may or may not be medically advisable when drying your patient after a sitz bath. However, wearing them may make the procedure less embarrassing for your patient and yourself.

THE SITZ BATH

Whether given in a sitz bath basin or a bathtub, water for the bath should as a rule be comfortably warm (see Bath Water Temperatures, Chapter 23) for the patient for the duration of the bath, which usually lasts for approximately 5 to 15 minutes.

For a prescribed *hot* sitz bath, water should be about 37.7° C/100° F at the start; then, over a period of about 3 minutes, it usually is raised to 41.1° or

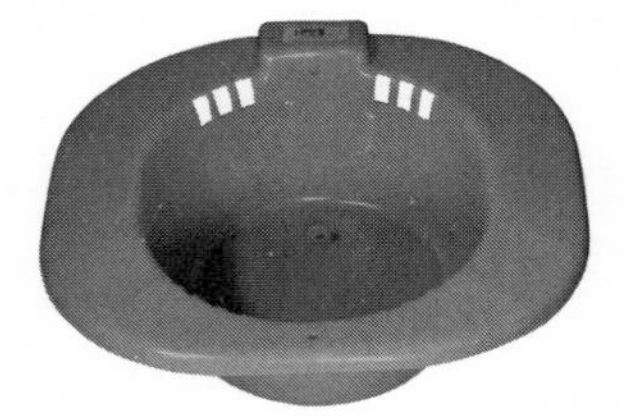

Fig. 24–1*a* *Sitz bath basin*

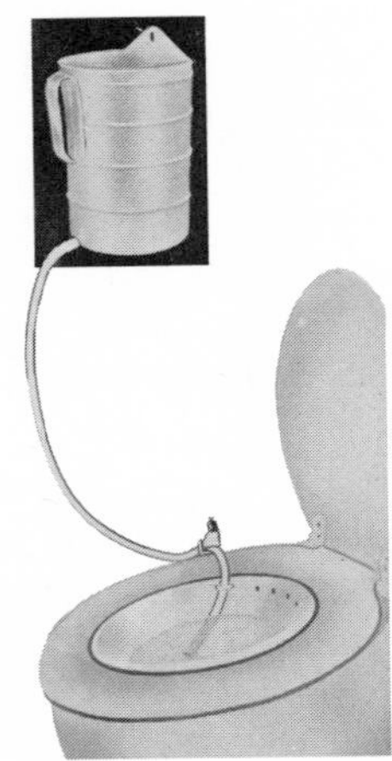

Fig. 24–1*b* *Sitz bath basin with water reservoir and tube*

48.8° C/106° or 120° F or as hot as the patient can tolerate. A hot sitz bath generally lasts for about 3 to 10 minutes—but first, be sure to ask the doctor!

For a medicated sitz bath, keep accurate record of how much water is put into the bathtub or water reservoir or other container, then stir in the medicine in the ratio or amount prescribed by the doctor.

The amount of water for a sitz basin bath usually is determined by the capacity of the water reservoir or other container and the basin. Water for a bathtub sitz bath generally is deep enough to cover a patient's thighs, buttocks, and abdomen below the umbilicus or navel.

25 The Enema

An enema is the instillation or injection of liquid, either plain or containing additives, into the rectum and colon (the large or lower bowel or intestine) to stimulate emptying of the colon, or to place in it medicine for therapeutic purposes. *To prevent possible severe internal injury to your patient,* take special care not to give a greater amount of liquid (or a stronger solution if additives are used) or use a greater pressure or force than specified by the doctor or your visiting nurse.

CLEANSING ENEMA

Briefly, the cleansing enema, the kind you will most likely give, is used either to liquefy the feces in the colon or to soften it enough for the patient to expel it with minimum discomfort. The enema water may or may not have an additive. Despite somewhat widespread self-prescribed home treatment calling for an enema on nearly any occasion because "it cleans the bowel and *that* can't do any harm," it should be given only on doctor's orders. The common excuse for giving an enema is "constipation." However, regular use of cleansing enemas may in time increase the occurrence and severity of the constipation it is intended to prevent or cure. Incidentally, constipation is not in itself a sickness but only a symptom of illness, and should be treated as such.

Cleansing enemas may be plain water, but more often contain a small amount of soap, baking soda, or table salt. Packaged castile enema soap and prepared enema solutions are available in many pharmacies and hospital supply outlets. Ask the doctor or your visiting nurse what additive and strength solution to use for your patient. Do not use too strong a solution; it could injure the intestinal mucous membrane or lining.

Soap Enemas *Soapsuds enema* is the term commonly used for soap enemas. It is, however, a misnomer, because the enema solution is a mixture of mild soap and water and should not have any suds.

Mild soaps, such as castile, are best for cleansing enemas. *Do not use detergents*—they are too irritating to the bowel.

Here are the proportions or mixtures of soap and water common for cleansing enemas; they may be used unless the doctor or your visiting nurse specifies other strengths. To prepare a soapsuds enema, place water in the enema solution container (see Equipment for Giving Soapsuds Enemas, below), add soap, mix. Do not mix or stir violently enough to whip up suds!

Liquid Soap: 1 part soap to 30 parts water; 30 ml. (milliliter) soap to 1 l. (1,000 ml.) water, or 1 oz. to 1 qt.

Soap Particles, Powder, Flakes: Use enough soap to make a milky solution. This usually is from 15–30 ml. soap to 1 l. of water, or 1–2 tbsp. soap to 1 qt. of water.

Bar Soap: Swish the bar of soap in 1 l. or qt. of water until a milky solution forms.

Packaged Liquid Castile Enema Soap: Usually available in 30-ml. or 1-oz. containers. Mix according to instructions on the label.

Packaged Cleansing Enema Solutions: Use only those recommended by the doctor or your visiting nurse, and prepare according to their instructions.

Amount of Enema It is important to use the proper amount of enema for your patient, as too much can cause cramping and discomfort, while too little can hinder the effectiveness of a cleansing enema. Be sure to ask the doctor what amount to use for your patient. However, as a basic guide:

Persons More than 12 Years of Age: Generally 1 l. or qt. of solution is satisfactory.

Children Between 1 and 12 Years of Age: Usually 500 ml. (½ l.) or 1 pt. of solution. For practical purposes, these quantities usually are prepared as needed with half the amounts of soap commonly used for larger quantities, above.

Infants Up to 1 Year of Age: These never should be given more than 300 ml. or 10 oz. of enema. NOTE: Instead of a soap solution, a mixture of 5 ml. of table salt to ½ l. of water (1 tsp. salt to 1 pt. water) usually is ordered.

Temperature of Enema For maximum stimulation of the colon without discomfort to your patient, the temperature of a soapsuds enema solution should be 41–43.3° C (106–110° F). The warmer it is, the greater its effect. For best results, determine the temperature of the solution with a thermometer.

Equipment for Giving Soapsuds Enemas For adults, and children more than 2 years old, the most convenient way to give an enema is with the modern, hospital-type disposable plastic enema kit, Fig. 25–1*a*, consisting of a solution container or bucket graduated in milliliters and ounces, and a hose with a stop-clamp; the free end of the hose usually serves as the rectal tip for giving a solid-stream enema. Also convenient but not always as practical (see Note I below) is the traditional home-style enema kit, Fig. 25–1*b*. It consists of a rubber bag container, rubber hose with stop-clamp, a large rectal tip with holes on the sides for a diffusion enema, and a small or short open end for a solid-stream enema, the kind more commonly given; an old-fashioned enema can may be used instead of the rubber bag. The infant syringe, Fig. 25–1*c*, is for giving enemas to children under 2 years of age; syringes are available in 1-, 2-, and 3-oz. (approximately 29.5-, 59-, and 88.5-ml.) sizes.

NOTE I: Rectal tips usually provided with home-style enema kits are made of hard rubber or plastic and are too short. They tend to be uncomfortable for the patient and do not go high enough in the colon for good results. The modern, flexible, and longer hospital-type plastic tubes are more satisfactory.

NOTE II: If the stop-clamp on the hose from a solution container does not completely stop the flow of liquid, double it back at a convenient point and fasten it with a spring-type clothespin.

NOTE III: In an emergency, an enema kit may be used for irrigating or giving a feminine douche, Chapter 26.

Practical substitutes for specialized enema equipment are:

1. A hot water bag that has a stopper with a hose connector and hose.
2. An irrigation or feminine hygiene or douche kit, Chapter 26, with a proper rectal tip.

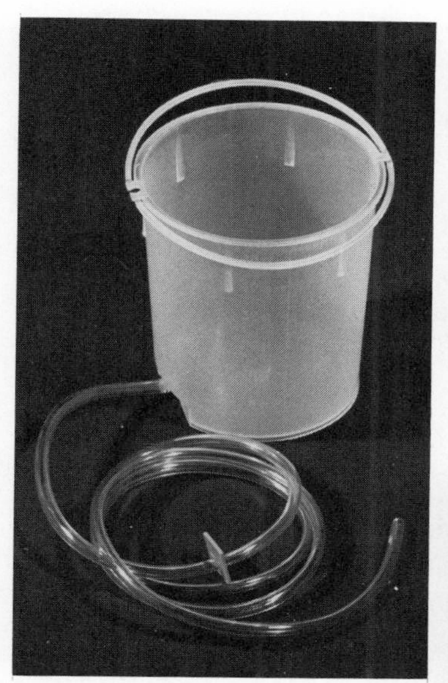

Fig. 25–1*a* *Modern hospital-type enema kit*

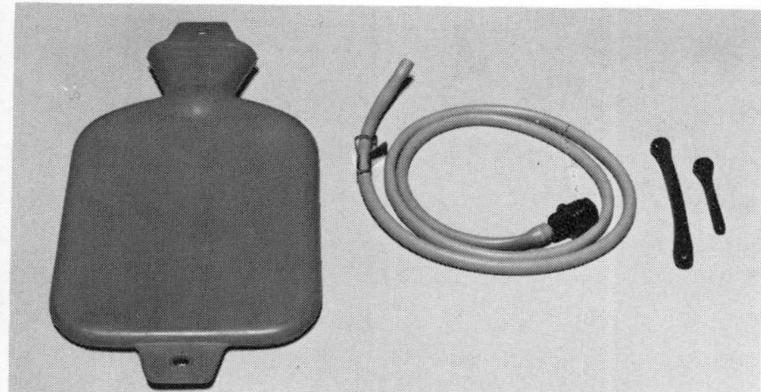

Fig. 25–1*b* *Traditional home-style enema kit*

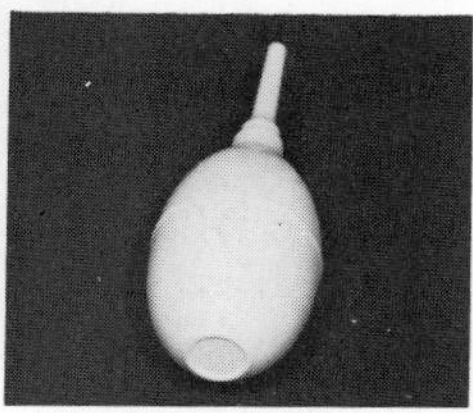

Fig. 25–1*c* *Infant syringe*

Fig. 25–1 *Equipment for giving enemas*

In addition to items specifically made for giving cleansing enemas, you need the following, which should be brought to your patient's bedside before giving the enema:

Bedpan (Chapter 8) for catching the expelled enema. However, it may be more practical to seat a child that you can carry on the toilet for expelling an enema—if the child can hold it until you get to the toilet!

Emesis basin (Chapter 8) to hold the rectal tip after giving the enema. Do not put the tip in the solution container.

Lubricant. Any medically accepted water-soluble lubricant or jelly can be used; Vaseline® is suitable, but difficult to clean off. Smear lubricant generously over the rectal tip to simplify insertion into the rectum and with less discomfort for your patient.

Toilet paper or paper towels for lubricating the rectal tip, and for wiping your patient after the enema is expelled.

Waterproof sheeting to place on the bedding under your patient. Or full-size sheets of newspaper may be used; eight to ten usually are enough. Newspaper is absorbent and holds spills well. Remove sheeting or newspapers as soon as possible after your patient expels the enema, or after cleaning the bed following a spill.

Large cloth towel to place on top of the waterproof sheeting or newspapers. Patients usually are more comfortable lying on toweling. Also, in case of a spill, toweling will keep liquid from flowing off the waterproof sheeting or newspapers onto the bedding.

Bath blanket (Chapter 8) or large beach towel to cover and protect your patient against exposure and chills.

Stand for holding enema solution container. If a commercial or hospital-type stand is not available, use a garment rack, floor lamp, or a photographer's light stand—anything high and sturdy enough to hold the container at the proper level (see Giving the Soapsuds Enema, below). String several loops of fairly heavy twine through the hole in the container and over an appropriate part of the stand; or hang the container to it with a hook made from a wire coat hanger.

Washing materials (warm water, soap, washcloths, hand towels) for cleaning patient after enema is expelled. If patient will clean self, provide an extra washcloth and towel for the patient to wash and dry hands.

Giving the Soapsuds Enema Except for a few important differences, cleansing enemas are given adults, children, and infants essentially the same way:

1. Bring all equipment and materials, including the prepared enema solution at the proper temperature, to your patient's bedside. Close all doors to the room, or arrange a screen or screens to give privacy to the bed area.
2. Have patient lie on the left side when possible, with the upper or right leg flexed or bent upward in a comfortable position, as in Fig. 25–2. Intestines normally offer less resistance to enema fluid when a patient lies on the left side. The upper leg is flexed for comfort and to open the buttocks for easier insertion of the rectal or enema tip.
3. Place the waterproof sheeting or newspapers, covered by the large towel, under the patient's buttocks. Cover patient with the bath blanket while fan-folding (Chapter 13) the top bedding to the foot of the bed.
4. Place bedpan on the bed near the foot.
5. Hang the enema solution container on the stand. It should be from 30–45 cm./12–18 in. above the patient's hips, as in Fig. 25–2*b*. Make sure that the stop-clamp on the enema hose works properly.

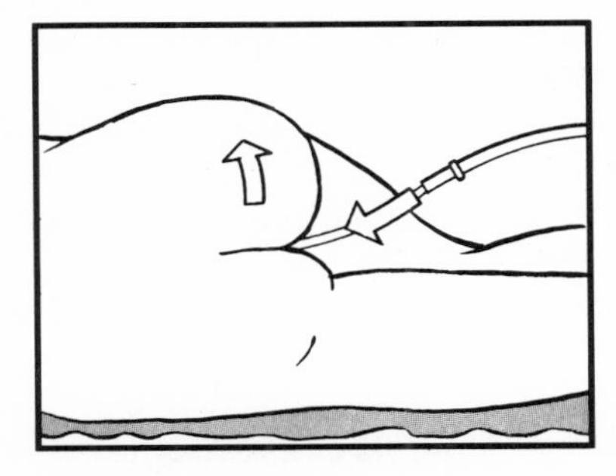

Fig. 25–2*a* *Inserting rectal tip into patient*

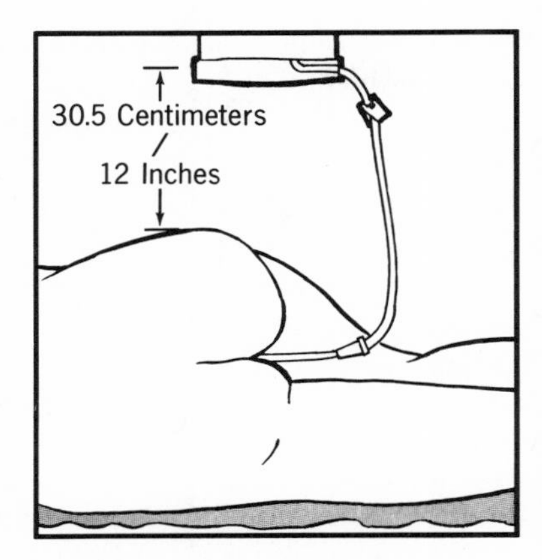

Fig. 25–2*b* *Giving enema*

6. Smear a generous amount of lubricant on toilet tissue or paper toweling and lubricate the first 5–10 cm./2–4 in. of the rectal tip.

7. Open the stop-clamp on the hose and run a little of the solution into the bedpan. This is to expel all air from the hose and warm the rectal tip. Close the stop-clamp.

8. Redrape or move the bath blanket to provide enough clear space for giving the enema. Do not uncover your patient more than is necessary.

9. Lift patient's upper buttock to expose the anus or rectum, as in Fig. 25–2*a*, enough for you to see what you are doing. Insert about 5 cm./2 in. of rectal tip slowly and gently. If it meets resistance, wait several seconds, let a small amount of solution flow inward, then insert tip at a slower rate than before. For a high enema, below, insert 12–20 cm./6–8 in. of tip.

NOTE: Often elderly people have poor control of the muscles that close the anus and cannot retain an enema. In such cases, give enema with the patient lying on a bedpan after insertion of the rectal tip. This lets any leakage drain into the bedpan without an embarrassing, messy situation for the patient.

10. When the tip is inserted the required distance, open the stop-clamp and let the enema flow in very slowly. If it flows too fast and causes cramping, pinch the hose with your thumb and forefinger to slow the flow until cramping stops.

11. When all the enema has been instilled or injected, close the stop-clamp, slowly remove the rectal tip, wrap it with paper toweling, and deposit in the emesis basin.

12. Help your patient onto the bedpan in a comfortable position for usual evacuation. Place several sheets of newspaper over the area of the lower abdomen, between the legs, and under the edges of the bedpan to act as a splatter board. Cover patient with bath blanket. As a general rule, a patient should be urged to try to retain a cleansing enema for about 5–10 minutes before expelling it. If your patient can go to the toilet for expelling the enema,

provide a folded washcloth or small towel to be held against the rectum to prevent dribbling on the way to the toilet.

13. Remove enema equipment. Prepare equipment and materials for cleaning the patient after expelling the enema.

14. When patient has finished expelling the enema, remove bedpan. Do preliminary cleaning with toilet paper, then bathe between the buttocks and the perineal area the usual way (see The Bed Bath, Chapter 23). If your patient does the cleaning and bathing, provide materials for washing and drying hands.

NOTE: Before emptying the bedpan, examine its contents. If you are maintaining nursing notes, record the color of the feces—light brown, black, tarry, clay colored, etc; its consistency—hard, formed, semiformed, liquid; whether there are undigested particles of food, mucus, etc.; the amount—small, medium, large. Report any unusual appearance to the doctor. A black, tarry stool, for example, indicates internal bleeding higher in the intestinal tract.

15. Remove bath blanket, replace upper bedding.

16. Remove protective toweling and waterproof sheeting or newspapers placed in Step 3 above. Remove all materials and equipment related in any way to the enema or cleaning after it, and clean and store them for future use.

17. Remove bed screens, if any, 1 above. Open doors as patient wishes and restore room to normal condition.

18. A room deodorizer may be used to eliminate the odor after an enema. If a deodorizer is not available, light several matches and let them burn for a few seconds.

The High Enema Occasionally a "high" enema may be prescribed for a patient. For a regular cleansing enema, the rectal tube or tip is usually inserted about 10 cm./4 in., 9 above. For a high enema, it is inserted 15–20 cm./ 6–8 in. with the intention of the fluid's reaching as high as possible into the transverse (crosswise) and ascending portions of the colon.

Enemas for Children and Infants The basic procedure for giving an enema to a child more than about 2 years old is essentially the same as for an adult; there are, however, important steps to take in preparing a child emotionally and mentally for an enema, 1 below. Basic procedure for giving an enema to an infant less than 1 year old is quite different from that for an older child or an adult.

Enema for a child:

1. Before attempting to give an enema to a child who is more than 2 years old, explain very carefully and clearly what you are going to do. You may need help in holding the child, but you will have much greater success if you can win the child's cooperation. Admit that there may be some discomfort and even a slight tummy ache, and promise that if there is, you will stop the flow of the liquid right away.

2. Proceed as in Giving the Soapsuds Enema, above, after preparing the prescribed amount of enema solution at the recommended temperature. Because children naturally do squirm about when in unusual positions, as a general rule it is not practical to try to give an enema to a child in your lap. Since you probably will need both hands to control the child, protect the bed with waterproof sheeting or newspapers and a towel the same as for an adult. Place the child on the bedpan, with enough pillows under the back for comfort. When actually giving the enema, it is quite important to allow it to run in very slowly so that the child will not experience cramping. At the first sign or complaint of cramping, stop the flow immediately. Let the child choose between going to the toilet or using the bedpan for expelling the enema.

Enema for an infant:

1. Equipment and material needed for giving an infant an enema are the proper amount of enema solution at the recommended temperature; a satisfactory changing table; extra diapers, preferably disposable; a small bulb syringe for administering the enema solution; and lubricant for the syringe tip.
2. To fill the syringe with enema solution, squeeze the bulb and place the tip in the solution, release the bulb so that the solution will be sucked up into it.
3. Place the infant, with a diaper under the buttocks, on the changing table. While holding the infant's legs out of the way with one hand, with the other pick up the syringe, hold it tip down over the solution container, and squeeze a few drops out the end to warm the syringe tip and expel any air in it. Insert the lubricated tip of the syringe about 3.75 cm./1½ in. into the rectum. Squeeze the syringe bulb slowly and gently to force liquid into the bowel. When finished, remove the syringe slowly and press the infant's buttocks together to help it hold the solution if possible. If the child is old enough and wants to be seated on a potty seat or toilet to expel the enema, do so. If not, allow enema and feces to be expelled into the diaper.

Baking Soda Enema In some cases, a baking soda cleansing enema may be prescribed. The usual solution is 5 ml. baking soda to 500 ml. warm water (1 tsp. baking soda to 1 pt. water). Administer it the same as a soapsuds enema.

Saline/Salt Enema Salt or saline solutions also are prescribed as cleansing enemas. Generally the solution is 5 ml. plain or iodized table salt to 500 ml. warm water (1 tsp. salt to 1 pt. water). Prepare and give the same as the soapsuds enema.

Harris Flush The Harris flush is not a cleansing enema in the strict sense, as its prime purpose is to help the patient expel gas. Plain warm water is instilled or injected into the colon to stimulate peristalsis (wavelike contractions of the intestines). Do not attempt this procedure without complete instructions by the doctor or your visiting nurse.

RETENTION ENEMAS

The solution used in retention enemas is meant to be retained by a patient until the prescribed amount of medicine has been absorbed by the walls of the colon. Prior to the retention enema a cleansing enema, above, may be given to help the medication be more readily absorbed by the colon. Retention enema additives must be ingredients that will not stimulate the nerve endings in the colon and so promote peristalsis. Retention enemas other than oil are not commonly given in home care of a patient. They should never be given without complete instructions by the doctor as to the liquid, additive, amount, how to give it, how long it should be retained by the patient, what to do if the patient expels all or part of it too soon. Even if you are experienced in giving cleansing enemas, you should have your visiting nurse demonstrate how to give a retention enema, since there are important differences in giving them. The more common types of retention enemas are the lubricating and the medicinal; the nutrient type is seldom used.

Retention Enemas for Children It usually is a very rare situation when a doctor prescribes a retention enema for a child. Because of such factors as the child's physical condition and maturity, age, and the purpose of the enema, you should expect detailed instructions on the amount of enema to be given, its composition and temperature. You also should be instructed by the doctor or your visiting nurse as to the equipment needed and the method of giving the retention enema. These may or may not be the same as or similar to the equipment and methods of giving children and infants cleansing enemas.

Lubricating Retention Enemas An oil retention enema is often given after surgery for hemorrhoids to soften the feces and lubricate the passage (anal canal) to the external orifice (anus, rectum). When there is an impaction or overloading of feces in the bowel, a lubricating or oil retention enema may be given, often followed sometime later by a cleansing enema.

Kinds of Oil Mineral oil and ordinary cooking olive and cottonseed oils are used for lubricating enemas.

Amount of Oil Enema Lubricating retention enemas for adults usually are 89–180 ml./3–6 oz. of oil. The actual amount to use will, of course, be specified by the patient's doctor or your visiting nurse. This is particularly important when treating infants and children.

Measure the amount of oil for a retention enema accurately. Much less than a specified amount generally will not be effective, while much more will tend to stimulate action of the colon walls and thereby cause premature expulsion of the enema.

Temperature of Oil Enema To minimize the stimulation of the colon and the discomfort of a patient, the temperature of an oil retention enema should be 37.6°C/100°F. At the start, a warmer enema may be more comfortable for the patient. But since it may stimulate colonic activity, the warmer enema can soon become more difficult and uncomfortable to retain. Determine the temperature of an enema oil with a thermometer; if you do not have one, spill a few drops of the oil on the underside of your wrist; if it feels comfortably warm but not hot, the oil temperature probably is satisfactory.

Equipment for Giving Oil Retention Enemas The equipment needed for giving oil retention enemas to adults is the same as for cleansing enemas (see Equipment for Giving Soapsuds Enemas, above) except that a complete enema kit and stand are not necessary; only the rectal tube or tip is used. Since such a small amount of liquid is given, much of it would be lost if placed in an enema container and run through the long hose to the rectal tip. It is far more practical to attach or hold a small kitchen funnel to the rectal tube or tip and pour the liquid into it.

If your patient is an infant or a child, ask the doctor or your visiting nurse what equipment to use for giving an oil retention enema.

Giving an Oil Retention Enema There are a few important differences between giving oil retention and cleansing enemas. In the following list of steps in giving oil retention enemas, references such as "Step 1" are to the steps in Giving Soapsuds Enemas:

1. With the exceptions of the complete enema kit, stand, and possibly the bedpan, bring together all the items needed for giving an enema; place patient in the proper position; cover patient; and set bedpan, if it will be used, in place, as in Steps 1 through 4.
2. Lubricate the end 18 or 20 cm./7 or 8 in. of the rectal tube or tip, Step 6.
3. Attach, or prepare later to hold, the small kitchen funnel to the open end of the rectal tube or tip. Put the warm enema liquid in a cup, preferably one that has a pouring lip.
4. Redrape your patient and insert the rectal tube or tip essentially as in Steps 8 and 9. Instead of inserting only about 5 cm./2 in. of tip or tube, insert 18 or 20 cm./7 or 8 in., unless it meets resistance or your patient suffers discomfort. In either case, wait several seconds, then try again to insert the tube higher; try this four or five times before quitting. If it is a matter of resistance rather than patient discomfort, try to move the tip or tube from side to side and possibly around the feces. If this is unsuccessful, give as much of the oil enema as possible, below.
5. Pour the oil into the funnel. Pour in a slow stream without ever completely filling the funnel. Pour the oil to run down a side of the funnel to permit air to escape as the oil runs into the tube or tip. There should be no cramping by your patient if you let the oil flow very slowly and do not give more than the prescribed amount. If your patient shows desire to expel the oil, stop the flow until there is no apparent desire to expel it.
6. When all the oil has been given, withdraw the rectal tube or tip slowly to avoid sudden stimulation of the rectal sphincter (muscles that close the anus or rectum). Cover the anus for 2 or 3 minutes with a pad of toilet paper, pressing it lightly to prevent premature evacuation or expelling of the enema solution. When the urge to expel weakens, have your patient lie flat on the back for about 30 minutes, after which any normal position may be assumed.

NOTE: If an oil retention enema was given to soften feces, a few hours later a voluntary evacuation or bowel movement may occur. If not, it may be necessary to give a cleansing enema; ask the doctor or your visiting nurse how long to wait before giving it.

7. After a retention enema has been completed satisfactorily, remove the equipment and clean your patient, as in Steps 12 through 17.

Medicinal Retention Enemas Under certain conditions, a doctor may prescribe medicine to be administered by rectum, or a medicinal retention enema. It might be done to a patient who is unable or refuses to take medicine by mouth. The doctor will instruct you fully as to the amount of medicine to be given, the solution to mix it in, and the length of time of retention. The method of giving the enema usually is the same as for an oil retention enema.

NOTE: Not all medicines can be given satisfactorily by enema, so do not try this method unless the doctor orders it.

Nutritional Retention Enema Despite sometimes widespread tales about people being kept alive by "nutrient" enemas, nowadays there are so many other ways of getting adequate nourishment into a patient that the enema is seldom used. A major reason for this is that digestion of nutrients takes place in the stomach and small intestine, not in the large one. But if a doctor orders nutritional enemas, you will be given complete instructions as to the ingredients, amount, temperature, necessary retention time, and so forth. The enema probably will be given the same way as an oil retention enema.

26 Douche/Irrigation

According to the standard dictionary, *douche* is a stream or jet of water or other fluid, or a current of vapor, applied to a part or a cavity of the body for hygienic or medicinal purposes. In practice, however, *douche* generally refers to females and is the short way of saying "vaginal douche." The other type of douche, in which water or other fluid or vapor is directed against wounds or infected areas of the body, is commonly called irrigation.

There are several kinds of douches and irrigations, some of which should be given by skilled nurses or technicians using highly specialized equipment. Those that you may have to give probably will be of a basically simple type. Even so, and particularly for the vaginal douche, have your visiting nurse show you step by step how to give them.

Most douche and irrigation fluids are water to which has been added an antiseptic, disinfectant, deodorant, astringent, or some other medication. Because irrigations and douches are applied to very sensitive parts of the body, be sure to follow exactly the doctor's or your visiting nurse's instructions as to the solution to be used, the amount, its temperature, and the pressure or force with which it should be applied.

Irrigations of the genitals and the rectal/perineal area may be given with your patient on a toilet or over a bidet, or lying in a bathtub or in bed, whichever is most convenient and practical. Most other irrigations may be given in bed or in a bathtub, or over a basin, bowl, sink, toilet, or bidet.

A douche should be given with your patient lying down, either in the bathtub or in bed on a bedpan, to enable the fluid to reach all parts of the vagina.

IRRIGATIONS

The most common irrigation is the cleansing type that should be given after every urination or bowel movement to clean the genitals and perineal/rectal area (see Giving the Tub Bath, Chapter 23) of all bedfast patients; of ambulatory patients following childbirth, curettement, genital, rectal, and other surgery in the perineal area; and during menstrual periods.

Other irrigations that you may be required to give will be to clean or medically treat sores or wounds (surgical or otherwise) on other parts of the body, such as arms, legs, etc.

Irrigation Solutions Plain water often is the required irrigation "solution." It may also be required that the water be sterilized either by boiling or by adding chemicals before use.

Common irrigation solutions are water to which an antiseptic or a disinfectant has been added. Place water at the prescribed temperature in the irrigation/douche solution container (below), add the antiseptic or disinfectant, and mix thoroughly. Be sure to use the exact amount of water or other fluid and additive; the doctor or your visiting nurse will clearly specify them in milliliters or in ounces.

NOTE: If irrigating with a syringe or squeeze-bottle instrument, such as the peri bottle (below), first prepare the solution, then fill the container.

Amount of Irrigation Solution It is important to use the proper amount of irrigation solution for your patient. With too little, cleansing or other treatment will not be thorough. If too much solution is prepared, there may be unnecessary waste. The doctor will prescribe the amount, or you will be able to judge for yourself after giving a few irrigations.

Temperature of Irrigation Temperature of a solution is of great importance for both its effectiveness and the patient's tolerance. Infected areas and tissues and those recently subjected to surgery, especially of the genitals and in the perineal area, may be extremely sensitive to heat. Most irrigations are given with a so-called hot solution, ranging from 36.7° to 40° C/98° to 104° F. Warmer or cooler solutions may be used if necessary for your patient's comfort. For practical purposes, and depending on how long in advance you prepare a solution, it should be a few degrees warmer than when it is to be used.

NOTE: "Scotch" irrigation, in which jets of hot and cold water are alternately applied, is sometimes prescribed. Complete instructions will be given.

Pressures of Irrigation Irrigations are commonly given by gravity-flow from elevated containers and by syringes such as the peri bottle, see Equipment for Irrigations, below.

With gravity-flow, the pressure or force of the flow of irrigation solution usually is prescribed as high or low: high, when the solution container is at least 61 cm./2 ft. above the area to be irrigated; low, when it is 31–46 cm./1–1½ ft. above the area. Pressure also may be prescribed by the height of the container; for example, it is to be 61 cm./2 ft. above your patient's hip.

When irrigating with a syringe or a peri bottle, squeeze it just hard enough to direct a steady flow of solution to the part of the body being treated. Do not squeeze any harder than is necessary, as with too much pressure or force the irrigating may injure tender tissue.

Types of Irrigation Flows Irrigating usually is done with a solid jet or stream of solution flowing from the end of a hose or from a single hole in the irrigation tip, Fig. 26–1*a*. A solid stream is easy to direct to a given point, confines the flow to a fairly small area, and makes less unnecessary mess. A circular flow, such as a fine spray coming from a number of small holes in the tip, spreads and may be difficult to confine to the area being treated. Of course, sometimes the fine or circular spray is preferred; if you lack the necessary tip, as a rule you can get a satisfactory flow by waving a solid jet spray around the area to be treated.

Equipment for Irrigations Since irrigating is done by spraying the solution on the body, an enema container with attachments, Fig. 25–1, a douche bag with attachments, or a peri bottle, Fig. 26–1, may be used. Irrigating is also done with bulb- and plunger-type syringes; however, as a rule they are more difficult for the average inexperienced nurse to use properly.

A stand to hold the solution container is needed. Any sort of sturdy enough stand, such as a garment rack, floor lamp, or photographer's light stand usually will do if it is high enough. String several loops of fairly heavy twine through the hole or handle of the container and over an appropriate part of the stand; or hang

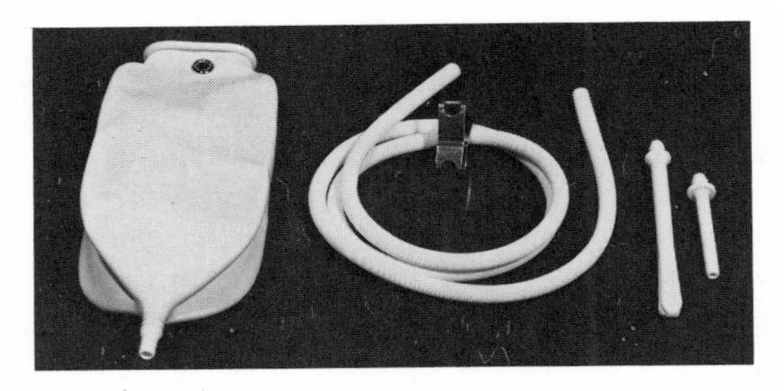

Fig. 26–1*a* *Irrigation or douche kit; from left to right: solution container, hose with stop-clamp, nozzle for circular or fine spray, nozzle for solid jet flow*

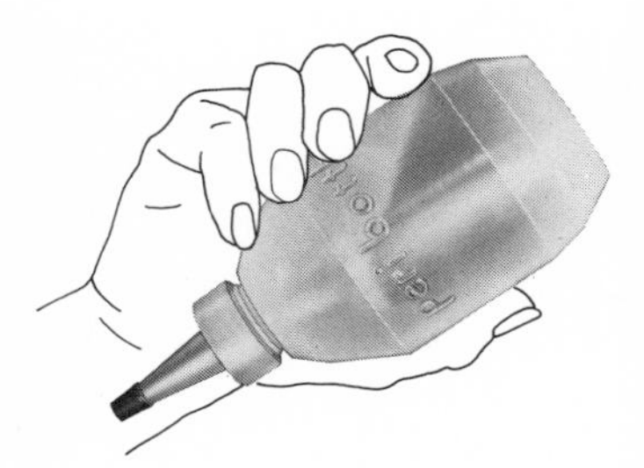

Fig. 26–1*b* *Peri bottle type of syringe held for self-irrigating by patient*

the container from the stand with a hook made from a wire coat hanger. Be sure that the container hangs at the proper height for irrigating your patient.

Rubber or plastic gloves, Chapter 8, as a rule are not medically necessary for giving an irrigation. But they may make the work less embarrassing for your patient and you.

To dry your patient after irrigation, you need a generous supply of cotton balls, pads, or squares. Use one for only one drying stroke, and immediately put it in the trash bag. Gauze pads are not recommended as they can irritate sensitive tissue.

In addition to items for irrigating in general, you need equipment and materials based on the part of the body being treated and the condition of the patient.

Arms, Face, Feet, Hands, Head, Legs, Neck, Shoulders. These irrigations often are done with the patient leaning or holding the afflicted part over a basin, sink, toilet, bidet, or bathtub.

Back, Belly, Buttocks, Chest, Hips. For these irrigations, patients may lean over a basin or sink . . . stand or sit in a shower stall or bathtub . . . or lie in a bathtub or a bed.

Genitals, Perineal/Rectal Areas. These irrigations frequently are done with the patient seated on a toilet or a bidet or in a bathtub, or lying in a bathtub or a bed. When irrigating in a bathtub following surgery or when there are painful sores in these areas, have your patient sit or lie on a rubber or soft plastic ring of the type used for a sitz bath, Fig. 8–17*b*.

Ambulatory patients who are to be irrigated in bed are treated basically the same as bedfast patients.

Bedfast Patients. A bath basin (Chapter 8) may be used for collecting liquid flowing off the body when irrigating the arms, faces, feet, hands, heads, legs, and necks of bedfast patients. A bath basin also may be used when irrigating the shoulders and other parts of the body, but a bedpan (Chapter 8) often is more comfortable for the patient, and easier for the nurse to handle. For irrigating in bed you also need:

Waterproof sheeting to place under your patient. Or full-size sheets of newspaper may be used; eight to ten generally are enough. Newspaper is absorbent and holds spills and splashes well. Remove sheeting or newspapers after irrigating.

Large cloth towel to place on waterproof sheeting or newspapers. Patients usually are more comfortable lying on toweling, and in case of a spill or splash it will help keep the liquid from running off the waterproof sheeting or newspapers onto the bedding.

Bath Blanket (Chapter 8) to cover and protect your patient against exposure and chills.

Irrigating Genitals and Perineal/Rectal Areas Give genital and perineal/rectal area irrigations on a toilet or a bidet, in a bathtub or in bed, whichever is more convenient for your patient and you.

Irrigating on a Toilet How practical this is depends on the area to be irrigated. There must be enough open space for you to reach between the thighs far and freely enough, without pressing on your patient, to direct the irrigation fluid as needed. However, if able and willing, let your patient do it.

Irrigating with an enema container, douche bag, or peri bottle is generally the practical and effective method. Pouring the solution over your patient from a pitcher usually is satisfactory only if the area to be treated is directly exposed. Irrigating by pouring the solution into a funnel connected to an irrigating hose requires either that your patient direct the spray or that you fasten the funnel and hose to a stand before starting to irrigate.

To irrigate:

1. *Bring all equipment and materials*, including the irrigation solution, into the bathroom.

2. *For irrigating the genitals and adjacent area*, seat your patient on the toilet just far enough toward the back of the seat so that, when the knees are spread apart, you can reach between the thighs and direct the spray. The patient's knees and buttocks should as a rule be spread as far apart as possible without causing severe discomfort.

3. *For irrigating the rectal area*, your patient should sit as close to the front of the toilet seat as is comfortable. The buttocks should be spread apart as far as possible without causing severe discomfort. During irrigation, and for the wiping and drying afterward, have your patient lean forward so that you can see to direct the spray as necessary.

4. *If storing the irrigation solution* in an enema container or a douche bag, hold or hang it at the prescribed height (Pressure of Irrigation, above).

5. *Hold the end of the irrigation hose or tip* several inches away from the area to be treated first and start the flow of the spray. Depending on how sensitive the patient's skin or tissue is, slowly or quickly bring the tip or hose close enough for the spray to irrigate satisfactorily. Work the spray around as necessary to try to dislodge feces, dried blood, or other matter stuck to the skin. If the irrigating hurts your patient, move the spray a few inches away, lower the solution container several inches to reduce pressure of the flow, or squeeze the syringe more gently. Continually moving the spray around instead of keeping it directed at one point usually is more comfortable for the patient. However, when feces, dried blood, etc., is stuck tight to the skin, it may be necessary to direct the flow at that point for 10 or 15 seconds to loosen it. If this fails to clean an area that has not had recent surgery or does not have an open sore, wound, or burn, you may try gently to wipe off the stuck particles with a ball or a small pad of wet absorbent cotton; do not use gauze pads, they can be very irritating to sensitive tissues.

6. *If irrigating for cleanliness* and/or to remove dried blood or other matter, when about two-thirds of the solution has been applied, stop the flow temporarily and examine the area being treated. If it is clean or nearly so, resume irrigation as a rinse or to complete the cleaning or removal of particles. Reexamine the patient after completing irrigation; if feces, dried blood, etc., still remains, prepare additional irrigating solution and rewash the area. As a rule, only two irrigations should be given at a time, since too much washing can in certain cases weaken damaged skin and tissue.

7. *After completing the irrigation,* put the equipment aside and dry your patient. Dry the genitals and perineal area with balls, pads, or small loose wads of sterile absorbent cotton. Make only one stroke with a piece of cotton, and deposit it immediately in the trash bag. Uninvolved wet areas may be dried with toilet tissue.

Irrigating on a Bidet Giving a plain water irrigation on a bidet is simply a matter of getting your patient satisfactorily positioned on the bidet and turning on the water. You must, of course, first determine the proper faucet settings for the temperature and pressure of the water flow (Temperature of Irrigation, Pressure of Irrigation, above); make final adjustments to suit your patient. Fluctuating the pressure, and possibly the temperature, instead of keeping the water flow constant may make an irrigation more comfortable for your patient. Irrigation on a bidet usually should last for about 5 minutes at most.

1. *When feces, dried blood, or other matter* sticks to the skin, it may be necessary to increase the water pressure appreciably for 10 or 15 seconds to help loosen it. Do not increase the pressure enough to hurt your patient, and do not maintain the higher pressure for longer than about 20 seconds. If this does not clean an area that is free of recent surgery or open wounds, sores, or burns, gently try to wipe off stuck particles with a ball or a small pad of wet absorbent cotton; do not use gauze pads, they often irritate sensitive tissue.
2. *When about two-thirds of the planned irrigation time has elapsed,* stop the flow and examine the area being treated. If it is clean or nearly so, complete the irrigation as a rinse, if your patient wants it, or to remove the last particles of soil. Examine your patient again after finishing irrigating; if particles of feces, blood, etc., are still there, renew irrigation for up to about 5 minutes at most.
3. *After completing the irrigation,* dry your patient as in 7, Irrigating on a Toilet, above.

Giving an antiseptic or medicated irrigation on the bidet may or may not be practical. It depends on how agile you and your patient are, and how well you can work together. It may be easier for both of you to irrigate on the toilet or in the bathtub.

Irrigating in a Bathtub Irrigating the genitals or perineal/rectal area is done in a bathtub as a rule only if the patient can lie on the bottom of it; if not, irrigating usually should be done in bed.

1. *Bring all equipment and materials,* including the prepared irrigation solution, into the bathroom.
2. *Before your patient enters the bathtub,* warm the bottom of it with a few inches of hot water, drain out, and dry tub. Instead of or in addition to warming the tub, spread a fairly thick bath towel over the bottom to go under the patient from head to hips.
3. *If irrigating after surgery* in the rectal area, or if for any other reason it is unusually sensitive, place a rubber or a soft plastic ring (Fig. 8–17*b*) for the patient's buttocks to lie on.

4. *Get patient into tub.* With the patient lying on the bottom of the tub, the knees should be elevated as high and spread as far apart as possible while keeping both feet flat on the bottom. Cover your patient from the shoulders to just above the pubic area with a bath blanket (Chapter 8) or a large beach towel.

5. *Irrigate* as in steps 3 through 7, Irrigating on a Toilet, above.

6. *Remove covering* and help patient out of tub.

Irrigating in Bed The main difference between irrigating the genitals and perineal/rectal area in a bathtub, above, and in bed is in preparing the patient:

1. *Bring all equipment and materials*, including the prepared irrigation solution at the proper temperature, to the patient's bedside. Close all doors and windows, or place a screen or screens to give privacy to the bed area.

2. *Have your patient lie in bed* in the same position as for irrigating in a bathtub, 4 above, except that a comfort ring is not needed.

3. *Place protective sheeting and towel* under patient. Set the bedpan under the buttocks to collect the irrigation flow-off.

4. *Fan-fold* (Chapter 13) the upper bedding to the foot of the bed. Cover patient with a bath blanket or large beach towel from the shoulders to just above the pubic area.

5. *Irrigate* as in Steps 4, 5, and 6, Irrigating on a Toilet, above. If instead of flowing into the bedpan the solution tends to splatter about, lower the solution container to reduce the force of the flow. If there is more solution than will fill the bedpan about two-thirds full, stop irrigating when it reaches that level, remove and empty the bedpan, replace and resume irrigating.

6. *When irrigation is finished*, remove bedpan, replace towel under patient if it is wet, then dry patient, Step 7, Irrigating on a Toilet, above.

7. *Remove all toweling* and protective materials from bed. Remove bath blanket or beach towel while drawing fan-folded bedding up over your patient.

8. *Remove all irrigation* equipment and materials from room, rearrange furniture and bedscreens, if any, for normal living.

Other Irrigations Irrigating areas on arms, legs, and other parts of the body is basically the same as for the genitals and the perineal/rectal area. It may be done with your patient leaning or holding the afflicted part over a basin, sink, bathtub, toilet, or bidet; or in a bathtub or in bed, whichever is most convenient and practical for both of you. For irrigating in bed, use whatever object—bedpan, emesis basin, plastic dishpan, etc.—is handiest for collecting the run-off liquid.

VAGINAL DOUCHE

The common vaginal douche (washing of the female vagina) may be given for cleansing, deodorant, antiseptic, stimulating, or hemostatic (to stop bleeding) purposes. Because the vagina, like many other parts of the body, usually cleans itself naturally, there is little reason for a normal healthy woman to use a vaginal douche. Also, a vaginal douche following sexual intercourse is not effective as a contraceptive.

For a vaginal douche to be most effective, the patient must lie either flat on her back, or with the hips slightly elevated as on a bedpan, so that the injected solution may go all the way to the upper end of the vagina. If she sits on a toilet or straddles a bidet for vaginal douching, as so often is done, it is unlikely that the douche solution will flow to all areas.

Vaginal Douche Solutions Common vaginal douche solutions usually are water to which a cleansing agent, deodorant, or medicine has been added. Place water at the recommended temperature in the solution container (see Temperature of Douche Solution, Equipment for Douche, below), add the prescribed ingredient, and mix thoroughly.

Since ingredients for douching may vary widely from one doctor to another, it is not practical to list or discuss them here. Many ingredients are items commonly found in the home, and others are simple, over-the-counter preparations. You will, of course, be given complete instructions for preparing the usable solution by the doctor or your visiting nurse.

Amount of Douche Solution Unless otherwise ordered, as a rule 1 to 2 l. or qts. of solution are used for a vaginal douche.

Temperature of Douche Solution Temperature of a douche solution is of great importance both for its effectiveness and your patient's tolerance of it:

Cleansing, Antiseptic, Deodorant Douches Temperature usually should be from 40.6°–44.4° C/105°–112° F.

Hemostatic, Stimulating Douches Temperature usually is from 47.8°–48.9° C/118°–120° F.

For practical purposes and depending on how far in advance you prepare a solution, it should be a few degrees warmer when prepared than when it is to be used.

Pressure for Douche A douche solution should flow slowly and at a low pressure or force. Generally the solution container should not be higher than about 61 cm./24 in. above the patient's hips. From this height, the solution flows with enough pressure or force to reach all parts of a recumbent patient's vagina. If the solution flows from a greater height, there is danger of forcing some of it into the cervix or uterus, possibly causing infection. For this reason, it is widely believed that vaginal douches should not be given with a syringe.

Douche Flow Vaginal douche solution usually flows from the openings on all sides of the douche hose or tip, Fig. 26–1*a*. To minimize the possibility of introducing the solution directly into the cervix or the uterus, there should not be a direct opening at the very end of the hose or tip.

Equipment for Douche Since a douche solution must be instilled or injected with some pressure to be effective, a douche bag with attachments, Fig. 26–1*a*, or an enema container with attachments, Fig. 25–1*b*, should be used, whichever you have or prefer. The douche bag comes with a douche tip; the enema kit may or may not have one. Do not use a rectal tip for a vaginal douche.

Rubber or plastic gloves usually are not necessary for giving douches, but wearing them may make the task less embarrassing for your patient and you.

To prepare your patient for a douche, and to dry her afterward, you need a generous supply of sterile "wipes" or "sponges" (cotton balls or pads). Use a wipe for only one cleaning or drying stroke, and deposit it immediately in the trash bag. If your patient has not had recent surgery in the vaginal area, or painful sores there, toilet tissue may be used for drying it.

In addition to items made more or less for vaginal douches, you will need for bedfast patients and others who are being douched in bed:

Bedpan (Chapter 8) for collecting liquid flowing from the vagina.

Waterproof sheeting or newspapers to place on the bedding under your patient; eight to ten full-size sheets of newspaper usually are adequate. Remove sheeting or newspapers after the douche is expelled from the vagina.

Large towel to place on waterproof sheeting or newspapers. Patients usually are more comfortable lying on toweling, and in case of a spill it will help keep the liquid from running off the sheeting or newspapers onto the bed.

Bath blanket (Chapter 8) or large beach towel to cover and protect your patient against exposure and chills.

Flexible padding (rubber or polyfoam) to put between the patient's back and the bedpan for comfort; a rolled towel may be used instead. Pads about 10 cm./4 in. square of 1.5 cm.-/½ in.-thick polyfoam usually are satisfactory.

Stand for holding solution container. A commercial hospital-type stand, garment rack, floor lamp, photographer's light stand—anything high and strong enough to hold the filled container at the proper height. String several loops of strong twine through the hole in the container and over an appropriate part of the stand; or hang the container to it with a hook twisted from a wire coat hanger.

Giving the Vaginal Douche When vaginal douching is done for normal cleansing or deodorizing, satisfactory results usually may be had with the patient seated on a toilet or straddling a bidet. But when done for therapeutic reasons, the patient should lie down, either in bed on a bedpan or in a bathtub, in order for the solution to have its most effective coverage.

Vaginal Douche on a Toilet If a patient is able to sit down on a toilet, as a rule she can insert the douche tip and hold it in place herself. For giving the douche:

1. *Bring all equipment and materials*, including the prepared solution, into the bathroom.
2. *The patient should sit* on the toilet just far enough toward the back of the seat so that, when her knees are spread apart, you can easily reach between the thighs and insert the douche tip in the vagina; however, if at all possible, the patient should insert the tip and hold it in place. As a rule, the

patient's knees should be spread as far apart as possible without causing severe discomfort.

3. *Hold or hang the solution container* at the prescribed height, see Pressure for Douche, above. Hold the tip in place for insertion in the vagina, and loosen the stop-clamp to allow enough solution to flow through the hose to expel all air from it. While rotating the douche tip back and forth, gently insert it into the vagina about 5–7.5 cm./2–3 in. Allow the solution to flow until the container is empty. Then gently remove the douche tip, put the equipment aside, and dry your patient. Dry the area around the perineum (external region between the vulva and anus) with sterile wipes or sponges. Press gently while wiping downward and toward the anus or rectum. Make only one stroke with a wipe or sponge, then deposit it immediately in the trash bag.

Vaginal Douche on a Bidet A vaginal douche over a bidet is given the same as when the patient is seated on a toilet, above.

Vaginal Douche in Bathtub or Bed Except for the actual washing process, vaginal douching is basically the same as irrigating in a bathtub or in bed:

1. *Bathtub*. For vaginal douching in a bathtub, proceed as in Steps 1–4, Irrigating in a Bathtub, except that the patient should, if possible, insert the douche tip and hold it in place.

2. *Bed*. For vaginal douching in bed, proceed as in Steps 1–4, Irrigating in Bed, except that for comfort a flexible pad may be placed between the patient's back and the bedpan.

3. *Cleaning before douching*. With the patient in position for douching, Fig. 26–2*a*, clean the labia (lips of the vagina) with sterile cotton wipes or sponges. Stroke down from the front toward the rectum. Press firmly, but not hard enough to hurt the patient. Discard each wipe or sponge after a downward stroke; do not stroke in an up-and-down motion.

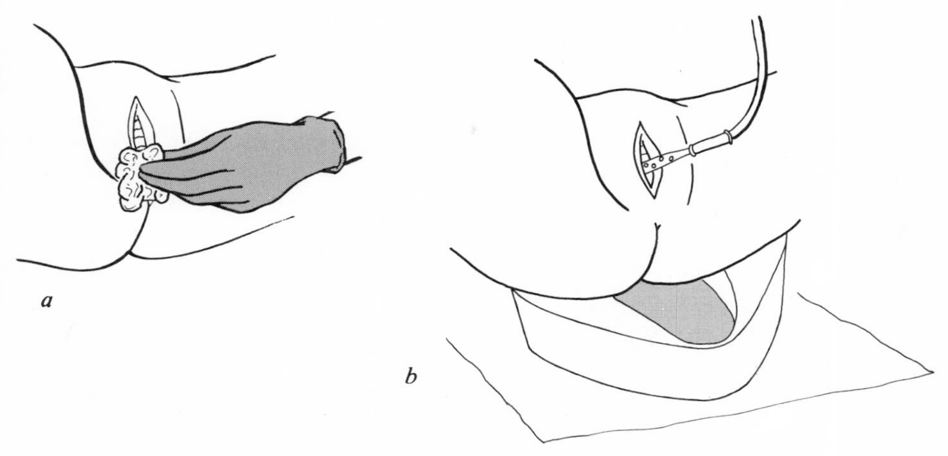

Fig. 26–2*a, b* *Vaginal douche with patient lying down*

4. *Prepare douche tip.* Before inserting douche tip, hold it over the bottom of the tub or bedpan and let enough solution flow to expel air from the hose and to warm the tip; about a quarter-cup of solution usually is enough. Pinch the tubing just above the tip to stop the flow and prevent waste of the solution.

5. *Insert douche tip.* Separate the labia to expose the vaginal orifice or opening. Rotate the douche tip back and forth while slowly, gently inserting it 5–7.5 cm./2–3 in. into the vagina, Fig. 26–2*b*, and directing it upward and slightly toward the patient's back.

6. *Douching.* Rotate the tip back and forth while the solution flows into the vagina. It should flow slowly rather than fast. If your patient complains that the solution is too hot or cold, stop the flow at once and check the temperature. If your patient complains of the force or pressure of the flow, lower the solution container until the flow is not uncomfortable. Shortly before the solution container is empty, stop the flow.

7. *Remove douche tip* from the vagina. Let your patient lie on the bottom of the bathtub or on the bedpan for a few minutes. Then assist your patient into a sitting position for the douche solution to be expelled. If your patient is bedfast and in a hospital bed, elevate the head of the bed.

8. *When expelling the douche stops,* dry the perineal area and vagina with sterile wipes or sponges as in Step 3 above.

9. *Bathtub.* If douching was in a bathtub, remove covering and assist patient out of bathtub.

10. *Bed.* If the douche was given in bed, remove protective toweling and waterproof material. Remove bath blanket while drawing fan-folded bedding up over patient. Remove douche equipment from room, restore room to normal condition.

27 Sleep, Rest, and Relaxation

It is generally agreed in medical circles that among the most effective remedies for illness and injury are sleep, rest, and relaxation. Natural sleep, rest, and relaxation are, of course, best; but sometimes they will not come to the aid of a patient without a little assistance from you, the nurse. There are also people who, in order to sleep, rest, or relax, need special therapy or medicine. Since many such treatments can be dangerous, inexperienced nurses should not give them without instructions by the doctor and, if at all possible, demonstration by the visiting nurse.

The most difficult part of learning what will best help your patient to sleep, rest, or relax is that so often what helps one person hinders another. Or, what helps Aunt Nell rest like a kitten makes Uncle Joe a nervous wreck. On the other hand,

Uncle Joe's jerky, jittery, disjointed words and actions may be very relaxing to him, while Aunt Nell's calm serenity may hide severe anxiety and fear. Part of your job as nurse is to help your patient find genuine rest and relaxation, and peaceful sleep.

SLEEP

There are two kinds of sleep: REM and NREM (nonrem). They alternate rhythmically throughout a person's entire sleep period.

REM Sleep REM sleep means "rapid eye movement" sleep. It is "active sleep," and the period in which a person dreams. During REM sleep the body is quiet, although small twitches of the muscles of the face and fingertips may be seen. Snoring stops and breathing becomes irregular—fast, then slow. Even though the sleeper's eyelids are closed you can see the movements of the eyes—side to side. During REM sleep the large muscles of the body are completely paralyzed—trunk, legs, and arms cannot move.

NREM Sleep NREM sleep is often called the quiet sleep period. It is characterized by slow, regular breathing and the absence of body movement. The body is not paralyzed, but does not move because the brain does not give any messages to the body muscles. It is mostly during NREM sleep that a person snores.

NREM and REM Sleep When we fall asleep, the first period of NREM sleep begins. It usually lasts for about 70–80 minutes. Following that is a period of REM sleep, which lasts about 10 minutes. Then another period of NREM sleep followed by one of REM. This cycle continues throughout the night, with the REM periods increasing in length as the hours progress. An adult who sleeps 7–7½ hours per night will as a rule spend 1½–2 hours in REM sleep, the periods in which dreams may occur.

Amount of Sleep Although each person requires a certain amount of sleep for good health, it changes from time to time. One of the most notable changes is in women during pregnancy; they commonly require 2 extra hours of daily sleep. The average daily amount of sleep needed:

Newborn infants	18–20 hours
Growing children	12–14 hours
Teenagers	10–11 hours
Adults	7–9 hours
More than 60 years of age	5–7 hours

NOTE: Females require more sleep than males.

The amount of sleep a person needs changes not only with age, but also in response to environment and especially to changes in environment. Noise or sound is particularly effective. Some people seem to have a natural need of a fairly high level of noise around them in order to sleep comfortably, while others need almost total silence; and people transferred from one sound environment to another commonly complain that the new one is too noisy or too quiet. Changes in temperature may also affect a person's sleep, although most people tend to adjust fairly quickly to normal or seasonal changes. Odor may or may not exert much influence on a person's sleep, although people accustomed to living in densely populated, highly polluted areas often complain of a "peculiar smell in the air" when arriving in an open-country, clean-air environment. Changes in these and other environmental factors tend to reduce the amount of time that a person sleeps—not the need for sleep—but as a rule the loss is only for a few days at most and not worth worrying about unduly.

When ill or injured, people commonly sleep a great deal more than they do normally. How much more they sleep depends on the nature of the sickness or injury, the patient's reaction to it, the treatment being given, and other factors; ask the doctor or your visiting nurse. The need for extra sleep decreases as a patient begins to recover from an ailment or becomes more aware of its probable course.

Sleep Patterns Most people have definite sleep patterns; that is, regular times of the night and day at which they become sleepy and wide awake. The majority of people are awake during the day and sleep during the dark hours. However, a very large segment of the population lives or would like very much to live the opposite way—sleep during the day, be awake at night! Whether this is an inborn trait or a habit due to years of working conditions, the fact is that to these "night owls" their hours of sleep and wakefulness are normal.

Occasionally patients change from their usual sleep patterns and sleep when they normally would be awake and cannot sleep at their usual sleep times. For example, a person who normally sleeps from ten o'clock at night to six o'clock in the morning may not, due to extra sleep during the day or evening, be sleepy at ten o'clock or, if sleepy, may sleep for only 3 or 4 hours instead of 8. Or a patient may go to sleep at seven instead of ten o'clock at night, and be wide awake from three o'clock on in the morning after a full 8 hours sleep. In either case the practical thing, unless the doctor forbids it, is to restore your patient's regular sleep pattern.

It usually requires conscious effort and may take several days to reprogram a person's sleep pattern. It basically consists of keeping patients awake during their normal wakeful hours and encouraging them through the regular sleep preparation, below, and particularly the back rub (Chapter 18), to sleep at their normal times. The key action in reprogramming is to keep your patient from sleeping or even napping after the midday meal, or what corresponds to it in the case of a night owl. During this time, schedule activities that will painlessly keep your patient awake. Give the daily bath. Remake the bed. Move your patient, if possible, into a different room. Have visitors if allowed. Talk about anything that interests your patient. Play games. In short, make every reasonable effort to keep your patient mentally and physically active. Avoid eye-tiring activities such as reading, sewing, or watching television for long periods of time. Preventing or correcting a patient's habit or pattern of sleeping at the wrong time is not always easy, but both of you will find it well worth the effort in the long run.

Getting Your Patient to Sleep During the early stages of a patient's sickness or postinjury period, there is usually no getting-to-sleep problem. Most people naturally do sleep more when they are disabled. Those who really cannot sleep due to shock, pain, fear, etc., usually are given the necessary sedation by the doctor. But as people recuperate, or perhaps simply become more accustomed to their ailment, they often just are not sleepy when they should be. Sometimes it is a problem of sleep pattern (above). Regardless, a regular preparation for sleep is helpful with many patients, and there are some nonmedical sleep aids to try before calling the doctor or your visiting nurse.

> NOTE: If the doctor has prescribed a sleeping pill, give it to your patient about 30 minutes before completing the regular preparation for sleep. It usually takes 20–30 minutes for a sleeping pill to take effect.

Regular Sleep Preparation The following schedule of preparatory work for getting a patient to sleep generally is convenient for both patient and nurse. But you may change it to meet your own circumstances.

1. *Warm beverage.* A warm, rather than hot or cold, beverage about 15 minutes prior to night bedtime often relaxes a patient. The beverage must, of course, conform to the patient's special diet, if any, Chapters 33–46 inclusive. Stimulating beverages such as coffee and tea generally are not as relaxing as milk, cocoa, mild soup, or other more readily digested liquid. However, although coffee seems to keep most people awake, many find that a cup just before bedtime is an excellent sleep aid; decaffeinated coffee lacks the stimulating effect. Some people believe hot toddies to be very good sleep aids; be sure to consult the doctor before giving your patient an alcoholic beverage.
2. *Snacks.* For many patients an easy-to-digest food, conforming to the special diet, if any, is a better sleep aid than a warm beverage. The warmth or coolness of a bedtime snack often is not as important to a patient as its taste and texture. However, as a rule highly spiced or seasoned foods are not as effective as somewhat mild, sweet, or semisweet ones. A small dish of ice cream, pudding, or fruit often has excellent effect.
3. *Toilet.* Patients who are able to should go to the bathroom for urination and bowel movement, washing hands and face, cleaning teeth and rinsing mouth. Provide these services for bedfast patients.
4. *Back rub.* The standard back rub (Chapter 18) is extremely relaxing at all times and is especially recommended as a basic part of preparing a patient for sleep.
5. *Bed.* Adjust the bed to the most comfortable position for your patient. Remove wrinkles in the sheets. Put additional blankets on the bed if needed. Reposition pillows for comfort.
6. *Sleep garment.* Find out if your patient wants a change of sleep garment before settling for the night.
7. *Bedside items.* Make certain that all items that may be needed during the night (facial tissues, bedside sack or wastebasket, bell, carafe of water and

drinking glass, lamp or light control, etc.) are within your patient's easy reach.

8. *Dentures.* Depending on your patient's normal behavior, provide a container with sufficient clean water for holding dentures overnight.

9. *Lights.* Turn the room lights out or down low, as your patient prefers, and leave your patient ready for sleep.

Sleeping Aids If the usual preparation for sleep is not effective with your patient, try one or more of the following nonmedical aids:

1. *Music.* Melodic, relatively soft-toned music of a romantic nature generally is a more effective sleep aid than a loud, brassy beat. A personal loudspeaker that fits under the pillow and connects to a radio or record or tape player often is more effective than a conventional radio or player loudspeaker.

2. *Eye-tiring activity.* Reading, sewing, and extensive watching of television usually have a harmless tiring effect on the eyes that helps induce sleep.

3. *Bath.* A bath (Chapter 23) and a freshly made bed may be the most effective ways of helping a patient go to sleep. It may, of course, be very inconvenient for your nursing, housework, or outside employment, and if so should be used only when all other nonmedical sleep aids fail. If your patient can take a tub bath, a 15-minute soak in warm—not hot—water should help induce sleep.

REST

Rest may be called a condition in which the body or mind is kept free of deliberate or intentional work or effort of any kind. Energy saved during a time of rest is used by the body and mind in their natural attempts to become and stay healthy. Therefore, the more your patient rests, the faster and easier recovery from sickness or injury usually is.

Getting your patient into a state of rest usually requires, especially at the start, quite a bit of work by both of you. Your tasks generally are: (1) convincing your patient that rest is possible and will occur; and (2) setting up and maintaining conditions that help your patient rest. Your patient's task is that of forcing body and mind into a state of inactivity or rest. The first several times they are tried, both tasks can be hard and discouraging.

In the early stages of a sickness, or shortly after suffering a serious injury, many people strongly doubt that any treatment will do much good. They often will agree that rest is one of Nature's best remedies, but this may be done to keep you quiet, to "stop you nagging" about resting. Depending on your patient's basic temperament as well as present physical and mental conditions, you may have to try almost every kind of reasoning, pleading, and threats to get your patient to at least try to rest, which is the all-important first step. There is no rule of thumb for what will work with a patient. Try any and every thing you can think of, but stop immediately any method that seems to upset your patient. Ask your visiting nurse for advice and suggestions.

Quiet surroundings are usually considered ideal for helping a patient rest. But there is such a thing as a room or house being too quiet, with so little noise that a patient becomes edgy and irritable. If, for example, your patient is accustomed to the normal hustle and bustle of family life and suddenly everyone whispers and goes on tiptoes, the lack of sound may be upsetting. Also, sick people often develop a nervous habit of expecting or listening for sounds of any kind, just something to hear; a radio, TV, or recorded music played somewhat softly often satisfies them. Sudden noises tend to startle people and should be prevented, or at least a patient should be warned if someone plans to turn on loudly a radio or such.

Getting into a State of Rest Putting body and mind into a state of inactivity or rest is not easy for some people. Various ways of relaxing (below) may help, but seldom are a complete solution. Since forcing oneself into a state of physical and mental inactivity is unusual, and frightening for most people the first few times they try it, you generally should suggest that your patient try it in easy stages:

> First the body goes to rest a little at a time, then the mind. Usually an easy way to put the body at rest is to start with the toes. Let them go limp; "tell" them that if they want to curl over limply, do it! Then let the feet go limp and rest any whichway, flopped over on the sides, away from one another, or against each other—just let the feet go into any position "they" want to. Then the lower legs, the knees, the upper legs, buttocks, lower back, waist, upper back and shoulders, neck, eyes, mouth, face; then the fingers, hands, wrists, lower and upper arms.

This method of letting adjacent parts of the body progressively go inactive, or to rest, works in most cases. Starting with the most distant part of the body—the toes—generally is more effective than starting with the fingers. Moreover, since it is a gradual process it tends to prevent the fear that so many people have of losing control of the body. When your patient's body seems to be at rest—you generally can tell by an unusual limpness of the hands and head—then suggest that:

> The mind should be let free to "wander as it will," not thinking of anything in particular, nor making any effort to reject or change a line of thought. Thinking of something pleasant or soothing is a good way to start the process of putting the mind to rest, but do not try to force any particular chain of thought or ideas. When talking with your patient during this procedure, speak slowly, softly, and in a soothing tone of voice.
>
> Patients must also be told that when they feel that they have had enough rest, they reactivate themselves by deliberately changing their position or moving around . . . making their bodies work again . . . forcing themselves to think about one particular thing for a few seconds.

Patients coming out of a period of rest often are amazed by how refreshed they feel—and that it happened in such a short length of time!

RELAXATION

Relax means to decrease or get rid of anxiety, intensity, nervousness, strain, or tension. Both rest and relaxation are highly beneficial to sick or injured people. But whereas *rest* means a state of inactivity, relaxation generally implies the doing of something that will take our minds off our troubles, or make them seem less important. Many people find that it is much easier to relax than to rest. There are many ways to relax; any activity, person, or object that eases a person's feeling of anxiety, etc., may be considered as being a good relaxant. One of the generally best relaxants, although seldom called that, is a "good listener."

The Good Listener Regardless of what they may say, most disabled people are full of worries. Worries and fears about their ailment, how long they will be laid up, their chances of recovery; worries about what their family and friends may think of them; fears about keeping their jobs, paying their bills, how much their disability will cost. Some patients discuss these problems frankly and at length with the doctor, visiting nurse, you, anyone within speaking distance. But intentionally or otherwise, they commonly hide some of their deepest worries. Also, there are patients who simply will not discuss their problems. Either way, you as their nurse are in a good position to learn of their fears—fears that may be hindering their recovery—just by being a "good listener."

Being a good listener is not spying. You should, of course, report to the doctor or your visiting nurse any fears or worries that seem to upset your patient. But your main value as a good listener is in giving your patient a chance to relax through talking about the things that are causing anxiety, nervousness, and tension. In most cases, just the act of talking about problems makes them less fearful, often to the extent that the patient realizes that a fear is pointless, and stops thinking about it. In many instances, in talking to a good listener a patient will reveal why a certain fear or worry exists. Knowing the real cause of a fear, an experienced doctor or nurse usually can help a person get rid of it or make it less frightening.

Being a good listener often is difficult. You should show interest in what your patient is talking about by asking pertinent questions from time to time, but you must not appear to be prying or spying. You should not antagonize your patient by pointing out that what is being complained about today was being highly praised yesterday. Nor should you in any way show a lack of interest in your patient's problems, aches, and pains, no matter how often you have been told all about them. Of course, these "don't's" are generalities; there are sick people who seem to thrive on being contradicted—you just have to know your patient. However, usually the most difficult part of being a good listener is that so often there are things other than the patient's condition, fears, and worries that you would like to talk about.

Relaxing Activities There are many activities that a patient can do, alone or with help, to relax. They may be divided into three general groups: passive, mild, and strong activities.

1. Passive activities are those requiring little or no effort, such as listening to the radio, watching television, being entertained by the family and visitors without trying to join in. Inexperienced nurses often become discouraged when a patient persists in passive activity. They should, however, keep in mind that there are many people who really would rather watch and listen than take an active part in conversation, games, etc. Also, a patient's physical or mental condition may be such that just lying back and listening is the most relaxing activity at the time. Of course, if passive activity continues longer than the patient's physical condition warrants, you should consult the doctor. Prolonged lassitude of this type may be a symptom of a mental depression.

2. Mild activities are those requiring relatively light exertion, such as reading, writing letters, sewing, knitting, playing cards and games, taking active part in family affairs and conversations, and so forth. As a rule, any mild activity can be relaxing and should be encouraged; but take care that it is not done for so long a time that it tires your patient. The other possible problem with a mild activity is boredom. A person can easily become bored with or depressed from reading, playing the same kinds of games, seeing the same people, and hearing the same talk day after day. Boredom can have a bad effect on a patient's appetite (Chapter 44) and general behavior.

3. Strong activities are physical or mental exercises, exacting crafts or hobbies or games, or anything that your patient would normally classify as work. If a strong activity appears to relax and soothe your patient, it generally should be encouraged, but only to the extent that it does not become exhausting. Although boredom may be a problem with a strong activity, as a rule a patient is first likely to become impatient, especially when working with a familiar craft or hobby, or anything else that normally would be done correctly and with little effort. Often a disabled person's inability to perform a familiar task perfectly causes deep discouragement and frustration; it may take you a long time and much work to help restore your patient's self-confidence. Ask your visiting nurse for advice and suggestions.

Change of Scenery In addition to the general types of relaxing activities above, there are the so-called basic relaxants that appeal to nearly every patient and at any time: the bath (Chapter 23), the back or body rub (Chapter 18), the freshly made bed (Chapter 13), and a change of scenery.

Just how much change of scenery you can give your patient depends on your patient's condition, your ability to move your patient if necessary, and equipment that may be available, such as a wheelchair (Chapter 8). Even if your patient must not get out of bed, you may provide a change of scenery by moving the bed for a different view out the window, or even just different walls of the room to see. If conditions permit, put a bird feeder or bath outside the window so your patient can watch the birds; it can be very relaxing as well as entertaining. Watching fish in an aquarium can also be relaxing. As a rule, any change of scenery, of something to look at, is welcomed by a bedfast patient.

Relaxing Persons Some people have a relaxing effect on sick or injured persons, others do not. Love has little to do with it. A wife may love her husband deeply, yet find that his efforts to comfort her when ill are anything but relaxing. A healthy wife's attempts to aid her injured husband may annoy him. On the other hand, just the presence of a child or a close or even casual friend may be extremely relaxing.

There is also a person's behavior. Some people tend to get bossy with the sick or injured. Others are too helpful, patronizing. Still other persons try to entertain by being cute and playful. These types of behavior may or may not relax your patient, and they may be relaxing at one time but very annoying at another. As a rule, all that you can do safely (without hurting the feelings of your patient or the other person) is to keep close watch on your patient, and at the first sign of irritation or tiredness get the other person away.

Relaxing Places Just as there are people, there are places that may relax your patient. It may be a particular room or the view from a certain window. It may be the way furniture is arranged, or how the window blinds are drawn or the drapes closed. It could be a picture on the wall; some people are made acutely uncomfortable by a picture that hangs at a sloppy slant instead of being level.

At the start of their disability, seriously sick or injured people seldom pay much attention to their surroundings. But as they become better, or more conscious of their disability, they also become more sensitive to everything about them—shapes, colors, sounds, odors, light, and darkness. There are several excellent texts dealing with the effects of colors, sounds, and shapes on men and women; they often react differently to a color, sound, or shape. If your patient has a long-term disability and does not seem to be at ease in the present surroundings, perhaps you should learn more about the effects of color, etc. But in most cases when a patient simply does not feel at ease in the present environment, the easiest solution is either to ask what seems to be the upsetting factor, or change a few things at a time until your patient does appear to be more at ease, comfortable, and relaxed.

Relaxing Things "Things," as opposed to people and places, can also irritate or relax a disabled person. It may be a decorative item, such as a bowl or vase or a table lamp, that because of its color, shape, or placement bothers your patient. Articles that appear to be unstable, about to topple over, commonly make people nervous, uneasy; but turn the item over so that it looks stable, and it may become attractive and relaxing.

In many cases, the "things" that upset a patient most are those which he or she should be able to use but cannot. A glass or cup that is too heavy, too large, or too small for disabled hands to grasp firmly. A light switch or lamp that is just out of reach of an immobile patient. Being unable to reach a pitcher of water or pour from it . . . or reading glasses or call bell . . . or other items which are needed for comfort or safety can be very disturbing to a patient.

NOTE: For elderly patients and those whose disability causes frequent need of a urinal or bedpan, be sure one is always within their easy reach.

Relaxing Routine Once a routine or schedule has been established, any deviations from it may be quite upsetting to your patient. On the other hand, some patients thrive on variations in routine. As a rule, it is not difficult to tell which pattern your patient prefers.

28 Exercising Your Patient

Exercise simply means muscular activity. Exercise may be mild or strenuous, such as wriggling fingers or toes (which for some patients can be very strenuous indeed), walking, turning over in bed, swimming, contracting and relaxing muscles without appreciable movement of the body, jogging, breathing deeply, dancing, golf, or any other sport or physical game or work. Exercise can be active, in which a person performs an activity with or without supervision or help. Exercise may be passive, as when it is given a patient by an operator (nurse, therapist, technician) without either the help or the resistance of a patient.

Lack of exercise can have a wide range of results, from mild discomfort to death.

Healthy people usually get all the exercise they need in normal living. It is difficult for them to get too little exercise; the fuzzy feelings of poor health often blamed on a lack of exercise generally are due to other causes. However, a reasonable amount of exercise in addition to that of normal daily living does tone up the muscles, improve circulation of the blood, stimulate the appetite, and sharpen the senses and the mind. As for reducing weight, exercise alone seldom is practical, since it stimulates the appetite and encourages the intake of more calories than it burns up. However, exercise may redistribute fat in certain parts of the body, and develop muscle tissue in the parts exercised.

> NOTE: Excessive exercise makes itself known by fatigue or unusual tiredness or weariness, and by soreness of muscles. As a guide for the future, you can tell that you have exercised too hard or too long if, 15 minutes after you stop, you still breathe heavily . . . or, if 2 hours after you stop, you still feel unusually weak or tired . . . or, you sleep poorly that night and the following day still are very tired.

LACK OF EXERCISE

A patient who is immobile for any length of time runs a great risk of developing *disuse* or inactivity disabilities such as muscle and joint degeneration or deterioration, and metabolic or body chemical and blood circulatory disturbances. The effects of these disuse disabilities can be severe, widespread psychological and physical deterioration and even death.

Common Disuse Disabilities Some of the common results of disuse are: (1) various kinds of atrophy, or wasting or withering of all or some parts of the body; (2) joint contractures, or shortening of the soft tissue structures around a joint; and (3) metabolic and circulatory disturbances, including stone formation in the kidney and bladder, rapid fall in blood pressure, formation of blood clots, constipation, and bladder and bowel incontinence or loss of control.

Atrophies Common atrophies resulting from lack of exercise are:

Muscular Atrophy: A decrease in the size and strength of a muscle because it has not been used for strenuous exercise at regular intervals.

Denervation Atrophy: A loss of nerve supply by a muscle. This atrophy cannot be reversed.

Disuse Atrophy: A decrease in the size of muscle fibers due to not having been contracted for a relatively long time. This atrophy is reversible, because if a muscle is exercised properly its fibers and the size of fibers will increase. But if the disuse atrophy is not reversed, additional weakness occurs and a vicious circle leading to physical and psychological deterioration follows.

Joint Contractures Joint contractures or shortening of soft tissue structures around a joint result in limiting the range of motion of a joint. It occurs when a joint is not frequently moved through its complete range of motion—up-down, front-back, right-left, and so forth. In elderly persons it may be impossible to reverse a joint contracture. With younger patients, stretching, placing the joint in a cast, or surgery usually will remedy the problem. If a contracture is painful, the joint frequently is not exercised because of the pain involved, and the contracture becomes worse.

A contracture reveals itself by its resistance when you try to move a patient's joint passively through its range of motion.

Although any joint can become contractured, it is most likely to occur to the hips, knees, and shoulders. These also are the most disabling contractures.

Metabolic and Circulatory Disturbances The lack of exercise can produce disturbances or changes in the body's chemical system and circulation of the blood that may require drastic medical or surgical means to remedy, and often prove fatal.

Common results of metabolic disturbances are:

1. *Osteoporosis* or increased porosity of bones due to loss of minerals, especially calcium, whenever immobilization or lack of movement limits muscular pull against a bone. Osteoporosis can be very painful and can cause fractures of bones and the formation of stones in the urinary tract—the kidneys, ureters (tubes carrying urine from kidneys to bladder), and bladder.
2. *Kidney and bladder stones* caused in whole or in part by the stagnation of urine in the kidneys or bladder. This happens when a patient lies too long on the back or does not change position often enough.
3. *Urinary tract infections*, especially in patients who do not completely empty their bladders.
4. *Constipation* and bladder and bowel incontinence or loss of control are due to disturbances of the metabolic system, and often go hand in hand with general psychological deterioration, below.

Common effects of circulatory disturbances due to lack of exercise are:

1. *A rapid fall in blood pressure* when a patient sits up or stands after being in a reclining position for a fairly long time. The patient will faint. If the blood pressure (Chapter 22) is too low, brain damage and even death can occur if the patient stays upright. This happens because, when a patient is immobile for a long time in a reclining position, blood collects in dilated

vessels of the abdomen and legs instead of being sent in normal amount to the brain. The rapid fall in blood pressure and its harmful effects can be prevented by gradually moving a patient from a reclining to a sitting position.

2. *Blood clots* can form in the leg veins of a patient who does not move around enough while lying in bed. Working their way through the body, the clots can in time cause pulmonary embolism (blood clots in the lungs), which can be fatal.

3. *Hypostatic pneumonia* can develop in a patient who remains in one position without turning for a relatively long period of time. To help prevent hypostatic pneumonia, have your patient take several deep breaths each hour for aeration and exercise of the lungs.

4. *Bedsores* (Chapter 15) due to remaining in one position without relieving pressure on the bony prominences of the body—the heels, back, head, shoulders, etc.

Psychological Deterioration Inactivity over a prolonged period of time coupled with an institutionalized way of living often triggers psychological deterioration. A patient may lose initiative and interest in surroundings. There may be personality changes, shown by a patient's becoming dependent, aggressive, or withdrawn. The first symptoms of psychological deterioration often are loss of appetite, inability to control bowels and/or bladder, and increasing inability to communicate.

PREVENTING DISUSE DISABILITIES

There are three basic therapeutic measures that are extremely simple but most effective in preventing disuse and the disabilities it brings. They are exercise, passive mobilization, and frequent change of position. In the following procedures, two or all basic therapeutic measures usually occur at the same time:

1. The simplest exercises for a bedridden patient are turning from side to side . . . from back to abdomen and abdomen to back . . . and moving up and down in bed. Done frequently all the time a patient is awake, they should provide enough exercise to prevent the disuse disabilities described above.

2. The patient who cannot actively exercise should be taught to move all joints through their full range of motion. If some parts are paralyzed, teach the patient to use other parts to move and position the limbs that are paralyzed.

3. When moving joints to prevent contracture, it is extremely important to move them through the complete range of motion. However, be careful not to force movement of a joint.

4. Any exercise a patient does must be strenuous, even though it may take only a few minutes to do. They ordinarily should be repeated several times a day—at least three times. Of course, what is "strenuous" for one patient may be too much for another and completely inadequate for still another. The doctor or therapist will prescribe and describe the exercises your patient should have.

5. A patient's position should be changed at least every hour, preferably more often. After lying in one position for 30 minutes, the pressure on the support area should be relieved for at least 1 minute. This allows blood to circulate in the affected tissues and should prevent pressure sores or bedsores (Chapter 15). Active changing of position also helps prevent muscular atrophy, joint contractures, and loss of minerals from the bones.

BOWEL AND BLADDER INCONTINENCE

Here are several suggestions to help alleviate matters for patients who have difficulty with bowel and/or bladder control:

1. Make certain that your patient has adequate intake of liquid and bulk to provide urinary output and bowel evacuation.
2. Develop a regular time each day for your patient's bowel evacuation.
3. Have your patient use a commode (Chapter 8) or the toilet instead of a bedpan or urinal whenever possible.
4. Avoid delay! Persuade your patient not to try to hold back when there is an urge to urinate or have a bowel movement.
5. Do not nag or keep after your patient to have a bowel movement. It is more important and usually more effective to stimulate normal bowel action by exercise and activity.
6. To help stimulate normal bowel function, encourage your patient to do all possible exercises and activities with the least help from you or anyone else.

EXERCISE AND YOUR PATIENT

The most effective exercises, especially for sick and injured people, are those that give satisfaction and pleasure. Satisfaction from feeling better generally, or from the sense of regaining the use, or preventing the loss, of a damaged part of the body. Pleasure from really liking the motions of an exercise and looking forward to more of it. The exercises, especially those of a therapeutic nature, prescribed by a doctor or a therapist usually are planned to encourage as well as help a patient physically.

Never give or let a patient take exercise as a form of punishment, as something that must be done like it or not! If your patient objects to exercising, take ample time to explain all about it—why any exercise and that particular one is necessary, what it is, and how its benefits may be seen or felt. If after that your patient still objects, it may be due to fear of pain. Promise that the exercise will stop the moment it does hurt too much—exercises often do hurt at the start!—and keep that promise. In an hour or so, try again.

A patient's refusal to do an exercise may also be due to believing that you are not really capable of supervising or giving it safely. Maybe you seem clumsy, or too weak or small. Postpone exercising until the visiting nurse or physical therapist shows you and your patient together how to do it, and supervises the two of you at least one time.

There are many kinds of both active and passive exercises. Some require highly specialized equipment, a physical therapist or trained technician, and are given in a hospital or a clinic. Other exercises, which may or may not require basically commonplace equipment, can be supervised or given safely by an inexperienced nurse after very little instruction. And there are, of course, many exercises that a patient can do with little or no supervision. For practical purposes, exercises may be divided into two basic groups:

1. *General Exercises.* These are exercises done to restore or maintain a general state of well-being, tone up the muscles, improve blood circulation, stimulate appetite, and sharpen the senses and mind. The exercises may be active or passive, and they may be therapeutic, below.

2. *Therapeutic Exercises.* Therapeutic exercises are those done for the purpose of preventing the loss (through atrophy, joint contracture, etc., above) of, or restoring normal use to, diseased or injured parts of the body. In most cases, they are carefully prescribed and graded by the doctor or physical therapist. Therapeutic exercises may be either active or passive; however, usually some assistance by an operator (nurse, therapist, technician) and/or equipment is required.

Active Exercises Active exercises are those that are done primarily by the patient, with or without supervision or help. The help may be, for example, a steadying hand by the nurse for getting out of bed or standing; a wheelchair, walker, crutches, or cane for moving about; a trapeze bar to enable a patient to move about in bed; a rubber ball to squeeze for exercising injured fingers and hand, and so on. The more of an exercise that a patient does without help, the better. However, you always should be close by, especially at the start of an exercise, to give prompt aid if needed and prevent an accident; for example, crutches are difficult to use at the start, and until your patient is accustomed to them, be ready to help in case a fall seems likely.

A problem with active-exercise patients is that they often tend to overdo it. In their joy at being able to get around, squeeze a rubber ball, tense and relax muscles, or use a trapeze bar to move about in bed they may do it so much that instead of strengthening they weaken themselves through excessive exercise. This should be especially guarded against for patients who have or are recuperating from:

Virus Infections, Heart Disease, Rheumatic Fever, Strokes, Fractures. These disabilities generally place more strain on organs and functions of the body than a patient realizes. To avoid serious complications, the limits of exercise prescribed by the doctor or therapist must be obeyed.

Passive Exercises Passive exercises are those that are given a patient by an operator (nurse, therapist, technician) with or without equipment and without the patient's help or resistance. Passive exercises are most commonly used for stroke patients, and those with spinal cord injuries and multiple sclerosis.

Stroke Patients When people are confined to bed for a long period of time, they are generally subject to disuse disabilities, above. It can happen to any bedfast patient; but it is most likely to happen to stroke patients who, because of injury to the brain, have actually lost the use of half of the body. Since they cannot move or exercise the affected joints, you must do it for them to prevent possible permanent injury and crippling.

The exercising of a stroke patient should start the day after the stroke. Exercise both sides of your patient. All these exercises can be done while bathing your patient, and should be repeated about every 2 hours until the doctor tells you that longer intervals will not be harmful. The sequence of exercises is the same as for bathing a patient in bed (Chapter 23); the difference is that you move a part of the body around as much as possible instead of merely holding it in place for washing. For example, when washing an arm, instead of simply holding it in a convenient position, move it straight up and down and above the head several times to exercise the shoulder joint; bend it several times to flex or exercise the elbow; bend and twist the wrist several times, curl and uncurl the fingers. Do the same with the legs to prevent stiffening of the hips, knees, ankles, and toes. While washing the head, neck, and face turn the head several times to right and left, forward and backward. As to the number of times you exercise a joint, generally the more times the better.

As a rule, you should change a stroke patient's position in bed at least once an hour—from lying on the back first to one side, then the other, then on the belly, then on the back—and every time you change your patient's position you should go through the routine of exercises the same as when giving the bath. Without such a continual program of exercises, a stroke patient's condition is not likely to improve. Of course, even with the best exercise program, total recovery from a stroke cannot be guaranteed; it depends on how severely the brain was damaged.

The Paralyzed Arm. A stroke patient's paralyzed arm usually is held close to the body. When you exercise it, be sure to move it out away from the body, both to maintain motion or prevent contracture of the shoulder and to allow air into the axilla or armpit. At other times, place a pillow between the body and arm so that air can continually get into the axilla. Without air, the skin becomes tender and raw, and painful sores can develop in a fairly short time.

PATIENT EXERCISE IN GENERAL

The kind of exercising that a patient should have depends on the patient's general condition, the illness or injury, and how severe it is. The patient who wants to exercise generally gets more benefit from it than the one who is opposed to or dislikes exercising. The benefits of an exercise program usually are more noticeable at the start than when a patient has been doing them for quite some time.

If a patient will be disabled for only a few days, an exercise program may not be necessary. But if an illness or injury will last more than about 7 days, and especially if the patient will be confined to bed most of the time, a program of exercises should be established and followed faithfully.

When possible, a patient in traction should have a trapeze bar (Chapter 8) as an aid to moving about in bed. Pulling on the bar provides excellent exercise for the arms, shoulders, and upper part of the body. If a leg is free to help in moving the body, it also will get excellent exercise.

The main purpose of exercise for ill or injured people is to prevent disuse disabilities, frozen or contractured joints, and permanent disabling, as well as to restore the body to maximum functioning as a whole. It is not to make big muscles.

29 Pain Pills

Antipain medicines can be habit forming, and people can become immune to their good effects. It is to try to prevent these undesirable results that doctors prescribe antipain medication only when it is really needed by a patient, and specify when and how much is to be taken.

> NOTE: By *pain pill* is meant an antipain medicine taken by mouth. Hypodermic injections must not be given by people who are not trained in the correct procedure. Improperly given injections can be dangerous.

HOW OFTEN

At the start of an illness, or following surgery, some therapy, or an injury, as a rule a doctor prescribes pain medication. The amount and frequency of dosage will be written on the prescription label. A common time period for pain medication is every 3 or 4 hours. Of course, other periods are often prescribed and sometimes the time of day is specified.

In case of severe pain, medication usually may be safely given up to 30 minutes ahead of the scheduled time. However, if medication is not effective for the allotted time, discuss it with the doctor. A stronger dose or a different medicine may be needed to control your patient's pain.

As your patient improves, or becomes less sensitive to pain, the doctor may specify that medication be given "only when necessary." This is often one of the more difficult decisions for an inexperienced nurse to make—should I give my patient a pain pill now?

You do not, of course, want your patient to suffer needlessly. On the other hand, you want to protect your patient against the possible bad side effects of pain pills. So it becomes a problem of deciding whether your patient really is in pain, and is it severe enough to warrant medication.

WHAT IS YOUR PATIENT'S PAIN?

Is your patient's apparent pain due to sickness or other disability, or to an attempt to hide worries and fears? In the first case a pain pill may be advisable. In the second case it may do more harm than good.

Pain Due to Ailment With some patients, it is extremely difficult to evaluate their ability to withstand pain and their need of pain medication. We all have our own levels of pain tolerance. Some people are very stoical, never flinching; others set up a terrific noise with a very minor discomfort. If your patient is your spouse or young child, you probably have a fairly accurate idea as to what kind of person you are nursing. This will help you decide the need for a pain pill.

Some signs to look for as evidence of genuine pain are:

Silence, unwillingness to talk.

Tenseness of the whole body, or of parts that are injured or ailing.

A facial expression indicating pain.

Dullness of the eyes.

The general body position; persons suffering real pain often curl up in the fetal position.

A patient who is comfortable and free of pain usually will move about freely, appear to be relaxed, and be more interested in general persons, places, and activities.

Even when patients are in real pain, you may make it more bearable by changing the subject from pains to things that interest them—hobbies, sports, friends, news, television, etc.

An Attempt to Hide Worries and Fears By the time patients have reached the stage of being given pain pills only when necessary, the pills may have become a sort of shield to hide troublesome worries and fears: How sick am I? . . . Am I getting any better? . . . What's really wrong with me? . . . Am I a hopeless burden? . . . Are they getting tired of me? Instead of asking you these questions, your patient asks for a pain pill. The longer your patient has been seriously disabled and needed your care, the more likely this is to happen. Also, it is much more apt to occur in patients with long-term illnesses or crippling accidents.

Giving a pain pill in such a case usually is no real help to your patient. In fact, if your patient's antipain medicine could be habit forming, the pill could do more harm than good. So if for any reason you suspect that the request for a pill may be based on worry or fear instead of true physical pain, ask your patient to describe it: Where is your pain located? . . . Is it sharp? . . . A dull ache? . . . Pulsating? . . . Steady? . . . A burning sensation? . . . Cramping? . . . When did it start? . . . Insist on definite answers, because you "will have to tell the doctor just what kind of pain you have."

Generally, if the "pain" is caused by worry or fear, a patient becomes somewhat vague as to the kind of pain and where it is centered. Also, if you carefully change the conversation from pain to the patient's condition and how much everyone is concerned, as a rule the more the patient talks about these matters the less mention there will be of pain.

The fact is that when a patient reaches the stage of being given pain pills only when necessary, often what is really needed and wanted is an opportunity to talk about troublesome worries and fears. A half hour of your time spent listening to your patient may do far more good, and ease far more "pain," than a box of potent pills. It is not always an effective treatment, but as a rule it is well worth trying.

30 Basics of Nutrition

Nutrition means the complete process of ingesting (taking in) and digesting (using) food substances or nutrients for the growth, maintenance, and repair of the body and its functions or activities. Food substances are any solid or liquid, including special preparations or formulae for feeding a patient intravenously, or by tube (Chapter 46).

In addition to the mechanical and chemical processings of food substances, nutrition deals with:

1. The foods themselves;
2. The combining of various food substances;
3. Foods that should or should not be taken by patients under various conditions (Diets, Chapters 32–46);
4. Selecting foods to make meals more attractive (Chapter 31);
5. Enticing or helping a patient to eat (Chapter 48); and,
6. If necessary, keeping a record of your patient's intake and output (Chapter 49).

DEFINITIONS AND DESCRIPTIONS

There are several texts dealing, in detail and in more or less nontechnical terms, with the many aspects of nutrition, most of which information is not necessary for nursing anyone at home. However, some such knowledge usually is desirable. So to help inexperienced nurses more readily understand the comments and instructions of a doctor, dietitian, nutritionist, or trained nurse, here, in alphabetical order, are brief basic definitions and descriptions of some of the materials and actions involved in nutrition.

ABSORB, ABSORPTION. The process by which a substance passes through a surface of the body into body fluids and/or tissue.

ACID. A chemical compound that, when dissolved in an ionizing solvent, yields hydrogen ions. Acids taste sour, unite with bases to form salts, and have, in general, chemical properties opposite those of alkalies. There are many acids in the body and they are essential to the metabolic process. The normal person may, as a rule, eat the so-called acid foods such as those high in protein.

ALKALI. A substance that can neutralize acids, and may combine with an acid to form a salt. Most fruits and vegetables are alkali-producing foods.

AMINO ACIDS. These are the basic parts of proteins and also are the end products of protein digestion. There are many amino acids, all of which are needed for metabolism and growth. Some amino acids come from nutrients and others can be produced by the body. There are ten "essential" amino acids. Proteins containing all the essential amino acids are called *complete* proteins; they are of animal origin, such as meat, milk, cheese, eggs. Those lacking one or more of the essential amino acids are called *incomplete* proteins; they are of plant origin, such as grains, legumes (beans, peas, etc.), nuts, seeds.

BASAL METABOLISM (See also Metabolism). Basal metabolism is the least amount of energy needed by a body, when at rest, to support all normal functions, such as digesting food, circulating blood, maintaining body temperature. Basal metabolism, often measured by a calorimeter, usually is expressed in terms of calories per square meter of body surface per hour. It should be measured when a body is:

1. *At digestive rest*, at least 12 hours after eating or drinking;
2. *At physical rest*, following restful sleep and without any exercise or other physical activity preceding the test; and,
3. *In a comfortable room temperature* between 16.7° and 30.5° C/62° and 87° F.

The normal range of basal metabolic rate (BMR) is +10 to -10. Factors influencing BMR are:

1. *Size*. Small people have higher rates than large people;
2. *Age*. BMR is lowest in newborn children, highest between ages 5 and 10 years, decreases fairly quickly till age 20, then decreases slowly until death;
3. *Sex*. Males have a 6 percent–7 percent higher BMR;
4. *Weight*. Thin people have a 50 percent higher BMR than stout people of the same size, age, and sex; and
5. *Endocrine glands* (thyroid, parathyroid, pituitary, etc., see Endocrine Glands). Disorders of the endocrine system can send a person's BMR far above normal (*hyperthyroidism*) or far below normal (*hypothyroidism*).

BASE. Essentially the same as an alkali, but has a bitter taste.

CALORIE. Calorie is a unit of heat commonly used to measure or express the energy or heat given by a food substance. Each food substance has a caloric rating; "counting calories" generally means controlling the amount of food intake, usually done to reduce caloric intake and thus reduce body weight. There are two calorie measurements: the large or kilocalorie, and the small calorie. The large Calorie, commonly used with matters of human nutrition, represents the amount of heat needed to raise the temperature of 1 kilogram (1,000 grams or 35.28 ounces) of water from 14.5° to 15.5° C. The *C* of large Calorie is capitalized to distinguish it from the small calorie, which is the amount of heat needed to raise 1 gram of water 1° C. The small calorie, also known as gram calorie and microcalorie, is abbreviated to "cal."

CARBOHYDRATE. A major class of food substances, containing carbon combined with hydrogen and oxygen in the same ratio as they are in water (2 parts hydrogen, 1 part oxygen). Carbohydrates are the so-called energy foods—sugars, starches, cellulose. Starches in particular are a major source of calories in most diets.

CELLULOSE. A fiber carbohydrate, containing many glucose (a sugar) units, that forms the fundamental material of the structure of plants. As a rule, cellulose is not changed chemically or absorbed by the body in the digestive process. Cellulose stimulates peristalsis (a progressive, wavelike movement in the hollow tubes of the body) and aids intestinal excretion.

CHOLESTEROL. A fat-related substance found in all animal tissues . . . egg yolks . . . in many plant oils that have been hydrogenated (see Fat) . . . and in the blood and many tissues of the human body. Cholesterol is produced within the body independently of food intake.

DEXTROSE. See Glucose.

DIET. Diet is the food substances consumed in the course of living. Special or prescribed diets (Chapters 33–46) are allowances or selections of particular foods and quantities of them to accommodate a state of health, sickness, or injury. Diet does not necessarily mean foods and amounts selected for the purpose of losing weight. Since *diet* actually means *food intake*, everyone is on a diet!

DIGESTION. This is the mechanical and the chemical breaking down of nutrients in the gastrointestinal tract (mouth, stomach, and intestine), and the changing of them into materials that can be absorbed by the body. Some substances, such as salts, certain sugars, and water, can be absorbed without being changed; but starches, fats, and most proteins cannot be absorbed until they have been reduced to their basic parts by the digestive juices.

ENDOCRINE GLANDS. These are ductless glands whose secretions or *hormones* partly control and regulate nearly all bodily functions. When an endocrine does not work properly, it produces too much or too little hormone. A very small change in hormone can have a major effect on bodily growth and development, resistance to fatigue, nutrition of tissue, sexual activity, and tone of muscles. Because a person's emotions as well as physical condition regulate the production of hormones, they can affect the relationships between body and mind. The seven most important and influential endocrine glands are the pituitary, thyroid, parathyroids, thymus, adrenals, islet cells in the pancreas, and gonads (male and female sex glands).

EXCRETION. The waste matter (feces, sweat, urine) expelled or cast out from the body. The end result of metabolism.

FAT. Fat is the most concentrated energy food. In a good, balanced diet fat usually furnishes 20 percent–25 percent of the Calories needed by the body. It is useful in many ways. Fat just under the skin is an insulating layer that prevents loss of body heat. Fat supports and protects certain organs, such as the eyes and the kidneys. It is a concentrated reserve of food, provides the fatty acids (below) needed for normal body growth and development, and is a vehicle for natural fat-soluble vitamins. Fat is an important part of cell structure. In the human diet, fat sources are:

Animal, such as lard, fat in meat;

Dairy products, mainly butterfat; and

Plant oils, such as corn, cottonseed, olive, peanut, soybean, etc. These often are hydrogenated or changed from polyunsaturated to a solid saturated fat by the addition of hydrogen.

Monounsaturated Monounsaturated is a class of long-chain carbon compound fats that has only one double bond in its molecule; when consumed, it tends to reduce the blood cholesterol level (see Cholesterol). Most monounsaturated foods are of plant origin.

Polyunsaturated Polyunsaturated refers to long-chain carbon compounds, a class of fats that has more than two double bonds in its molecule and that, when consumed, tends to reduce the blood cholesterol level (see Cholesterol). Polyunsaturated foods are mainly of plant origin.

Saturated Nutritionally, *saturated* means an organic compound, usually a fat, which when consumed tends, because of its molecular structure, to increase or maintain the level of blood cholesterol. Saturated fats are mainly of animal origin and in dairy products, and commonly are created by the hydrogenation of polyunsaturated foods.

FATTY ACID. This is any of a type of organic acids derived from saturated or unsaturated hydrocarbons (chemical compounds made of hydrogen and carbon only). Unsaturated fatty acids are important in the metabolism of cholesterol (see Fat: Polyunsaturated, Saturated).

GLUCOSE. The sugar glucose (also called dextrose and d-glucose) is a product of the digestive breakdown of carbohydrates. Absorbed from the intestine into the blood, glucose is known as "blood sugar." Both too much and not enough glucose in the body are caused by and also can cause serious illness.

HEMOGLOBIN. The iron-containing pigment of red blood cells that carries oxygen from the lungs to body tissue.

HORMONES. See Endocrine Glands.

HYDROGENATE. See Fat.

INGESTION. Ingestion is the taking of materials, particularly nutrients, into the gastrointestinal tract (mouth, stomach, and intestine), or the process by which a cell takes in foreign particles. Nutrients also may enter the body intravenously.

INORGANIC. A substance not of animal or plant origin.

INTRAVENOUS FEEDING. A means of providing the nutritional needs of a patient by injecting solutions into a vein. People have been nourished for months by this process.

KILOCALORIE. See Calorie.

METABOLISM (see also Basal Metabolism). The term *metabolism* takes in all mechanical and chemical changes constantly occurring in all body cells during all periods or stages of life. In a narrower and more everyday sense, metabolism deals with the changes or conversions of the chemical energy in nutrients into the mechanical or physical energy used, or the heat given off, by the body. The two fundamental processes of metabolism are:

Anabolism: The construction or building-up process of converting ingested nutrients into the necessary parts of elements for cell growth and repair; and

Catabolism: The opposite of anabolism is the disintegration or breaking-down process of substances into simpler substances, the end products usually being excreted from the body.

MINERALS. Minerals are inorganic substances. They are essential parts of all cells . . . regulate the activity of muscular and nerve tissues . . . are necessary for a proper acid-base balance . . . are essential for the secretion of glands . . . and are important in the metabolism of water and in the regulation of the volume of blood. Mineral salts and water are excreted daily from the body, and must be replaced through food intake.

MONOUNSATURATED. See Fat.

NUTRIENT. A food substance, either solid or liquid, that supplies the body with necessary elements is a nutrient. The better-known necessary elements are vitamins, minerals, fats, carbohydrates, proteins, water, sugars, starch, and chemicals such as oxygen, nitrogen, carbon, potassium, sulfur, sodium, chlorine, and trace minerals.

ORGANIC. Nutritionally, an organic substance is one derived from animal or plant life.

OXYGEN. Oxygen, a colorless, odorless, tasteless gas found free in the air, is a basic part of animal, mineral, and plant substances. Oxygen enters into all metabolic activities of the body. Red blood cells (see Hemoglobin) carry oxygen to all parts of the body to support metabolism. An interruption of oxygen supply to tissue damages it.

PERISTALSIS. Peristalsis is the progressive, wavelike movement that occurs involuntarily in the hollow tubes of the body, such as the intestine, and forces their contents onward.

POLYUNSATURATED. See Fat.

PROTEIN. Protein is the principal source of energy and heat for the body. Proteins are essential for the growth, maintenance, and repair of body tissue. Proteins make up the greater part of plant and animal tissue.

Amino acids (see) represent the basic structure of proteins. Other substances in proteins are carbon, hydrogen, iron, nitrogen, oxygen, phosphorus, and sulfur.

In the body, proteins are oxidized and liberate heat. One gram of protein supplies 4 Calories of heat. The amount of protein a person needs depends on age and on the intake of other nutrients. The amount needed usually decreases with age. Among factors causing an increase in the amount of protein needed are a person's increase of physical work, and convalescence from sickness, surgery, or severe injury.

ROUGHAGE. Indigestible plant fibers that act as a stimulant to aid intestinal peristalsis.

SALTS. A salt is a chemical compound resulting from the interaction between an acid and a base. Salts and water are the inorganic or mineral parts of the body. They have specific roles in the functions of cells, and are essential for life. Salts in the nutritional sense should not be confused with the salts, such as Epsom and Glauber's, used for stimulating bowel movement.

SATURATED. See Fat.

SPARER. A sparer is a substance that, although itself destroyed by *catabolism* (see Metabolism), reduces catabolic action on other substances. *Protein sparers* are carbohydrates and fats in a diet that keep tissue protein from being used for energy.

STARCH. Starch, a complex carbohydrate found in plants, is an excellent source of body energy. All starches except cellulose must be changed, by metabolism, into sugar before they can be absorbed by the body.

SUGAR. Sugars are simple carbohydrates generally having a sweetish taste. Sugar is an excellent form of quick energy because it is absorbed directly by the body. There are many forms of sugar—beet sugar, cane sugar, blood sugar, maple sugar, milk sugar, brain sugar, liver sugar, malt sugar, etc. Eating too much sugar in the form of candy or sweets commonly is associated with overweight, but is not the cause of overweight. Reducing diets usually demand a reduction of sugar intake.

TRACE MINERALS. The many inorganic elements that are in the body in extremely small amounts are called *trace* minerals. Among the essential trace minerals are cobalt, copper, fluorine, manganese, molybdenum, and zinc.

UNSATURATED. See Fat.

VITAMINS. A vitamin is any of a group of organic substances (except proteins, carbohydrates, fats, minerals, organic salts) that are essential for normal metabolism, growth, and development of the body. Vitamins are not sources of energy, nor are they a major substance of the body; but they are vital for normal bodily activities and the maintenance of health. Vitamins are mainly controllers of metabolism, and are found in all organs and cells.

Vitamins usually are classified by being soluble in either fat or water:

Fat-Soluble Vitamins: A, D, E, K. These are fairly stable (not easily decomposed) in general cooking. But prolonged exposure to higher than normal cooking temperatures will destroy them.

Water-Soluble Vitamins: C, and the B Complex group. These are easily destroyed by oxygen, alkalies, and high temperatures. For this reason, Vitamin C foods should be cooked in as little water as possible for as short a time as possible; steaming and microwave cooking are recommended. Baking soda should not be added to preserve vegetable color in cooking. Fruit juices should not be left uncovered.

WATER. Water is the principal chemical part of the body, making up about 75 percent of it. It is essential for metabolism within cells, as it is the medium in which chemical reactions can take place. Outside of cells, water is the main transportation agent of the body. Excessive intake of water can lead to water intoxication and death; excessive loss of water, to dehydration and death.

CLASSES OF FOOD SUBSTANCES

Food substances are grouped into six classes: carbohydrates, fats, proteins, minerals, vitamins, and water.

CARBOHYDRATES. The following are common food substances that either primarily are, or contain relatively large amounts of, carbohydrates:

Alcoholic beverages, all.

Breads, all kinds, including biscuits, muffins, rolls, waffles, etc.

Cakes, Cookies, Pies, all.

Candy, chewing gum, all regular kinds; see labels of others, such as diet, sugar-free, etc.

Condensed milk, sweetened.

Cereals, all cooked, dry.

Fruit, all, canned, cooked, fresh, frozen.

Jam, jelly, all regular kinds; see labels of others, such as diet, imitation, etc.

Macaroni, noodles, spaghetti, etc.

Rice, all kinds.

Soft drinks, all regular kinds; see labels of others, such as diet, sugarfree, etc.

Sugar, honey, all kinds.

Syrups, all, natural, artificial.

FATS. Common foods with a high fat content, which may be polyunsaturated or saturated, are:

Polyunsaturated

Plant oils: Corn, cottonseed, olive, peanut, safflower, soybean, sunflower.

Saturated

Animal: Bacon, beef fat, lard, poultry fat, red meats, seafood, salt pork.

Dairy products: Butter, butterfat, cheddar and other cheeses, egg yolks.

PROTEINS. The following common foods have high protein value (for complete, incomplete protein see Amino Acids).

Complete Proteins

Animal origin: Fish, meat (beef, lamb, pork, veal), poultry (chicken, turkey, etc.).

Dairy products Butterfat, cheese (cheddar, cottage, etc.), eggs, ice cream, milk, yogurt.

Plant origin: Soybeans.

Incomplete Proteins

Plant origin: Dried beans, lentils, peas, nuts.

MINERALS. The following minerals are found in relatively high content in these common foods:

Calcium: Cheese, milk; yogurt; greens such as collard, kale, mustard, turnip; sardines, canned salmon with bones.

Iodine: Seafood contains considerable iodine. Commercially iodized table salt is the chief dietary source of iodine.

Iron: Dried fruit; egg yolks; leafy green vegetables; legumes (dried beans, peas, etc.); meat (beef, lamb, pork, veal); organ meats, especially liver; seafood; whole wheat.

Phosphorus: Found in the same foods as calcium. Therefore, if calcium needs are met, phosphorus needs usually are, too.

Potassium: Fruit, such as bananas, dried prunes, oranges; leafy vegetables; legumes (beans, peas, lentils, etc.); meat (beef, lamb, pork, veal); whole grains (oats, rye, wheat, etc.).

Sodium: Beets, carrots; common table salt; eggs; meat (beef, lamb, pork, veal); milk; spinach and other leafy greens.

VITAMINS. Here is a list of the more common vitamins and the foods containing them:

Vitamin A: Butter; carrots; cheese; eggs; greens such as parsley, spinach, swiss chard; liver; margarine; milk; winter (yellow) squash.

Vitamin B_1 (Thiamin): Beef; lean pork; legumes (beans, lentils, peas, etc.); liver; whole or enriched grains.

Vitamin B_2 (Riboflavin): Beans; milk; organ meats (heart, kidney, liver); peanuts; peas.

Vitamin B_6 (Pyridoxine): Corn; meat, especially kidney, liver; wheat; yeast.

Niacin (a vitamin of the B complex group): Brewer's yeast; fowl; green vegetables; liver; meat.

Pantothenic Acid (a vitamin of the B complex group): Broccoli; cheese, eggs; kale; kidney; lean beef; legumes; liver; skim milk; sweet potatoes; yeast; yellow corn.

Vitamin C: Asparagus; broccoli; cabbage; citrus fruit (oranges, grapefruit, lemons, lime); green and yellow vegetables; green peppers; kale; melons; strawberries; sweet potatoes, turnip greens; white potatoes.

Vitamin D: Irradiated milk; fish liver oils; fortified margarine.

Vitamin E: Cereals (all kinds, cooked, dry); eggs; leafy vegetables; milk; muscle meats (chops, roasts, steaks); vegetable oils; wheat germ.

Vitamin K: Small amounts of Vitamin K are in leafy green vegetables such as cabbage, cauliflower, kale.

WATER. Necessary water is consumed in its free state, as a major part of common beverages (coffee, tea, soft drinks, soups), and as essential parts of animal and plant or vegetable foods.

BASIC FOOD GROUPS

Food substances are divided into four basic groups, each of which should be in the daily diet of a normal, healthy person. In a prescribed diet some or all of the foods in a group may be reduced, eliminated, or greatly increased over the normal amount, depending on the condition and needs of a patient. The four basic food groups are: dairy products, meats, fruit and vegetables, and breads and cereals.

DAIRY PRODUCTS. Milk and milk products are essential to a balanced diet because of their high calcium, protein, and riboflavin contents.

Children need calcium for growing bones and teeth. Adults need calcium to maintain bones and teeth, to help their nerves and muscles function normally,

and their blood to clot properly. The average daily requirements of milk, based on the number of 356.6-ml. (8-oz. or 1-cup) servings per day is:
Children under 9 years of age—2 to 3 servings
Children 9 to 12 years—3 or more servings
Teenagers—4 or more servings
Adults—2 or more servings
Pregnant women—3 or more servings
Nursing mothers—4 or more servings.

MEAT GROUP. This group includes eggs, fish, meat (beef, lamb, pork, veal), poultry (chicken, turkey, etc.); dried beans and dried peas; and peanut butter. The meat group supplies the protein that is essential for the body cells to live, reproduce, and repair themselves.

Normally there should be two or more servings daily from the meat group. A serving usually counts as:
57–85 gm./2–3 oz. of cooked lean meat, poultry, or fish; or,
2 eggs; or,
237 ml./8 oz./1 cup of cooked dried beans or peas; or,
118 ml./4 oz./4 tbsp. peanut butter.

FRUIT AND VEGETABLES. A balanced daily diet includes four or more servings of 118 ml./4 oz./½ cup servings of raw or cooked fruit or vegetables. As well as vitamins and minerals, fruit and vegetables help provide the roughage or bulk needed by our digestive systems. They are also a good source of iron, especially the green leafy vegetables (broccoli, spinach, swiss chard, turnip greens, etc.), and dried fruit such as apricots, prunes, and raisins.

Daily there should be citrus fruit (an orange or tangerine, or ½ grapefruit) or a tomato to supply Vitamin C. Instead of fruit or a tomato, 118 ml./4 oz./½ cup of juice may be used. Vitamin C must be supplied daily since it is not stored by the body.

Three or four times a week a balanced diet includes a dark leafy or deep yellow vegetable, or a yellow fruit, to maintain the necessary level of Vitamin A.

BREADS AND CEREALS. The foods in this group contribute important amounts of the B vitamins as well as protein, iron, and food energy. There should be four or more servings of breads or cereals daily. Typical servings are:

1 tortilla; or,
1 slice bread; or,
28 gm./1 oz. dry or ready-to-eat cereal; or,
118–177 ml./4–6 oz./½–¾ cup of cooked cereal, cornmeal, grits, macaroni, rice, or spaghetti.

DIETS IN GENERAL

Starting with what well may have been the granddaddy of all diets, "feed a cold and starve a fever" or "starve a cold and feed a fever," there have been near countless diets designed to prevent or to cure practically every ailment or injury known to mankind. Some diets undoubtedly worked wonders with some people. And just as undoubtedly, some patients recovered in spite of their diets. Unfortunately, many well-meaning people "prescribe" a diet on the basis of what it is reported to have done for other people, not on the basis of what food substances it may deny or overload a patient.

The diet information in Chapters 33 through 46 deals only with generalities—what foods usually are allowed or banned by a particular diet, and why. The doctor or dietitian will, of course, furnish a list of do-eat and don't-eat foods based on the specific condition of your patient. It may or may not agree with other diets you have heard of. Regardless, it is the diet that you must serve your patient. If it does not seem to agree with your patient, or your patient sincerely dislikes it, then ask the doctor or dietitian or your visiting nurse for suggestions for making it more acceptable or palatable to your patient. If these changes do not work, then ask for a complete change of diet.

31 Choosing Foods for Diets

When choosing foods for conventionally consumed diets (Chapters 32–45), always be guided by what will make attractive, enticing balanced meals. Sick people often have delicate appetites and tend to be finicky about food. If meals do not attract them, they tend to lose what little appetite they have or, if they do eat, they may not get the full benefits of their food. On the other hand, a plate or meal of attractive foods often makes a sick person want to eat, and enjoy every morsel! Preparing meals on the basis of attractiveness is mainly a matter of planning ahead.

Four factors that control the attractiveness of a plate of food or an entire meal served course by course are:

eye appeal or the color, shape, and amount of food;
nose appeal or the aroma of food;
mouth appeal or flavor and consistency; and
personal likes and dislikes.

To a person who can see, eye appeal and personal like and dislike are about equally strong factors in making food attractive or unattractive. However, eye appeal often can get a person to at least try a food usually disliked, and it can make a person refuse a favorite food. Nose appeal or aroma and being told what a food is will replace eye appeal for a person who cannot see.

As well as choosing foods for greatest appeal, use as many as necessary of the little extras in serving (Chapter 48) to help get your patient to enjoy and actually look forward to meals.

EYE APPEAL

Whether you actually serve a meal or have to leave one prepared in advance for self-serve, the first thing your patient does is look at it. If anything looks unappetizing or unattractive, your patient, who may have been eager to eat a few minutes ago, may suddenly lose interest in food. The eyes did it.

The eye appeal of a plate of food or of an entire meal served course by course is controlled by color and amount. Food must be attractive on both counts if it is to whet or sustain a patient's appetite. If the colors are uninteresting or the amounts so large as to be frightening, a patient often loses all desire to eat.

Attractive Colors The key to making meals color-attractive is variety of color, shape, and texture, achieved primarily by selecting foods that are not basically the same or very similar in appearance either naturally or by preparation. For example, a plate of sliced breast of chicken, whipped potatoes, and white asparagus could be, to many sick persons, a totally uninteresting white blah. Diet permitting, you possibly could make the meal more attractive by spooning brown gravy over the chicken ... putting a pat of butter or yellow margarine on the mound of potatoes and a few sprigs of parsley around it ... and running two or three ribbons of mayonnaise or yellow salad dressing across the asparagus and topping them with generous sprinklings of paprika or a slice of pimiento.

However, simply decorating foods with sauces and seasonings, as above, is not always the best, let alone practical, way to prepare color-attractive meals. Relatively small splashes of color do not always adequately disguise or conceal the basic color. And your patient may not care for the gravies, sauces, and seasonings allowed by a diet, or soon tire of them. So when possible, choose foods that are in themselves basically different colors and will not be changed by cooking. In the all-basic-white meal mentioned above, change any two of the foods in order to get a practical variety of color. Instead of breast of chicken, serve thigh or other dark meat. Instead of white potato, serve yams, sweet potato, or yellow corn. Instead of white asparagus, serve the green, or serve garden peas or any other green vegetable.

In most cases, you can be fairly sure of getting a good variety of color for a plate or for an entire meal by choosing any green vegetable, a white- or yellow-group (which includes light oranges and browns) vegetable, or fruit that contrasts with the color of the meat, poultry, or fish. Since the color green is fairly attractive to most people, generally you will be safe by serving a light and a dark green vegetable instead of one of the white or yellow groups.

As a rule, artificial food coloring is accepted by a sick person only for certain kinds of dessert and, possibly, cottage cheese. However, since most people associate certain flavors with colors, food coloring alone may not be satisfactory. Rice pudding, bread pudding, plain tapioca, and other basically white desserts may be colored yellow (lemon flavor), orange (orange), green (mint, pistachio), pink (mint, peach), and so forth. If you are not sure of your patient's favorite colors, or perhaps feel that the same foods may have been served too often, serve a new color-flavor without mentioning it and see how your patient accepts it.

Another factor that has an important part in food coloring is the light by which a patient eats. Normal so-called white daylight or artificial light is no problem; foods have their so-called normal colors. But colored light, either artificial or daylight coming through colored windows or through curtains, can completely destroy the attractiveness of many foods.

Attractive Amounts You should not, as a rule, serve food in large portions, no matter how hungry your patient seems to be. Large portions often frighten a sick person, especially one who has been on a restricted diet, or is really not very hungry at the moment, or is just not interested in food. Also, a large portion may make your patient eat more than is wanted to keep you from thinking that your food is not liked. So regardless of the extra work it may cause, always serve small portions and let your patient know that more is available. If you offer it or your patient asks for more, fine. But let your patient decide—without urging!

It is fairly common at the onset of an illness or shortly after major surgery or a severe injury, for a patient to eat much less than the doctor recommends (Chapter 47). In this case, instead of serving three regular-size meals a day, serve five or six small ones with the amounts of food reduced to what the patient can and will eat. Permissible snacks should, as a rule, be available at all times.

How Food Is Served The overall effects of eye appeal often depend on how meals are served. The chance of unattractive colors and frightening amounts is greatest when all items except bread, spread, and beverage are served on the same plate at the same time. The chance of poor eye appeal, particularly due to frightening amounts of food, usually is least when an entire meal is served at one time but in many separate dishes; for example, a fairly small or luncheon-size dish for the meat, fish, or poultry . . . small sauce or vegetable dishes for vegetables and soft desserts . . . separate salad or bread-and-butter dishes for bread, salad, and firm desserts. It is extra work for you, but serving a meal course by course has several advantages:

A lack of variety in color and shape may not be very noticeable;

Your patient has better opportunity to ask for "seconds"; and

Since foods are served as your patient is ready for them, hot foods will be hot, and cold foods will be cold!

NOSE APPEAL

Nose appeal or the aroma of food is, of course, of prime importance to people who cannot see. But although it generally is far less important to people who can see, food odors and their effects should not be ignored. Odors do not have to be strong to be effective. In fact, very weak or so-called subtle odors commonly arouse more eater interest than strong ones—possibly a case of "the strong odor tells you what food it is," but "the weak odor makes you ask." Also, strong odors may have a reverse effect and actually turn off the appetite, particularly if the patient is very ill.

You should select foods to create an appetizing parade of savory aromas. However, several factors can make this extremely difficult:

A strong odor usually completely overpowers a weak one; for example, the odors of fried onions and of mushrooms.

The stronger a food odor is, the longer it generally lasts.

Hot foods usually give off stronger odors than cool or cold ones.

The attractiveness of a food odor often is due, to great extent, to seeing the food itself. For example, the smell of searing meat may not be attractive unless you see the steak.

People often like the collective odor of a prepared combination of foods without really liking the odors of any of the foods involved. Your patient, for example, might not like the odors of garden peas, onions, bay leaf, carrots, potatoes, salt, pepper, and beef—but love the savory odor of beef stew!

All these possibilities of food odors can be so difficult to plan and handle that often the only practical solution is to settle for a few odors that you know your patient likes. And if the odors of food cooking disturb your patient, keep the kitchen door closed and open a window, or turn on the exhaust fan to remove the odors.

Real and artificial flavorings, especially those with distinctive and fairly strong odors, can do much to make relatively uninteresting foods appetizing, and keep a food from becoming tiresome. Eggs, for example, are to many people an uninteresting food and easily become monotonous. But there are many seasonings that can give eggs nose and taste (below) appeal—celery salt, onion salt, grated cheese, prepared salad seasonings, ketchup, plus scrambling eggs with a small amount of condensed soup, and so forth. Custard, plain puddings, cakes, and other soft desserts can be varied by flavoring them with vanilla, lemon, mint, butter-rum, orange, etc.

When serving a patient who cannot see, be sure to name and describe each food the first time it is served so that the patient can make a simple association between food and odor.

MOUTH APPEAL

The mouth appeal of foods depends on the eater's likes and dislikes of their consistency and actual taste, and the temperatures at which they are served. Select permissible foods according to your patient's likes and dislikes, and make enough variations in preparing and seasoning them to keep your patient from becoming bored with eating.

Consistency The overall consistency of a food—its degree of firmness, thickness, density, smoothness, stringiness, etc.—as a rule greatly influences a person's like or dislike of it. For example, the consistency of cooked liver may be positively revolting to the same people who thoroughly enjoy liverwurst; and some people think cooked okra is a slimy slick mess while others relish it. If not by word, then by acceptance or rejection of various foods you soon can tell which consistencies your patient likes and dislikes.

Fortunately, consistencies of most foods can be changed rather easily. Treatment before cooking may do it, such as pounding meat with a special mallet or with the edge of a plate to tenderize it. Cooking itself may change consistency, like changing hard, crisp apples into soft, mellow applesauce. Simple treatment after cooking can change consistency, such as mashing or whipping boiled potatoes, grinding cooked meat to make hash, slicing meat extra thin or across the grain to "tenderize" it.

Being able and willing to change consistencies of foods is commonly accepted as one of the signs of a good cook. Knowing how to cut meat across the grain is a sign of a good carver. When buying meat or poultry, ask the butcher how it should be cut or sliced for maximum tenderness or ease of eating.

Taste Seasonings—and there is an almost limitless number of them singly and in combination!—can do more than anything else to change commonplace foods into mouth-watering delicacies—and make delicacies and commonplace foods completely unappetizing. It depends, of course, on how strongly the eater likes or dislikes the seasonings used. Because of this, aside from specialty items, such as chili con carne for example, foods in hotels, restaurants, hospitals, etc., often are served very bland so that each person can season according to taste. Home-cooked foods, however, usually are seasoned during preparation or when "dishing up" according to established family likes, leaving it to each person to add salt, pepper, ketchup, grated cheese, lemon juice, pickle relish, and so forth.

Whether you should season foods for your patient is for the two of you to decide. Do not be surprised, however, if later your patient decides to change the agreement. At the start of an illness or following major surgery or a severe injury, most people take little interest in food and eat what is given them almost regardless of its seasoning. But as their disability stabilizes, they tend to become more finicky or picky-picky about what tastes good and what does not. Save both of you work and worry by seasoning food exactly as your patient wants, or serve the seasonings apart from the food and let your patient apply them. Of course, the kind and amount of seasonings must be within the limits, if any, of your patient's diet.

Cooking and Seasoning The natural flavor and the effects of seasonings are more noticeable with vegetables than with other foods.

Most vegetables should be steamed, as this method minimizes the vitamins and minerals lost by cooking, and enhances the flavor.

Many doctors, dietitians, and nutritionists believe that it is far better and much healthier to eat vegetables without salt. Cooking vegetables without salt tends to keep them from becoming tough.

If you season your patient's meals, do it after the foods—vegetables in particular—are cooked. As a rule, the taste of the seasonings will be more noticeable, hence less will be needed. Also, there will be fewer, if any, adverse effects on the food.

Temperature Most people, especially when incapacitated, have very strong feelings about how hot or cold their foods should be. They want their hot foods served hot, and cold foods cold. Food served at a so-called wrong temperature they find unappetizing, often to the point of not eating it.

To help hot foods stay hot and cold foods stay cold when served, first heat or chill the dishes. Plates that cannot be warmed safely in an oven usually may be warmed enough by being soaked in hot water for a few minutes. Chill dishes in the refrigerator for about an hour before mealtime, or soak them for several minutes in cold water containing several ice cubes. To keep foods appetizingly hot or cold for very slow eaters, it may be necessary to serve foods in thermal or "heat-holding" containers, such as infant's plates with compartments for storing hot or cold water, or the vacuum-type or double-walled cups often used for transporting hot and cold foods.

PERSONAL LIKES AND DISLIKES

The presence or absence of the various appeals, above, of a food may be completely overcome by a patient's personal like or dislike of it. If the doctor tells you that it does not matter one way or the other if your patient has a particular food, then serve it or not just as your patient asks. However, there are many cases, especially in the more restrictive diets, in which a certain food should either be taken or avoided regardless of a patient's likes or dislikes, and this can be a difficult problem for you to solve.

There are people who, no matter how a meat, fish, fruit, vegetable, or beverage is prepared, will refuse to take it. Or if they swallow it, will feel sick to the stomach or even vomit. With some people this is a genuine strong aversion to a food, and a natural defense reaction. The dislike may be lifelong and normal, or it may be due to sickness. But in either case it should be respected; ask the doctor, dietitian, nutritionist, or your visiting nurse for satisfactory alternate foods or formulas. It also is not uncommon for sick people to form very strong dislikes of foods as the stages of a sickness change, or of foods that have been served too often.

There also are people who believe they dislike something they have never tasted. Sometimes this belief is so strong that it should be treated the same as an honest strong aversion to food. However, often you can persuade a patient to try a food in order to "humor" or please you—with your promise not to serve it again unless asked. Also, although this has a certain element of risk, you may get your patient to try a "never-tasted-but-know-I-don't-like-it" food by calling it by a name other than its usual one; for example, instead of "yogurt" call it Bulgarian buttermilk, fermented milk, madzoon, or matzoon; or serve cold potato cream soup as "vichyssoise."

Another problem eater is the person who is accustomed to and likes a very limited menu, and does not care to change it. The so-called beef-and-potatoes-and-pie eater, for example. As long as these people are sick enough to take only slight interest in food, there is no real problem. But as they improve in health, it often takes the combined efforts of the doctor, visiting nurse, closest and dearest relatives and friends to persuade them to eat as they should.

Often the most difficult problem eater to handle is the one who demands—no other word for it—foods that the doctor or dietitian has forbidden. If a commonsense explanation of why such foods are forbidden does not satisify your patient, the practical solution is to make sure that none of them is available.

If you even suspect your patient of strong likes and dislikes of foods, then for the good of your patient and to strengthen your authority as nurse, be sure that you are present when the doctor, dietitian, or visiting nurse explains why some foods are forbidden, and the probable harm they may do if the patient takes them.

AND FINALLY...

Choosing, preparing, and serving foods with the eye, nose, and mouth appeals that your patient likes is much more than something done just to please someone who is sick. Every patient has certain rights, which should not be violated. Among them is the right to refuse special diets as well as individual foods.

As nurse, it is your responsibility to make certain that the doctor has explained thoroughly to your patient the consequences of refusing or eating certain foods. But a dying person or a very old one may feel or even say, "What difference does it make?" and eat anything, or starve, regardless of its probable effect.

Difficult as it may be for you to accept this kind of action from a rational person, you must accept your patient's wishes and decision. It is, after all, your *patient's* decision and life, not yours.

32 The General Diet

Except for a few restrictions, the patient who is on a general, normal, or regular diet can eat and drink just about every food substance. The few limitations concern selecting foods to make a balanced, healthy diet (Chapter 30) . . . foods that the patient is able to consume . . . and practical amounts. If a patient starts making unreasonable—and unhealthy!—dietary demands, point out that many people have eaten themselves off general and onto highly restrictive, specialized diets (Chapters 33–46).

A suggested 7-day general diet menu is given later in this chapter. Remember that the foods are only suggestions, based on a balanced diet; feel free to change them, with the doctor's, dietitian's, or nutritionist's consent, to meet your patient's likes and dislikes. You should also ask your visiting nurse for food suggestions based on the meat, produce, etc., that are available in your shopping area.

> NOTE: Regardless of what your patient's favorite foods are, do not serve them day after day or even on the same day of every week. Try to make each day a new adventure in eating. With the variety of foods in the suggested menu and your own good ideas for changing foods from day to day, your patient should never feel like saying, "It must be Sunday, there's chicken for dinner."

BALANCED DIET

In planning a diet, it is important to plan the whole day's menu or food intake at a time. That way it is easy to be sure of providing your patient with the basic nutrients necessary for good health.

There are four basic food groups, treated in detail in Chapter 30. Briefly, here are the groups and minimum daily servings recommended for the average person. The quantities for your patient will, of course, be given you by the doctor or dietitian.

Dairy Products: Milk, cheese, ice cream, and other milk products. Children more than 9 years old should have three or more 237-ml./8-oz. glasses of milk per day; smaller servings for younger children. Teenagers should have four or more full servings, and adults two or more.

Meat Group: This includes meats, fish, poultry, eggs, and cheese, with dried beans and peas, and nuts as alternates. Two or more servings from this group should be given daily.

Fruit, Vegetables: This group includes citrus fruit, tomatoes, and dark green or yellow vegetables. There should be four or more servings from this group each day.

Breads, Cereals: In this group are whole-grain breads, cereals; enriched or restored macaroni, noodles, spaghetti, etc.; rice. Serve four or more foods from this group each day.

Of course, some juggling of foods and amounts usually is unavoidable, especially when caring for a patient at home. But as a rule, anyone who is on general diet can tolerate temporary deficiencies or excesses without serious reaction. Most general diet patients can consume, without discomfort, many of the so-called ethnic foods that are highly seasoned, very starchy, have a high animal fat content, are pan fried, and so forth. However, these and rich foods in general should be served only as a treat, or on special occasions, and be followed by meals that are carefully balanced.

WHAT A PATIENT CAN EAT

Regardless of what your general diet patient wants or what foods are readily available, be sure to select those that actually can be eaten. Sometimes a person well enough internally to be on general diet is physically unable to handle certain foods. For example, a person with a badly broken jaw might, a few days after breaking it, be put on general diet; it certainly would be foolish as well as downright mean to serve steak, corn on the cob, or anything else that needs strong chewing and biting. Chopped meat, whipped potatoes, and soft spring peas would be much better.

HOW MUCH

Even though your patient is on general diet, keep in mind that disabled people often do not have large appetites, and that small servings (Eye Appeal, Chapter 31) may be necessary. However, important as it is to get a patient to eat enough, it is just as important to prevent overeating. The tendency to overeat is especially common among people who have led physically strenuous lives and regularly enjoyed large meals with, as a rule, too much starch (bread, potatoes, corn, doughnuts, etc.), so-called meals that "stick to the ribs." When disabled and less active, these people generally still want the same hearty meals—and without their former hard work, they may soon become dangerously overweight.

EXAMPLE OF 7-DAY MENU FOR GENERAL DIET

Amounts or quantities of food substances are not suggested, because the doctor, dietitian, or nutritionist will specify them according to your patient's age, physical activity, and general overall condition. Following the basic meals are recipes for preparing several easy-to-make, nourishing between-meal drinks.

NOTE: Between-meal and bedtime snacks are optional.

DAY No. 1

BREAKFAST

Grapefruit
Shredded wheat with milk, sugar to taste
Egg
Toast with butter or margarine
Glass of milk, or
Coffee, tea with cream, sugar to taste

MIDMORNING

Banana milk

LUNCH

Celery sticks
Tuna fish sandwich
Tapioca pudding
Glass of milk, or
Coffee, tea with cream, sugar to taste

MIDAFTERNOON

Orange chiller

DINNER

Swiss steak with gravy
Boiled potatoes
Green beans
Carrot-apple salad
Ice cream
Glass of milk, or
Coffee, tea with cream, sugar to taste

BEDTIME

Apricot milk

DAY No. 2

BREAKFAST

Glass of orange juice
Cooked rolled oats cereal with milk, sugar to taste
Whole-wheat toast with butter, margarine, jam
Glass of milk, or
Coffee, tea with cream, sugar to taste

MIDMORNING

Maple milk

LUNCH

Vegetable soup
Soda crackers
Fruit—fresh pear in season
Cookies
Glass of milk, or
Coffee, tea with cream, sugar to taste

MIDAFTERNOON

Peach cooler

DINNER

Roast beef
Baked potato
Broccoli
Tossed salad: lettuce, tomato, cucumber, bell pepper
Baked apple
Glass of milk, or
Coffee, tea with cream, sugar to taste

BEDTIME

Pineapple-lemon shake

DAY No. 3

BREAKFAST

Stewed prunes
Waffles with butter or margarine and syrup, jam or jelly
Ham
Glass of milk, or
Coffee, tea with cream, sugar to taste

MIDMORNING

Molasses milk

LUNCH

Egg salad sandwich on whole-wheat bread
Sliced tomatoes
Cookies
Glass of milk, or
Coffee, tea with cream, sugar to taste

MIDAFTERNOON

Spiced peach blossom

DINNER

Sliced roast veal
Zucchini squash and onions steamed together
Potato salad
Slice of watermelon, fresh, frozen, or canned fruit
Glass of milk, or
Coffee, tea with cream, sugar to taste

BEDTIME

Banana-orange shake

DAY No. 4

BREAKFAST

Orange juice
Applesauce
Bran muffins with butter or margarine, jam or jelly
Egg
Glass of milk, or
Coffee, tea with cream, sugar to taste

MIDMORNING

Vanilla milk

LUNCH
Split pea soup
Crackers
Liverwurst slices
Peaches, fresh, frozen, or canned
Glass of milk, or
Coffee, tea with cream, sugar to taste

MIDAFTERNOON
Banana milk

DINNER
Macaroni and cheese
Steamed Swiss chard
Bell pepper, carrot and celery sticks
Cookies
Glass of milk, or
Coffee, tea with cream, sugar to taste

BEDTIME
Milk Graham crackers

DAY No. 5

BREAKFAST
Strawberries, fresh or frozen
Cooked cereal
Egg
Biscuits, butter or margarine, honey, jam, jelly
Glass of milk, or
Coffee, tea with cream, sugar to taste

MIDMORNING
Glass of orange juice

LUNCH
Pineapple and cottage cheese salad
English muffin, butter or margarine
Cookies
Glass of milk, or
Coffee, tea with cream, sugar to taste

MIDAFTERNOON
Apricot milk

DINNER
Meat loaf
Rice
Baked squash (banana, butternut, or acorn)
Green salad
Apple crisp
Glass of milk, or
Coffee, tea with cream, sugar to taste

BEDTIME
Maple or coffee milk

DAY No. 6

BREAKFAST
½ cantaloupe or fresh, frozen, or canned fruit
Whole-grain dry cereal
Toast with butter or margarine
Glass of milk, or
Coffee, tea with cream, sugar to taste

MIDMORNING
Crackers with butter or jelly and fruit juice

LUNCH

Minestrone soup
Crackers
Plain cake
Glass of milk, or
Coffee, tea with cream, sugar to taste

MIDAFTERNOON

Orange chiller

DINNER

Chili con carne
Hot French bread, plain or garlic butter, margarine
Tossed salad
Fruit
Glass of milk, or
Coffee, tea with cream, sugar to taste

BEDTIME

Spiced peach blossom

DAY No. 7

BREAKFAST

Glass of cranberry juice
Egg
Link sausages
Whole-wheat toast, butter or margarine, jam, jelly
Glass of milk, or
Coffee, tea with cream, sugar to taste

MIDMORNING

Graham crackers

LUNCH

Toasted cheese sandwich
Sliced tomatoes
Melon; fresh, frozen, or canned fruit
Glass of milk, or
Coffee, tea with cream, sugar to taste

MIDAFTERNOON

Maple milk

DINNER

Baked ham
Scalloped potatoes
Spinach
Molded carrot and pineapple salad
Custard
Glass of milk, or
Coffee, tea with cream, sugar to taste

BEDTIME

Plain cake

SUGGESTED BETWEEN-MEAL DRINKS

In a covered container and refrigerated, these drinks can be stored safely for 3 or 4 days.

APRICOT MILK DRINK

1 355-ml./12-oz. can apricot nectar
355 ml./12 oz. milk
Dash nutmeg

Combine milk and fruit juice, top with dash of nutmeg. 4 servings.

BANANA MILK DRINK

1 ripe banana
237 ml./8 oz./1 cup cold milk

Mash banana, put in blender with milk, blend smooth, serve.

BANANA ORANGE SHAKE

1 177-ml./6-oz. can frozen orange concentrate
2 ripe bananas, mashed
1.5 l./1½ pts. vanilla ice cream, softened
1.5 l./6 cups cold milk

Place thawed orange juice concentrate, bananas, and ice cream in large (3.79-l./4-pt.) bowl. Beat until thoroughly blended. Continue beating and gradually add milk. Beat until smooth and frothy. 12 generous servings.

ORANGE CHILLER

1 l./5 cups liquid nonfat milk
1 180-ml./6-oz. can frozen orange juice concentrate
88 ml./3 tbsp. sugar

Pour half of milk into a large jar or pitcher. Add juice concentrate and sugar. Mix well. Add rest of milk, chill thoroughly. Stir well before serving. Makes 1.37 l./1½ qts.

PEACH COOLER

2 eggs, separated
Pinch of salt
59 ml./2 tbsp. sugar
178 ml./6 oz./¾ cup peaches, fresh, frozen, or canned
15 ml./1½ tsp. lemon juice
Few drops almond extract
237 ml./8 oz./1 cup milk
.25 l./½ pt. vanilla ice cream

Beat egg whites and salt until they hold soft peaks. Add sugar gradually, continue beating until stiff and glossy. Combine egg yolks, peaches, lemon juice, and almond extract, mix well. Add milk and ice cream, beat until smooth. Fold in egg whites. Serve in tall, chilled glasses. 4 to 5 servings.

PINEAPPLE-LEMON SHAKE

1 390-ml./13-oz. can crushed unsweetened pineapple and syrup
1 l./2 pts. vanilla ice cream
.5 l./2 cups cold milk
39 ml./4 tsp. lemon juice

Combine all ingredients in blender or mixing bowl. Beat for about 2 minutes, till frothy and smooth. Makes 4 servings.

SPICED PEACH BLOSSOM

.2 l./6 oz./¾ cup mashed peaches
89 ml./3 tbsp. sugar
Pinch of salt
89 ml./3 tbsp. lemon juice
2.5 ml./¼ tsp. each cinnamon and nutmeg
592 ml./2½ cups milk
.25 l./½ pt. vanilla ice cream

In blender combine peaches, salt, sugar, spices, and lemon juice. Blend well. Stir in cold milk. Pour into tall glasses, top with scoops of ice cream. 3 to 4 servings.

Milk Variations

To vary the taste of milk, to 1 l./1 qt. of it add any of the following:
5 ml./1 tsp. vanilla extract.
2.5 ml./½ tsp. imitation maple flavoring.
89 ml./3 tbsp. light molasses and a dash of cinnamon or nutmeg.
39 ml./4 tsp. instant coffee. If sugar is allowed, sweeten to taste.

33 The Liquid Diets

There are two kinds of liquid diets: clear and full. Both usually are given in six feedings a day, in amounts recommended by the patient's doctor, dietitian, or visiting nurse, and according to the patient's willingness to take and ability to tolerate or accept them. Liquid diets usually are prescribed for very limited lengths of time. Protein, vitamin, and mineral supplements generally are prescribed with clear, and may be ordered with full, liquid diets.

A liquid diet should, of course, be given only when so ordered by a patient's doctor, dietician, or nutritionist. Detailed information will be given as to how long your patient should be on the diet, the foods and beverages allowed and their amounts, how they should be prepared, and the items that should not be given. Most items allowed by liquid diets are stocked in regular food stores and markets; your visiting nurse probably can advise you where to buy any special items.

Liquid diets may be fed by a straw or spoon, or cup or glass, depending on your patient's condition and preference.

In addition to the usual utensils for preparing food, you should have a high-speed blender or similar food machine for pureeing and liquefying; and for straining, a fine-mesh wire strainer or preferably a triple thickness of lintfree cloth such as cheesecloth or a well-used dish towel, or a jelly bag.

Temperature is important for feeding liquid diets. If a soup should be served hot, serve it hot! Your patient may have to wait a few minutes for it to cool sufficiently, but in most cases soup served lukewarm is unappetizing. The same is true of a food or beverage meant to be served cold—serve it cold! If your patient does not consume a serving within about 10 minutes, it may be advisable to serve it in a thermal or "heat-holding" container, such as an infant's plate with a compartment for hot or cold water, or the vacuum-type or double-walled cup often used on picnics.

Examples of clear and full liquid diets are at the end of this chapter.

FOODS FOR THE CLEAR LIQUID DIET

A clear liquid diet usually consists of regular liquids such as water, coffee, tea . . . strained clear fruit and vegetable juices . . . seasonings such as sugar, salt, and pepper, all to be taken only as prescribed by the diet instructions.

Broth: Clear meat, poultry, or fish broth may be seasoned with pepper and salt (artificial salt, if prescribed) to taste. Bouillon cubes or powder, canned consomme, meat and poultry extracts may be used to prepare broth. If broth has noticeable globules of fat when it cools, and your patient is also on a low-fat or low-cholesterol diet (Chapters 41, 42), remove as much fat as possible by passing an ice cube through the fatty deposits several times. The fat will congeal and stick to the ice long enough for you to wipe it off quickly.

Carbonated beverages: Serve any carbonated beverage allowed by the diet instructions.

Coffee, tea: These may be weak or strong, served hot or cold and plain or seasoned, as your patient wants; with sugar (artificial sweetener, if ordered by the doctor) and milk, cream, or a nondairy product if approved by the doctor or dietician.

Juice: Any fresh, frozen, cooked, or canned fruit or vegetable juice that is allowed. To eliminate pulp or other fiber that might injure your patient, strain the juice through a fine-mesh wire strainer, through a triple thickness of lintfree cloth such as cheesecloth or a well-used dish towel, or through a jelly bag. Suggested fruit juices are: orange, grapefruit, pineapple, cranberry, apple, prune, boysenberry, apricot nectar, pear nectar. For vegetable juices: carrot, celery, mixed vegetable, tomato.

Water: Water usually may be given hot or cold, as often and in any reasonable amount that your patient wants.

FOODS FOR THE FULL LIQUID DIET

A full liquid diet, which can be nutritionally adequate, generally is more satisfactory to the patient than a clear diet. The full liquid diet usually is for a patient whose main problem is not being able to chew, and may be continued until that condition passes. In addition to the items allowed by the clear liquid diet, above, a full liquid diet contains, in general, any food that can be strained or liquefied to a satisfactory consistency.

Cereal, gruel: Cooked, soft white cereals, such as Cream of Wheat or Farina, thinned with milk or cream to a consistency that your patient can readily tolerate.

Custard: Plain or any flavor, but without solid particles of fruit.

Eggs: Soft-boiled only.

Eggnog: Any flavor.

Gelatin: Any flavor, but without solid particles of fruit. As thick or thin as your patient wants and can tolerate.

Ice cream: Real, imitation ice cream, or ice milk, provided it does not contain solids such as nuts, fruit bits, candy chips, etc.

Malted milk, milkshakes: Any flavor, as thick as your patient wants and can tolerate. Make only with permitted kinds of ice cream, ice milk, etc., above.

Plain pudding: Any flavor, but without solid particles of fruit, nuts, candy chips, etc. As thin or thick as your patient likes and can tolerate.

Soup: Any strained cream or clear soup; be sure all solids are removed. In summertime a soup served cold may be very appetizing and refreshing.

Tapioca pudding: Any flavor, but without solid particles of fruit, candy chips, etc. Dilute with cream or milk according to your patient's ability to eat.

EXAMPLE OF CLEAR LIQUID DIET

The amounts in a clear liquid diet may or may not be specified; it depends on the condition of a patient. Often an amount is given as, for example, "1 cup or more," with the understanding that you will try to get your patient to take at least the minimum amount. Sometimes it will be necessary to change an item from one so-called mealtime to another, or perhaps even add a meal, in order to get the necessary food into your patient. These changes should, of course, be done only with the consent of the patient's doctor, dietician, or nutritionist.

BREAKFAST

Chicken broth, hot
Orange juice
Coffee or tea, plain, or with sugar and cream or milk

MIDMORNING

Pear nectar

LUNCH

Beef broth, hot or cold
Apple juice
Coffee or tea, plain, or with sugar and milk or cream

MIDAFTERNOON
Boysenberry juice

DINNER
Fish broth, hot
Carrot and celery juice
Strawberry gelatin
Coffee or tea, plain, or with sugar and cream or milk

BEDTIME
Tomato juice

EXAMPLE OF FULL LIQUID DIET

The amounts of foods are treated the same as for a clear liquid diet, above.

BREAKFAST
Orange juice
Chicken broth
2 Soft-boiled eggs
Milk
Coffee or tea, plain, or with sugar and milk or cream to taste

MIDMORNING
Grapefruit juice

LUNCH
Cream soup
Apricot nectar
Tapioca pudding
Milk
Coffee or tea, plain, or with sugar and milk or cream to taste

MIDAFTERNOON
Cranberry juice

DINNER
Beef broth
Apple juice
Custard pudding
Milk
Coffee or tea, plain, or with sugar and cream or milk to taste

BEDTIME
Milkshake

34 The Naturally Soft or Light Diet

As a rule, the last special diet for postoperative patients before going on general diet is the naturally soft or light diet. It consists of foods that are naturally soft in consistency, as opposed to those that are made soft by grinding, pureeing, or other mechanical means (Chapter 35). Naturally soft diets usually exclude rich, strongly flavored, and highly spiced foods that could cause digestive distress. Within these limits, there is a wide range of balanced foods to please almost any patient.

It commonly happens that patients who have advanced from the liquid (Chapter 33) to the naturally soft diet are now more aware of food and responsive to it and how it is served (Chapters 31, 47, and 48).

Your patient should, of course, be on a naturally soft diet only when it is ordered by the doctor, dietitian, or nutritionist. Dietary instructions will list the foods and beverages allowed and the amounts, how they should and should not be prepared, items that should not be given, and as a rule a daily or weekly menu. Most food and beverages you need for a naturally soft diet are carried by regular food stores and markets; your visiting nurse probably can suggest several places to shop for special items that may be wanted.

A sample 1-day naturally soft diet is at the end of this chapter. Keep in mind that the foods listed are only suggestions, based on a balanced diet (Chapter 30). Feel free to change them, without changing the food balance (for example, substitute canned pears for canned peaches), to meet your patient's likes and dislikes, and to prevent boredom with food and eating. You also should ask your visiting nurse for suggestions, based on the meat, fish, produce, etc., now available in your market area.

FOODS ALLOWED BY NATURALLY SOFT OR LIGHT DIETS

All the food items in liquid diets (Chapter 33) are allowed by naturally soft diets, but usually in a firmer consistency and greater quantity. In most cases, food may be prepared any way except by frying. Mild seasonings generally are permitted.

Gravies, cream sauces, and dessert toppings usually are allowed by naturally soft diets. But since they may tend to increase your patient's weight, ask the doctor, dietitian, or visiting nurse what kinds of gravies, etc., and amounts are suitable for your patient.

Foods and beverages in addition to those in liquid diets that usually are allowed by naturally soft diets are:

Breads: Enriched white.

Butter: Fresh, salted.

Cakes: Plain.

Candy: Hard, to be held in mouth while melting.

Cereals: Cooked refined, such as oatmeal, Cream of Wheat, cornmeal, porridge; usually thicker than in liquid diets.

Chicken: Baked, broiled, roasted; not fried.

Cookies: Plain.

Cottage cheese: Creamed, regular, or low fat; large or small curd.

Crackers: Soda.

Cream sauce: Mildly seasoned.

Dessert toppings: Meringue, whipped cream, commercial toppings; may be mixed with small bits of cooked fruit.

Eggs: Soft-cooked, poached, scrambled; not fried.

Fish: Baked, broiled, poached; not fried.

Fruit: Bananas, ripe, raw; canned, cooked apricots, apples, applesauce, pears, peaches, prunes.

Gravies: Pan, milk; not from fried foods.

Ice cream: Real, imitation, ice milk; all flavors, including those containing small bits of cooked fruit.

Juices: All cooked fruit, vegetable; uncooked orange; juices need not be strained.

Macaroni, spaghetti: Seasoned with butter, margarine, mild cheese, cream sauce.

Margarine: Enriched.

Meat: Tender beef, lamb, veal; baked, broiled, roasted; not fried.

Milk: Whole, low fat, or skim; buttermilk.

Potatoes (no skin): Baked, boiled, creamed, mashed, scalloped; not fried.

Puddings: Plain, or mixed with small bits of cooked fruit.

Rice: Polished, boiled.

Seasonings: As allowed by doctor or dietician: table salt, pepper, grated mild cheese; celery, garlic, onion salts, powders; commercial seasoning salts.

Soup: All kinds; need not be strained unless solids are too hard or large for patient to eat.

Turkey: Baked, broiled, roasted; not fried.

Vegetables: Cooked and pureed beets, carrots, peas, potatoes (without skins), spinach, string beans, turnips, squash (acorn, banana, butternut, Hubbard, zucchini).

Yogurt: Plain; may be mixed with small bits of cooked fruit.

FOODS USUALLY AVOIDED BY NATURALLY SOFT OR LIGHT DIETS

The foods to be avoided in naturally soft diets are those that tend to form gas (any fried food) and those containing tough fibers.

Cereals: Whole grain.

Corn: Except cornmeal.

Fruit: Raw, except ripe bananas, orange juice.

Potato: Skins.

Vegetables: Raw.

EXAMPLE OF NATURALLY SOFT OR LIGHT DIET

The amount of each food and beverage prescribed by the doctor, dietitian, or nutritionist will be based on your patient's sex, age, general build, and overall condition. When making substitutions, as a rule the amount as well as the food balance should be maintained; for example, substitute 1 cup of cooked apricots for 1 cup of applesauce.

BREAKFAST

Orange juice
Soft-boiled egg
Enriched white bread, toast
Enriched butter, margarine
Applesauce
Milk
Coffee, tea, plain, or with sugar, cream or milk as desired

MIDMORNING

Grapefruit juice

LUNCH

Creamed tomato soup
Pureed beets
Cottage cheese
Enriched white bread
Cherry gelatin dessert
Milk
Coffee, tea, plain, or with sugar, cream or milk as desired

MIDAFTERNOON

Milkshake

DINNER

Chicken broth
Baked chicken
Baked potato (do not eat skin)
Pureed spinach
Plain cake
Milk
Coffee, tea, plain, or with sugar, cream or milk as desired

BEDTIME

Yogurt with pureed canned peaches

35 The Mechanically Soft Diet

The mechanically soft diet is for persons who, from the digestive standpoint, are capable of eating any food allowed by a general diet, but have temporary or permanent difficulty in chewing and/or swallowing. It is not, as a rule, a starvation diet in any sense of the word, although amounts of certain foods may at times be limited.

In most cases, the foods allowed by a mechanically soft diet are the same as those in a balanced general diet (Chapters 30, 32), but are chopped, ground, or pureed to a consistency that a patient can chew and swallow without pain or other distress. Generally you should serve the coarsest food that your patient can tolerate, to give the greatest stimulation to the upper part of the digestive tract.

A mechanically soft diet should of course be used only as ordered by a patient's doctor or dietitian. Detailed information as to the duration of the diet, the items and portions allowed, and those to be avoided will be given, along with daily or weekly menus. Foods and beverages for most mechanically soft diets are stocked by regular food stores and markets. Your visiting nurse probably can give you helpful suggestions for shopping for special or unusual foods that may be ordered.

A 1-day sample menu for a mechanically soft diet is at the end of this chapter.

PREPARING FOODS FOR MECHANICALLY SOFT DIETS

To eliminate the extra work of having to cook special foods for your patient:

Fruit, Vegetables: If you have a blender or similar food machine, prepare fruits and vegetables the normal way, then grind or puree them separately in the blender or other machine. Reduce foods only to the coarsest consistency that your patient can tolerate. A baby-food grinder usually may be used in place of a blender.

Meats: After cooking meat the regular way, put it through a meat grinder. Grind only to the coarsest consistency that your patient can eat.

Instead of your processing foods to a thin enough consistency for your patient to eat, it may be more practical to use commercial baby, infant, and junior prepared foods. However, since they often are too bland for adult tastes, it may be necessary to season them for nose and mouth appeal (Chapter 31).

EXAMPLE OF MECHANICALLY SOFT DIET

Because of the difficulty of eating, it is often advisable to serve patients on a mechanically soft diet four, five, or even six small meals a day instead of the so-called three normal ones. If this is not practical or your patient really does not want so many meals, serve as much as your patient can comfortably accept at the three regular meals, and provide an ample supply of snacks for between-meal munching.

Whether or not amounts of foods and beverages are specified on a mechanically soft diet usually depends on a patient's general condition, sex, build, and age.

BREAKFAST

Orange juice
Applesauce
Cooked enriched cereal with cream or milk and sugar to taste
Soft-boiled egg
Milk
Coffee, tea, plain or with milk, cream, sugar as desired

LUNCH

Cream of celery soup
Baked potato, no skin
Roast beef, ground after cooking; add beef gravy for flavor
Pureed string beans, carrots
Molded gelatin salad
Ice cream
Milk
Coffee, tea, plain or with milk, cream, sugar as desired

DINNER

Tomato juice
Rice, cooked soft
Chicken, ground after cooking
2 pureed vegetables (beets, peas, squash, broccoli, etc.) in equal amounts
Custard dessert
Milk
Coffee, tea, plain or with cream, milk, sugar as desired

36 The Bland or Ulcer Diet

Before the development of many modern medicines and medical treatments, a *bland* or *ulcer* diet commonly was imposed on persons afflicted with ailments such as ulcers in the digestive tract, especially peptic or "stomach" ulcers . . . colitis or inflammation of the colon . . . and gastritis or inflammation of the stomach.

The purposes of the bland diet were to minimize the mechanical irritation of the digestive tract, to dilute or weaken stomach juices, and to help neutralize the contents of the stomach, which are acid.

Because all foods, including water, stimulate the secretion or flow of digestive juices and increase stomach acidity, the foods allowed on the standard bland diet were about as bland or unirritating (and generally uninteresting) as possible. Very few of the goodies that most of us take for granted, and few if any seasonings, were allowed to make the bland diet more appetizing. It may well have been that the bland diet gave birth to one idea of a diet: "Make a list of all the things you like to eat—and don't eat 'em!"

Briefly, an oldtime bland or ulcer diet allowed mostly soft foods such as ripe bananas, milk, strained cooked fruit juices, white bread, cooked white cereals, cream or cottage cheese, eggs, fish, gelatin, lean meats (often scrapped), creamed and thin soups, cooked and strained vegetables.

Usually not allowed by the bland or ulcer diet were, in most cases, alcoholic or carbonated beverages, coffee, strong tea, whole-grain bread or cereal, cheddar or other strong cheese, rich desserts, frosted cakes or cookies, most raw fruit, nuts, seasonings, spices, raw or cooked but not strained vegetables, tobacco in any form.

Modern medical care has, in most cases, eliminated need of the bland or ulcer diet. Of course, sometimes the doctor or dietitian will ban certain foods or beverages, or allow them only in small amounts. By following these usually mild restrictions, most persons being treated for peptic ulcers, colitis, gastritis, and so forth can enjoy nearly normal balanced meals.

If your patient rebels against the medical treatment and, probably, mild restrictions in diet, it may be well to ask the doctor or dietitian for a sample old-fashioned bland or ulcer diet menu, and let your patient see how much worse meals could be.

37 The Low-Residue Diet

The purpose of the low-residue diet is to reduce the unabsorbed residue of food remaining in the intestines after digestion has taken place. This diet is prescribed especially for patients with intestinal or rectal diseases, or who have had rectal surgery. It should be a balanced diet (Chapter 30) of foods that are low in bulk and are easy to digest. A low-residue diet is not, as a rule, a starvation diet in any sense of the word, although the amounts of certain foods may at times be limited.

As is the case with all special diets, the low-residue should be used only as specified by a patient's doctor or dietitian. You will be given complete information as to how long your patient should be on the diet, the items and portions allowed, and those to be avoided. Also, you probably will be given daily or weekly menus. Make sure that they contain foods that are readily available in your shopping area, and priced within your means. Your visiting nurse very likely can give you excellent shopping suggestions.

Foods and beverages for low-residue diets generally are carried by regular food stores and markets. When buying a packaged item, read the label carefully to see if all the ingredients are allowed your patient. Do not buy packaged foods or beverages that fail to list their ingredients.

Exact amounts usually are not as important with low-residue as with low-calorie (Chapter 39) diets. But when certain portions are specified by volume or weight, you should measure them with reasonable accuracy.

An example of a 1-day low-residue diet is given at the end of this chapter.

FOODS ALLOWED BY LOW-RESIDUE DIETS

As a rule, all the following foods and beverages can be included in low-residue diets. Nearly all must be cooked. Frying is a no-no for low-residue diets, but any other method of cooking that your patient wants usually is satisfactory.

Beverages: Decaffeinated coffee, tea with cream, sugar; fruit drinks; strained fruit juice; cooked, canned vegetable juice.

Bread: Enriched white, rye breads, rolls, crackers.

Butter: Salted, unsalted; very small amounts.

Cake: Plain.

Cereal: Cooked fine white, such as Cream of Wheat, cornflakes, puffed rice, puffed wheat.

Cheese: Cottage, mild American, cream cheese.

Cookies: Plain.

Crackers: Soda, made from enriched white flour.

Cream: In small amounts, with coffee, tea.

Custard

Desserts: Cake, cookies plain; bread pudding; custards; gelatin; rice, tapioca puddings. No fruit or nuts added.

Eggs: Any way except fried.

Fruit: Fresh—banana, cantaloupe, honeydew melon, watermelon, grapefruit or orange sections without membrane. Cooked, without skins—applesauce, apricots, peaches, pears.

Gelatin: With cooked fruit mixed in if desired.

Jellies: All.

Juices: Cooked or strained raw fruit; cooked vegetable.

Margarine: Very small amounts.

Milk: Boiled or cooked, as in cream soup.

Noodles: Small amounts.

Potatoes: Small amounts, not fried.

Rice pudding: With cooked, strained fruit mixed in if desired.

Seasonings: Salt, sugar in small amounts. Mild flavorings, such as vanilla. No "seed" seasonings.

Sherbet: All fruit flavors.

Spaghetti: Buttered, seasoned.

Soup: All kinds, creamed, clear.

Sugar: Small amounts.

Tapioca pudding: With strained cooked fruit mixed in if desired.

Vegetables: Small amounts, cooked and strained or pureed. Baked potato without skin. Cooked juices. Asparagus tips, beets, eggplant, pumpkin, squash, green and yellow beans, carrots, peas, spinach, canned tomatoes.

FOODS TO AVOID IN LOW-RESIDUE DIETS

It is most important for comfort as well as health that persons who have had recent rectal surgery avoid certain foods. The following foods tend to irritate and strain the lower digestive tract, and usually are forbidden by most low-residue diets:

Beverages: Iced drinks, carbonated beverages, unboiled milk and milk drinks, coffee except decaffeinated.

Bread: Whole wheat.

Cereal: All whole-grain and coarse cereals, especially bran and wheat.

Fats: Lard and all other fats except minimal amounts of butter, margarine.

Fried foods: All.

Fruit: All fresh fruit and juices except those listed under Foods Allowed, above.

Meats: Smoked, fried, highly seasoned processed meats.

Melons: All except those listed under Foods Allowed, above.

Milk: Use only in cooking; cheese.

Nuts: All.

Potato: Skins; sweet potatoes, yams.

Raisins

Rice: Whole grain.

Vegetables: All raw vegetables, juices except those listed under Foods Allowed, above.

EXAMPLE OF A LOW-RESIDUE DIET

Low-residue diets prescribed by a doctor or dietitian usually specify the amounts of certain foods and beverages based on the age, sex, general condition and so forth of the patient. You should measure them with reasonable accuracy, although as a rule it need not be as accurate as for a low-calorie diet.

BREAKFAST

Fruit juice, strained, and/or pureed cooked fruit
Fine, white cooked cereal, such as Cream of Wheat, with sugar and small amount of cream
1 or 2 eggs, not fried
Slice enriched white bread with minimal amount butter or margarine, and jelly
Decaffeinated coffee, weak tea as desired, sugar

MIDMORNING

Strained fruit juice
Soda crackers

LUNCH

Lean, tender meat, any way except fried
Potato or rice, any way except fried; or spaghetti
Vegetables, pureed
Slice enriched white bread, minimal amount butter or margarine, and jelly as desired
Dessert—Pureed fruit; gelatin; or custard
Decaffeinated coffee, weak tea as desired, sugar

MIDAFTERNOON

Strained fruit juice
Plain cookies

DINNER

Lean meat, any way except fried
Buttered rice
Any two cooked and strained allowable vegetables
Slice enriched white bread, minimal butter or margarine, and jelly
Dessert—Pureed fruit, gelatin, sherbet, rice pudding, or plain cake
Decaffeinated coffee, weak tea as desired, sugar

BEDTIME

Strained fruit or vegetable juice

38 The High-Calorie Diet

High-calorie diets, for persons who are underweight or malnourished, feature foods that are high in carbohydrates, proteins, minerals, and vitamins (Chapter 30). Sugar and fats are added as a patient wants and can tolerate them. Supplemental vitamins often are prescribed. The goal of a high-calorie diet usually is to increase a patient's daily caloric intake by 25 percent to 50 percent above what is usually eaten.

Depending on your patient's condition and ability to tolerate food, instead of three meals a day with between-meal and bedtime snacks, you may have to serve several small meals relatively often. But as a rule, this is necessary for only a fairly short period of time.

A high-calorie diet should, of course, be given only as ordered by your patient's doctor or dietitian. You should receive full instructions covering how long your patient probably will be on the diet, the foods and portions allowed, and those to be avoided. You also should be given daily or weekly menus. Be sure they contain foods that are readily available in your shopping area. Your visiting nurse probably can give you many helpful shopping suggestions.

A sample 2-day high-calorie menu is at the end of this chapter. Remember that these foods and meals are only suggestions, based on a balanced diet (see Basic Food Groups, Chapter 30); feel free to change them, with the doctor's permission, to satisfy your patient. You should also ask your visiting nurse for menu suggestions based on the meat, fish, produce, etc., that are available in your area.

WHAT A HIGH-CALORIE DIET IS

Basically, a high-calorie diet is a regular or general diet (Chapter 32) with high-caloric foods added. This can be done many ways.

You can increase calories by adding sugar to fruits and juices . . . giving your patient whole instead of skim or nonfat milk . . . adding powdered milk to soups, and to baked goods such as breads, cakes, and cookies . . . using cream and extra butter or margarine when preparing mashed potatoes . . . adding 2 ml./2 tbsp./¼ cup powdered milk to normal recipes for biscuit, muffin, pancake, and waffle batters . . . adding marshmallow and extra sugar and powdered milk when preparing hot cocoa . . . topping desserts such as custard, fruit cobbler, rice and other puddings with sweetened whipped cream . . . pouring liberal servings of tasty sauce on ice cream and puddings.

You can also easily increase your patient's caloric intake by serving richer and possibly larger than customary between-meal and bedtime snacks. These might be a milkshake . . . ice cream with cake or cookies . . . an eggnog . . . custard . . . a dish of gelatin with sweetened fruit and a creamy topping, and so forth.

Some No-No's Since the main purpose of a high-calorie diet is to increase your patient's caloric intake, as a rule you should not serve:

Artificial sweeteners
Diet-type beverages
Low-calorie desserts, mayonnaise, packaged fruit, puddings, salad dressings
Low-fat cottage cheese, milk
Nonfat milk
Skim milk, buttermilk

SAMPLE 2-DAY HIGH-CALORIE DIET MENU

High-calorie diets usually specify the minimum amount of each food your patient should have. If your patient cannot tolerate three so-called normal meals a day but must eat more often, ask the doctor or your visiting nurse how to divide and serve the foods. Regardless of whether you make up or are given your patient's menu, it usually should be changed so that the same foods are not served too often or on the same days of the week. A sure sign of your failure to change foods sufficiently is when your patient says something like, "It must be Monday, hash for dinner."

DAY No. 1

BREAKFAST

Fruit juice, any kind, with sugar added
Cereal, cooked or dry, with cream and sugar
Eggs
Bread or toast, enriched white or whole wheat, butter or margarine
Jam, jelly, honey, or fruit butter
Glass of whole milk, or
Coffee, tea with cream and sugar to taste

MIDMORNING

Dish of fruit with cream and sugar

LUNCH

Cream of tomato soup with butter, margarine
Cheddar cheese
Potato with butter, margarine
Beets with salad dressing or mayonnaise
Bread with butter, margarine
Glass of whole milk, or
Coffee, tea with cream, sugar to taste

MIDAFTERNOON

Dish of ice cream

DINNER

Roast turkey with gravy
Dressing
Creamed spinach
Candied yams
Molded gelatin salad with mayonnaise or dressing
Carrot cake
Glass of whole milk, or
Coffee, tea with cream, sugar to taste

BEDTIME

Eggnog made with extra cream and sugar

DAY No. 2

BREAKFAST
- Fruit juice, any kind, with added sugar
- Scrambled eggs
- Ham
- Enriched biscuits with butter and honey
- Glass of whole milk, or
- Coffee, tea with cream, sugar to taste

MIDMORNING
- Fruit gelatin with cream

LUNCH
- Cream of asparagus soup
- Tuna sandwich on enriched white or whole-wheat bread
- Sweet pickles if desired
- Chocolate pudding with whipped cream
- Glass of whole milk, or
- Coffee, tea with cream, sugar to taste

MIDAFTERNOON
- Custard pudding

DINNER
- Meat loaf (with powdered milk added)
- Baked potato with sour cream and butter
- Creamed carrots
- Waldorf salad (apples, celery, raisins, nuts)
- Plain cake
- Glass of whole milk, or
- Coffee, tea with cream, sugar to taste

BEDTIME
- Hot cocoa with cream and marshmallow, cookies

39 Low-Calorie Diets

There are many low-calorie and other diets for reducing a person's weight. The type of low-calorie diet most widely favored by the medical profession consists of a balanced daily intake made up of items in all four of the basic food groups (Chapter 30), but in sharply limited quantities. Basically the same diet or menu is used regardless of the weight-reducing problem, the differences being in the number of calories allowed; for example, bread, fruit, eggs, milk, meat, and vegetables are allowed in both 800- and 1,500-calorie diets, but in greater amounts in the higher-calorie one. Simply because most medically approved low-calorie diets are balanced, there is a tendency for the followers to lose weight at a slower rate than with so-called crash diets. For the same reason—balanced food intake—a person generally can follow these diets for a longer time with less discomfort or "yearning for forbidden foods"! Also, remaining on a balanced diet will give longer-lasting results.

In most cases, preparing a low-calorie diet is a matter of simple arithmetic based on the number of calories somebody needs daily to maintain current weight, and how many "deficit" or fewer calories per day are needed to lose weight at a desired rate. For example, somebody weighing 68–72.5 kg./150–160 lbs. needs 2,200 calories per day to maintain that weight. For a loss of .45 kg./1 lb. per week, a deficit of 500 calories per day is necessary, thus reducing food intake to 1,700 calories per day. The daily diet then consists of permitted foods and beverages in quantities that total no more than 1,700 calories.

Generally a daily diet is divided into three meals, two relatively small and one large, but this is not a necessity. If your patient is accustomed to more or fewer daily "meals" of various sizes, divide the daily total accordingly. Snacks must, of course, be included in the daily total number of calories. However, there are foods and beverages that do not contain calories, and these usually are allowed in any reasonable amount that a patient wants.

Examples of possible 1-day menus for 1,000- 1,200-, and 1,500-calorie diets are given at the end of this chapter. Keep in mind the food items are only suggestions, based on a balanced diet, and may be changed according to your patient's desires.

Low-calorie diets, like all other types, should be used only as ordered by a doctor. Your patient's doctor or dietitian will give you details as to the total number of calories allowed each day, how many days to keep your patient on a diet, the kinds and amounts of foods and beverages allowed, special directions for preparing foods when necessary, and, usually, sample daily or weekly menus. Be sure that the food list contains items that are readily available now in your market area and priced within your budget. Your visiting nurse probably can give you worthwhile shopping suggestions.

As a rule, the items needed for a low-calorie diet are available at regular food stores and markets. In the case of canned and packaged foods, be sure to read the labels for the exact contents (principal item, preservatives, flavorings, etc.), and number of calories per serving. Buy only products that give this information.

BASIC ALLOWABLE FOODS

Generally all the following foods and beverages are allowed in low-calorie diets. However, some items and the amounts allowed are based on the daily caloric intake prescribed for your patient.

Beverages: Plain regular and decaffeinated coffee, tea, Postum and similar grain beverages. Skimmed milk, see below.

Butter: See Fat, below.

Bread: Whole-grain, enriched white; may be replaced by cereal.

Cereal: Cooked, such as oatmeal, porridge, Cream of Wheat; dry such as Grapenuts, exploded enriched rice, etc.; may be substituted for bread.

Cheese: Low-fat cottage (not creamed); may substitute for meat, fish, poultry.

Eggs: Any way except fried with butter, fat, shortening, etc.; may be fatfree fried in a "no stick" pan.

Fat, Oil, Butter, Margarine, Mayonnaise: Separately or in other foods; may be allowed in limited amounts in diets of 1,000 or more calories per day.

Unsaturated oils (see Fat, Chapter 30) and products made from them generally are preferred.

Fish: See Meat, below.

Fruit: Raw, all kinds, unsugared. Canned, cooked, all kinds, but only those that have been prepared without sugar.

Margarine: See Fat, above.

Mayonnaise: See Fat, above.

Meat, Fish, Poultry: All, any way except fried; may be replaced by cheese. NOTE: Do not eat the skin of fowl or any of the fat on any meat.

Melons

Milk: Nonfat, skimmed, buttermilk made from skimmed milk; fatfree powdered milk; plain yogurt (may be seasoned by adding fresh or unsweetened fruit, berries). Within the amount allowed by a diet, skimmed milk may be fortified by adding up to an equal amount of powdered milk to make a thicker, richer-tasting beverage with greater protein content.

Poultry: See Meat, above.

Salad dressing: Sugarless.

Starch: Potato, yam, corn, lima beans, green peas, winter squash may be allowed, depending on the total number of calories desired.

Vegetables: Raw, salads, cooked green, yellow vegetables; clear soup. NOTE: Salads made from raw vegetables and sugarless dressing are not counted in the total caloric intake.

FREE FOODS

Free foods are those that can be used in unlimited amounts in most low-calorie diets. Some of these are:

Bouillon: Fatfree only.

Coffee: Plain.

Flavorings: Cinnamon, lemon, lime, mint, nutmeg.

Gelatin: Unsweetened.

Pickles: Dill, unsweetened.

Renin tablets

Seasonings: Celery salt, chili powder, garlic (powder, salt), horseradish, mustard (sugarless), onion (minced, powder, salt), paprika, parsley, pepper (black, red), salt.

Tea: Any kind, plain.

THE "MAYBE" FOODS

"HEALTH," "NATURAL," "ORGANIC," "DIET," "LOW-CALORIE," "INSTANTS," "JUICE DRINKS." These types of specially grown, produced, formulated, or processed foods and beverages may or may not be allowed in your patient's low-calorie diet. Before serving them, consult the doctor or dietitian. As a rule, it will be enough to merely ask about the item by its brand name. But in the case of foods or beverages that are new on the market, get a container that lists the ingredients, nutritional factors, and serving suggestions.

The composition of specialty foods and beverages may at times be changed. Therefore always compare the label of a fresh supply with that of the product you have been allowed to serve. Report any differences to the doctor or dietitian before serving it to your patient.

FORBIDDEN FOODS

Forbidden foods and beverages are those not allowed in most low-calorie diets. Some of them are:

Alcoholic beverages
Cakes
Candy
Chewing gum
Condensed milk
Cookies
Honey
Jams, see The Maybe Foods, above
Jellies, see The Maybe Foods, above
Pies
Soft drinks, see The Maybe Foods, above
Sugar
Syrup

EXAMPLE OF 1,000-CALORIE DIET

A prescribed diet of this type usually lists the caloric value of each item and of suggested or allowable substitutes.

BREAKFAST

59 ml./2 fl. oz./¼ cup low-fat cottage cheese, or 1 egg
237 ml./8 fl. oz./1 cup cooked cereal
118 ml./4 fl. oz./½ cup skimmed milk
½ small cantaloupe
1 slice bacon, broiled, very crisp, almost charcoal
Coffee, tea as desired, no milk, cream, sugar

LUNCH

Tuna salad made with 57 gm./2 oz. tuna (preferably waterpack), lettuce, celery, onions, cucumbers, radishes, 5 ml./2 tsp. mayonnaise
1 slice bread, whole wheat
30 ml./2 level tbsp. raisins
Tea, with lemon

DINNER

57 gm./2 oz. roast chicken, no skin
114 gm./4 oz. spinach or Swiss chard
114 gm./4 oz. cooked cauliflower
Green salad made with lettuce, green pepper rings, celery, sugarless French dressing; as much as patient wants
2 medium-size apricots, fresh or water-pack canned
Coffee, tea, plain, as desired

EXAMPLE OF 1,200-CALORIE DIET

The caloric value of the specified amount of each item usually is listed as part of the menu prescribed by the doctor or dietitian. Because of the greater number of calories allowed, the 1,200-calorie diet usually offers more leeway in making substitutions than the 1,000-calorie diet.

BREAKFAST

118 ml./4 fl. oz./½ cup unsweetened orange juice, fresh, frozen, canned
1 egg, not fried
1 slice toast
.6 gm./1 tsp. margarine
Coffee, tea as desired, plain

LUNCH

86 gm./3 oz. sliced turkey
1 slice bread or 1 plain yeast roll
Celery, radishes as desired
½ grapefruit
237 ml./8 fl. oz./1 cup skimmed milk
Coffee, tea, plain, as desired

DINNER

86 gm./3 oz. lean roast beef
1 medium potato boiled or baked
227 gm./1 cup cooked spinach
114 gm./½ cup carrots, cooked or raw
½ medium banana
Coffee, tea, plain, as desired

BEDTIME

237 ml./8 fl. oz./1 cup skim milk
3 soda crackers

EXAMPLE OF 1,500-CALORIE DIET

The caloric value of each item in the amount specified usually is given as part of a prescribed menu. Since more calories are allowed, a 1,500-calorie diet usually allows more freedom in substitutions than a 1,200-calorie diet.

BREAKFAST

2 5-inch-square by ½-inch-thick waffles with sliced strawberries or other fruit
28 gm./1 oz. lean ham, not fried
118 ml./4 fl. oz./½ cup plain skim yogurt
227 gm./1 cup strawberries, fruit, plain
Coffee, tea, plain, as desired

LUNCH

86 gm./3 oz. lean ground beef, not fried
1 hamburger bun
1 medium tomato, raw
Above, with dill pickle and mustard to taste may be made into a conventional hamburger
118 ml./4 fl. oz./½ cup plain skim yogurt
1 medium-size pear, raw or waterpack canned
Salad made of endive, raw cauliflower, 6 nuts, sugarless dressing; as much as patient wants
Coffee, tea, plain, as desired

DINNER

86 gm./3 oz. baked salmon
227 gm./1 cup spaghetti, plain
113 gm./½ cup cooked mushrooms, not fried
118 ml./4 fl. oz./½ cup skim milk
1 medium banana
.6 gm./1 tsp. butter
Salad made of watercress, radishes, celery, sugarless French dressing; as much as patient wants
Coffee, tea, plain, as desired

BEDTIME

237 ml./8 fl. oz./1 cup skim milk

40 The High-Protein Diet

The purpose of a high-protein diet is to aid the body in the growth and repair of tissue that has been wasted by disease or malnutrition. Clinical studies show that a high-protein diet can help prevent bedsores (Chapter 15) and speed the healing of them.

A high-protein diet is needed when there is a depletion or loss of protein in the body from any cause such as nutritional preparation (a special diet) before surgery . . . liver diseases including cirrhosis and hepatitis . . . and general malnutrition. The goal of a high-protein diet is to increase a patient's protein intake to two or more times that supplied by a normal diet having protein of high value.

A high-protein diet is essentially a normal or general diet (Chapter 32) with an increased amount of protein. However, the carbohydrates and fats usually are sharply reduced and the protein foods increased proportionately, as the purpose of a high-protein diet is to build or repair body tissue and not necessarily increase body weight; in fact, a sharp increase of weight could be harmful.

As with any type of medication, a high-protein diet should be used only as directed by your patient's doctor or dietitian. Your instructions will list the foods and portions allowed, the foods that should not be given, and how long your patient may be on the diet. In most cases, you will also be given daily or weekly menus. Be sure that they list items that are readily available in your shopping area, and priced within your budget. Most visiting nurses can give worthwhile shopping tips and suggestions.

To help keep a patient from gaining too much body weight, high-protein diets usually specify the maximum allowable amounts of certain foods and drinks. These should be measured with reasonable accuracy, although you generally need not be as accurate as when measuring for a low-calorie diet.

The items in the sample menus below are only suggestions, based on a balanced diet (Chapter 30). They may be changed to other allowed items to please your patient; but first ask the doctor or dietitian, or your visiting nurse.

Whether you make up your patient's diet or are given it, change it so that the same foods are not served on the same days of the week, or too often. If your patient says something like, "It must be Friday, fish again!" you should know that it is high time to change your menus.

SAMPLE 4-DAY HIGH-PROTEIN MENU

This sample menu provides approximately 130–140 gm./4.5–4.9 oz. of protein per day. If more is required, you usually add cottage or other nonfatty cheese, eggs, cocoa, dextrose or maltose, and additional casein. Also, commercially prepared powdered protein supplements can be added to milk and eggnogs. The addition of 75 ml./5 tbsp. of nonfat dry milk to 237 ml./8 fl. oz./1 cup of milk doubles its amount of protein.

The dairy product and meat groups (see Basic Food Groups, Chapter 30) provide the greatest amounts of protein. Rely heavily on these to supplement the regular or general diet (Chapter 32) when planning a high-protein diet:

Dairy Products	*Meat Group*
Cheese, cheddar, cottage	Beans, peas, dried
Ice cream	Beef
Milk	Eggs
Yogurt	Fish
	Lamb
	Nuts
	Pork
	Poultry
	Veal

DAY No. 1

BREAKFAST

1 orange or ½ grapefruit
118 ml./4 oz./½ cup enriched cereal with low-fat milk, sugar
2 eggs, any way except fried
1 slice whole-wheat bread or toast
15 ml./½ oz./1 pat butter or margarine
237 ml./8 oz./1 cup low-fat milk, or,
Coffee, tea with milk, sugar to taste

MIDMORNING

237 ml./8 oz./1 cup low-fat milk

LUNCH

120 gm./4.25 oz. or more meat, fish, or fowl
100 gm./3.5 oz. potato or rice any way except fried, dried beans, or spaghetti
100 gm./3.5 oz. vegetable salad (peas, carrots, beans, lettuce, tomatoes), low-fat dressing
1 slice whole-wheat or enriched white bread, toast
15 ml./½ oz./1 pat butter or margarine
118 ml./4 oz./½ cup canned, fresh, or frozen fruit
237 ml./ 8 oz./1 cup low-fat milk, or,
Coffee, tea with milk, sugar to taste

MIDAFTERNOON

237 ml./8 oz./1 cup low-fat milk

DINNER

120 gm./4.25 oz. or more meat or equivalent
100 gm./3.5 oz. potato, any way except fried
100 gm./3.5 oz. vegetable of choice
1 slice whole-wheat bread or toast
15 ml./½ oz./1 pat butter or margarine
118 ml./4 oz./½ cup milk-base dessert, such as pudding, ice cream, etc.
237 ml./8 oz./1 cup low-fat milk, or,
Coffee, tea with milk, sugar to taste

BEDTIME

237 ml./8 oz./1 cup eggnog made with low-fat milk, egg, sugar, flavoring

DAY No. 2

BREAKFAST

237 ml./8 oz./1 cup fresh berries
118 ml./4 oz./½ cup rolled-wheat cooked cereal with milk, sugar to taste
2 eggs, soft-boiled
1 slice whole-wheat toast
15 ml./½ oz./1 pat butter or margarine
237 ml./8 oz./1 cup low-fat milk, or,
Coffee, tea with milk, sugar to taste

MIDMORNING

237 ml./8 oz./1 cup low-fat milk, flavored

LUNCH

120 gm./4.25 oz. or more sliced cold roast beef
100 gm./3.5 oz. potato salad
100 gm./3.5 oz. sliced tomatoes, cooked carrots
1 whole-wheat or enriched white roll
15 ml./½ oz./1 pat butter or margarine
2 halves canned pears
237 ml./8 oz./1 cup low-fat milk, or,
Coffee, tea with milk, sugar to taste

MIDAFTERNOON

237 ml./8 oz./1 cup low-fat milk

DINNER

120 gm./4.25 oz. or more baked filet of sole
100 gm./3.5 oz. creamed potatoes
100 gm./3.5 oz. broccoli
1 slice enriched white bread or toast
15 ml./½ oz./1 pat butter or enriched margarine
118 ml./4 oz./½ cup custard pudding
237 ml./8 oz./1 cup low-fat milk, or,
Coffee, tea with milk, sugar to taste

BEDTIME

237 ml./8 oz./1 cup eggnog made with low-fat milk, egg, sugar, flavoring

DAY No. 3

BREAKFAST

½ grapefruit
118 ml./4 oz./½ cup cereal (dry wheat biscuits) with milk, sugar to taste
2 eggs, scrambled
1 slice whole-wheat bread or toast
15 ml./½ oz./1 pat butter or margarine
237 ml./8 oz./1 cup low-fat milk, or,
Coffee, tea with milk, sugar to taste

MIDMORNING

237 ml./8 oz./1 cup low-fat milk, flavored

LUNCH

120 gm./4.25 oz. or more ground beef patty
100 gm./3.5 oz. baked beans
100 gm./3.5 oz. tossed salad (lettuce, tomatoes, cucumbers, onions, avocado) with dressing of choice
1 slice enriched white bread or toast
15 ml./½ oz./1 pat butter or margarine
4–6 halves canned apricots
237 ml./8 oz./1 cup low-fat milk, or,
Coffee, tea with milk, sugar to taste

MIDAFTERNOON

237 ml./8 oz./1 cup milkshake or malted milk made with ice milk

DINNER

177 ml./6 oz./¾ cup cream of celery soup
120 gm./4.25 oz. or more baked chicken
100 gm./3.5 oz. mashed potatoes
100 gm./3.5 oz. steamed carrots
1 slice whole-wheat bread or toast
15 ml./½ oz./1 pat butter or margarine
118 ml./4 oz./½ cup cherry cobbler dessert
237 ml./8 oz./1 cup low-fat milk, or,
Coffee, tea with milk, sugar to taste

BEDTIME

237 ml./8 oz./1 cup milkshake made with ice milk

DAY No. 4

BREAKFAST

177 ml./6 oz./¾ cup orange juice
118 ml./4 oz./½ cup cooked oatmeal cereal with milk, sugar to taste
2 eggs, poached
1 slice whole-wheat bread or toast
15 ml./½ oz./1 pat butter or margarine
237 ml./8 oz./1 cup low-fat milk, or,
Coffee, tea with milk, sugar to taste

MIDMORNING

237 ml./8 oz./1 cup low-fat milk

LUNCH

120 gm./4.25 oz. creamed chicken over 100 gm./3.5 oz. noodles
100 gm./3.5 oz. carrots, raisin, apple salad with mayonnaise
1 slice enriched white bread
15 ml./½ oz./1 pat butter or margarine
237 ml./8 oz./1 cup low-fat milk, or,
Coffee, tea with milk, sugar to taste

MIDAFTERNOON

237 ml./8 oz./1 cup ice milk

DINNER

177 ml./6 oz./¾ cup cream of mushroom soup
120 gm./4.5 oz. or more roast lamb
100 gm./3.5 oz. baked potato
100 gm./3.5 oz. peas and onions
1 whole-wheat roll
15 ml./½ oz./1 pat butter or margarine
1 baked apple
237 ml./8 oz./1 cup low-fat milk, or,
Coffee, tea with milk, sugar to taste

BEDTIME

237 ml./8 oz./1 cup yogurt with fruit

41 The Low-Fat Diet

Digesting fats is difficult for many people, especially those with gallbladder or liver disturbances. In addition to medication, these patients usually are put on a low-fat diet that sharply restricts the use of butter, cream, eggs, and fats, but has little or no restriction of carbohydrates and protein. Some fats are, of course, required; the doctor or dietitian will prescribe what kinds and amounts your patient should have.

Because so much of the so-called good taste of many foods is due to their fat content, a low-fat diet may not at the start be very appetizing unless extra care is taken in choosing foods and serving them (Chapters 31, 47, and 48).

As is the case with any kind of medication, a low-fat diet should be used only as ordered by your patient's doctor or dietitian. You will receive full instructions as to the items and amounts allowed, those that should not be given, and how long your patient probably will be on the diet. As a rule, you also will be given daily or weekly menus. Make sure that they include items that are readily available in your marketing area. The dietitian or your visiting nurse can give you some helpful shopping information.

Below is a list of common food items usually allowed and banned by low-fat diets. Following this is a sample menu, based on a balanced diet (Chapter 30). Keep in mind, however, that these food items and meals are only suggestions or possibilities, and should not be used without the approval of your patient's medical advisors.

BASIC LOW-FAT DIET FOODS

Since a low-fat diet may be prescribed for weight control as well as, or instead of, digestive problems, be sure to find out what amounts your patient may have. In addition to the commonly allowed and banned foods, there is a group of "maybe's"—items that are often allowed by about as many doctors and dietitians as forbid them. In the following list, all items are freely allowed unless some sort of restriction or limitation is given.

Beverages: Plain coffee, coffee substitutes, tea; skim milk; buttermilk made from skim milk.

Bread: Whole-grain, enriched white; serve plain or toasted.

Bouillon, Broth: Fatfree types; avoid or skim fats from other bouillons, broths.

Cereal: Any kind, cooked or dry. Season to taste with nonfat or skim milk, sugar.

Desserts: Angel food cake, plain cake; fruit, see below; sherbets, fruit ices; puddings made with skim milk; gelatin.

Eggs: Whole eggs usually are strictly limited, but egg whites may be used as desired.

Fats, Oil, Shortenings: The use of most of these is limited to a bare minimum in a prescribed low-fat diet. The allowed items usually are soft margarines (liquid oil generally is listed on the label as the main ingredient); nonhydrogenated corn, cottonseed, safflower, soybean oils. AVOID: Butter, cream, most cream substitutes, hydrogenated margarine or shortening (read the package label carefully), lard, nondairy cream containing coconut oil, olive oil, peanut oil.

Fish: All except shellfish usually allowed. Broil, bake, poach (in nonfat milk). Low-fat cheese (made from skim milk), and low-fat cottage cheese often are substituted for fish.

Fowl: All poultry usually allowed except duck, goose. OMIT: fat, skin of all fowl. Same substitutes as for Fish, above.

Fruit: Nearly all fresh, frozen, canned, cooked fruit, fruit juice allowed, usually as much as a patient wants and can tolerate. AVOID: Avocado, olives; any item, such as raw apple, that may be gas-forming for your patient.

Meat: Low-fat diets usually allow *lean* pieces of beef, Canadian bacon, ham, lamb, pork, veal; bake, broil, stew, but do not fry. Same substitutes as for Fish, above. OMIT: Bacon (except lean Canadian), corned beef, frankfurters, fat or fatty (marbled) meat, fat adhering to meat (as in chops, steaks, roasts), gravies, regular hamburger, luncheon meats (cold cuts), meat drippings, organ meats (heart, liver, etc.), so-called prime cuts, salt pork, sausage.

Melons: Usually allowed if not gas-forming for your patient.

Milk: Skim or nonfat milk usually allowed, but often in limited quantity. AVOID: Whole milk, low-fat milk; see Fats, above.

Miscellaneous: Condiments, herbs, lemon juice, relishes, seasonings in general, sour pickles, spices usually are allowed in any quantity a patient wants and can tolerate.

Poultry: See Fowl, above.

Starch: Pasta (macaroni, noodles, etc.), potato, rice, sweet potato, yams usually are allowed served plain or with tomato sauce.

Vegetables: As a rule, you can serve as many raw or cooked vegetables as your patient wants and can tolerate. Use as wide a variety as your marketing area allows, being sure to include green leafy and yellow vegetables. Omit, of course, any vegetable that is gas-forming for your patient.

The "Maybe" Items Although there are many "diet" foods, beverages, and seasonings on the market, most of them are neither commonly accepted nor rejected by the medical world. There are, for example, about as many doctors who recommend as those who forbid the use of artificial sweeteners. Also, changes in the composition or manufacture of an item can alter a doctor's opinion of it and whether your patient should have it. Make it a point always to ask your patient's doctor or dietitian if a particular food, beverage, or seasoning may be used; be sure to give the brand name of the item. Among the common "diet" items found in regular food stores and markets are:

- Artificial salt, sweetening
- Cake, cookie mixes
- Cereals
- Fruit, fruit juice; fruit drinks
- Margarine
- Meat, meat substitutes
- Sherbet
- Soft drinks, carbonated, plain
- Vegetables

EXAMPLE OF LOW-FAT MENU

The quantity of each food allowed would, of course, be based on your patient's sex, age, general build, activity, and overall physical condition.

BREAKFAST
Citrus fruit
Cereal, whole grain or enriched, with skim milk, sugar
Egg, not fried
Bread, whole wheat or enriched white
Margarine, enriched
Skim milk, or
Coffee, tea with skim milk, sugar to taste

MIDMORNING
Skim milk

LUNCH
Cottage cheese
Potato, rice, or spaghetti
Salad with lemon or vinegar dressing
Vegetable
Bread, whole wheat
Margarine, enriched
Fruit
Milk, nonfat or skim; or,
Coffee, tea with skim milk, sugar to taste

MIDAFTERNOON
Citrus fruit

DINNER
Lean meat, fish, or fowl
Potato, plain (no butter or margarine)
Bread, whole wheat
Margarine
Dessert: fruit, or angel cake
Milk, nonfat or skim; or,
Coffee, tea with skim milk, sugar to taste

BEDTIME
Skim milk

General Daily Consumption From the following food groups, a total day's food consumption should be:

- Fruit—3 servings
- Vegetables—3 servings of 237 ml./8 oz./1 cup
- Cereals (include bread, pasta)—3 servings
- Desserts—2 servings
- Fats—3 servings
- Meat, fish, or fowl—118 ml./4 oz./½ cup
- Beverages—as desired

42 The Low-Cholesterol Diet

> NOTE: The basic theory of cholesterol in the body as presented here is widely but not universally accepted by the medical profession. If your patient's doctor subscribes to this theory of cholesterol, and saturated and polyunsaturated fats (Chapter 30), this chapter should be of great help in caring for your patient and explaining the need for the diet. However, do not be surprised if the doctor or dietitian prescribes a different diet.

Cholesterol is a fat-soluble substance present in body cells, animal fats, and tissues. There appears to be a relationship between the amount of cholesterol in a person's system and the condition of the person's heart; but it is not agreed whether a high level of cholesterol causes a heart condition, or is the result of a heart condition. However, it is generally agreed that a high level of cholesterol in a person should not be allowed to exist over a long period of time.

Although cholesterol is produced by the body, it is widely believed that most of the dangerously excessive amount comes from food. Some sort of "fat" is in most of our foods, and most fats are directly related to high and low cholesterol levels. Also, there are *cholesterol-rich* foods, primarily egg yolks, organ meats (heart, liver, etc.), and some shellfish. These are not fatty foods in the usual sense of the term, but are fairly high in a cholesterol that can be transmitted to the blood. The low-cholesterol diet is an attempt to prevent the accumulation of a high level of cholesterol in a person's blood by sharply reducing or even eliminating the intake of saturated fats, usually by replacing them with polyunsaturated fats, and avoiding cholesterol-rich foods.

Low-cholesterol diets can be every bit as varied and tasty as so-called regular meals. Most vegetables and fruit, certain fish and poultry, lean meats, some dairy products, breads, and cereals are allowed IF they are not prepared or served with saturated-fat foods; for example, cereal must not be served with cream or whole milk, but skim milk or nonfat milk is all right.

Sometimes a "low-fat–low-cholesterol" diet is prescribed. Basically this is a diet containing only foods that are allowed by a low-fat diet (Chapter 41) and a low-cholesterol diet. A food allowed by one diet but not by the other should not be used.

Your patient should, of course, be given a low-cholesterol diet only as ordered by the doctor. The dietitian will give instructions as to how you should or should not prepare certain foods as well as the foods and amounts that are allowed, and those that are not allowed. There should also be daily or weekly menus. Read them carefully, to be sure they contain foods that are readily available in your shopping area. The dietitian or your visiting nurse probably can give you some helpful shopping suggestions.

BASIC LOW-CHOLESTEROL DIET FOODS

Here are the foods usually allowed, and not allowed, in a low-cholesterol diet. Following this listing is a sample 7-day menu, based on a balanced diet (Chapter 30) of allowable low-cholesterol foods. When shopping for your patient, always study the labels carefully to determine if the ingredients are suitable.

BEVERAGES. Coffee, coffee substitutes, tea seasoned to taste with liquid or powdered skim or nonfat milk (see Milk) and a sweetener (see Sugar) usually are allowed in low-cholesterol diets. Also allowed are skim milk buttermilk, fruit ades (lemonade, orangeade, etc.), fruit and vegetable juices; and carbonated and plain soft drinks that are not made with hydrogenated oil. Low-cholesterol diets often limit or forbid alcoholic beverages.

BREADS. Any enriched white or whole-grain bread (including nonfat or very low-fat biscuits, French bread, muffins, rolls, etc.) is allowed in low-cholesterol diets, provided it is not made with butter, lard, or any form of whole egg or of coconut oil. Many bakeries feature bread items made with suitable vegetable oil and other allowable foods instead of saturated fats. There seldom is much difference in taste between these and high-cholesterol products.

BUTTER, see Milk.

CAKES, COOKIES. Same restrictions as for Breads.

AVOID: Packaged cake, cookie mixes. Most of them contain butter, lard, coconut oil, and sometimes powdered whole eggs or egg yolks.

CEREALS. Most low-cholesterol diets allow cooked whole-grain cereals (oatmeal, rolled oats, porridge, wheat, etc.) and dry cereals (cornflakes, exploded wheat and rice, etc.), seasoned to taste with reconstituted powdered skim or nonfat milk (see Milk) and a sweetener (see Sugar) or fruit.

DESSERTS. Desserts generally allowed by low-cholesterol diets are:

Angel food cake (see Cakes).

Bread pudding, if made with an allowed bread (see Breads) and skim milk.

Cornstarch, gelatin, rice, tapioca, and other cooked puddings made with liquid or powdered skim or nonfat milk (see Milk).

Fruit, canned, cooked, fresh, or frozen.

Sherbet, ices, unless made with animal fat or with any form of coconut oil. (Most commercial products contain coconut oil.)

All the above can be prepared and served in many ways to avoid food monotony for your patient. For example, colors and flavors of gelatin can be mixed, in plain or in whipped layers, with or without fruit, and served alone or with a wedge of angel food cake.

OMIT: Any cake, pudding, or other food made with chocolate, and instant puddings and other foods that contain animal fat, any form of coconut or coconut oil, or any hydrogenated oil or shortening.

DIET SPECIALTIES. Diet whipped cream, diet dessert topping, nondairy "creamers," artificial sweeteners, and similar items commercially developed for the "diet" market may or may not be allowed in your patient's diet. Many of these items contain coconut oil, often in relatively large amounts; other common ingredients are animal fat and hydrogenated oil. If you cannot tell from the listed ingredients on the package label whether your patient may have a particular product, ask the doctor, dietitian, nutritionist, or your visiting nurse. Be sure to specify the product by its brand or trade name and, if necessary, show a label from it.

EGGS. Egg whites in any form are allowed by most low-cholesterol diets. Cholesterol- and saturated-fat-free egg substitutes are widely available. As well as being suitable for breads and most other baked items, egg substitutes can make tasty scrambled eggs, crepes, omelets, almost everything that usually is made with whole eggs. Since powdered eggs have basically the same properties as fresh eggs, only the powdered whites are suitable for low-cholesterol diets; they are excellent for meringues.

| NOTE: A limited number of whole eggs, 2 or 3 per week, commonly is allowed.

FAT, SHORTENING. Because of high saturated-fat and cholesterol contents, animal fat in any form is held to a minimum in low-cholesterol diets.

Animal fat may be visible, such as so-called marbling . . . the layers of fat around chops, roasts, steaks . . . in a mixture of foods made into sausage and variety or luncheon meats . . . and lard shortening.

Animal fat may be nearly invisible, as in fatty meats such as Canadian bacon, ham, and other forms of pork . . . and in organ meats such as heart, kidney, liver, etc.

Many vegetable fats (see Oil) usually are allowed in low-cholesterol diets.

FISH. Most low-cholesterol diets are liberal in the use of fish, except some shellfish. As a rule, you may serve your patient canned, fresh, or frozen fish . . . baked, broiled, or poached in nonfat milk . . . provided it is cooked without whole eggs, saturated fat, hydrogenated shortening (see Oil), or most forms of milk.

There are many herbs, seafood, and other commercial seasonings suitable for fish. A few drops of lemon juice sprinkled on fish usually enhances its flavor. There are several homemade sauces that are easily adapted to fish (see Salad Dressings).

AVOID: Shellfish, such as abalone, clams, crab, crayfish, lobster, oysters, prawns, scampi, shrimp, etc., until after consulting with your patient's doctor or dietitian.

OMIT: Cream sauce, tartar sauce made with mayonnaise, drawn butter, mayonnaise, and any sauce made with animal fat and/or whole eggs and/or any type of cream or whole milk.

FLAVORINGS. Cinnamon, lemon, lime, nutmeg, orange, peppermint, vanilla, etc., are great aids in varying low-cholesterol diet desserts. But remember that cooking can change the taste of some flavorings.

OMIT: Chocolate, coconut in any form.

FRUIT, MELON. Except for coconut, nearly all canned, cooked, fresh, or frozen fruit and melons are allowed in most low-cholesterol diets. "Diet" packs have less sugar content, and in some cases are preferred to standard fruit packaging; ask your patient's doctor or dietitian about them. Powdered skim milk and homemade yogurt (see Milk) are common fruit toppings.

OMIT: Nuts, avocado.

JAM, JELLY. All jams and jellies, except those containing any form of coconut, usually are allowed in low-cholesterol diets. Your patient may prefer diet jams and jellies (see Diet Specialties) because of their low sugar content.

As well as being conventional spreads, jams and jellies are good for flavoring cottage cheese (see Milk). Some jellies, such as mint and orange, are often served with meat and fish.

JUICE, JUICE DRINKS. Provided they do not contain any form of coconut or a hydrogenated oil, fruit and vegetable juices and juice drinks are allowed in most low-cholesterol diets. Juice drinks have less real fruit or vegetable than a standard juice, and usually have more artificial flavoring and coloring.

"Slush," a snack and dessert generally liked by children, is easily made at home by freezing fruit juice or drink to a thick, mushy consistency. You can add body and nourishment to slush by whipping fresh or powdered egg white into the liquid before freezing it.

MARGARINE. Since there are so many margarines, be sure to examine the list of ingredients on a package before buying it for your patient. Margarines made from corn, cottonseed, safflower, and soybean oils usually are acceptable for low-cholesterol diets. However, margarines may or may not be made from 100 percent polyunsaturated vegetable oils (see Oil); they may contain coconut, peanut, or hydrogenated oils. The "soft" margarines usually have less saturated fat than the others.

Many people dislike the taste and odor of margarine in any form and at any time. Others do not object to it cold, but do not like it warm, as on hot biscuits or toast, or in cooking. If this is so with your patient, try disguising margarine with jam or jelly when serving it as a spread, and by using stronger seasoning when cooking. However, most people who are on low-cholesterol diets accept margarine, adapt themselves to it, or simply ask you not to serve it.

MEAT. Because of its high animal-fat content, meat consumption in low-cholesterol diets generally is limited to lean beef, lamb, and veal served only two or three times a week. How you select a meat, prepare it for cooking, and cook it often can somewhat reduce its saturated fat and cholesterol contents.

Selection. When visible fat (see Fat) can be trimmed off, as from chops and steak, the remaining meat, if not too heavily marbled, usually is acceptable. Trim off fat before cooking. But invisible fat, as in pork and organ meats, cannot be trimmed off and is extremely difficult to reduce adequately by cooking. Lean ground round usually is allowed in low-cholesterol diets; the many ways in which it can be served makes it generally popular with patients and nurses. It should, however, be ground to order, after all the fat is trimmed off, from *lean round steak* that you select. Do not buy hamburger that is already ground, since it may be nearly half fat; cooking will not remove or reduce the fat sufficiently.

Cooking Meat. How you cook meat, rather than how long you cook it, is the key to reducing the fat content:

When broiling, roasting, or baking meat, place it on a rack so that the melted fat will drain off.

Broil instead of pan-fry meats such as lean ground round, and chops and steak after removing all visible fat.

Do not baste meat with fat drippings. Instead, baste with wine or tomato juice.

Stews, soup stock, boiled meat, any cooking in which fat melts into the liquid or gravy should be done at least a day before you plan to serve it. When the food is cold, or fast-chilled in the refrigerator, skim off the hardened fat.

Gravies. Gravy made from fat or fatty drippings, and cream gravies, are not allowed by most low-cholesterol diets.

However, tasty meat gravy can be made from the liquid left after the fat is skimmed off. If it is not practical to wait for the fat to harden for skimming, pass an ice cube quickly (to minimize melting) through the fatty liquid several times; rinse off the coating of fat that hardens onto the cube. Repeat this procedure until there is no glitter of fat on the liquid. Some ice will melt into the meat liquor, but water is less harmful than saturated fat.

MILK, MILK PRODUCTS. Because of animal-fat content, cream, whole milk, canned milk, condensed milk, butter, ice cream and milk, most cheese except uncreamed low-fat cottage cheese, and dishes prepared with any of these foods are not allowed in most low-cholesterol diets.

Butter. Instead of butter, use a suitable margarine (see Margarine), disguised if necessary to make it more palatable for your patient.

Skim Milk. Liquid and powdered skim milk are generally permitted as is cheese made only from skim milk. Powdered skim milk is a very useful product, and most dieters accept it in a fairly short time. Tasty cold and hot drinks may be made by mixing powdered skim milk with water and a flavoring; for richer drinks, use twice the recommended amount of milk powder.

Puddings (see Desserts) may be made with liquid or powdered skim milk—and tastefully decorated with a dessert topping that resembles whipped cream made from powdered skim milk; recipes for this usually are on commercial packages of powdered skim milk.

Certain nondairy products (see Diet Specialties) are acceptable.

NONDAIRY PRODUCTS, see Diet Specialties.

NUTS. Nuts may be good snacks and, chopped or grated, handy toppings for puddings and fruit desserts. But first be sure to ask the doctor or dietitian if your patient may have them.

OIL, SHORTENING. Nonhydrogenated corn, cottonseed, safflower, sesame, soybean, and sunflower oils, and nonhydrogenated shortenings made 100 percent from them, are generally allowed in low-cholesterol diets. They may, however, be forbidden in a low-fat diet (Chapter 41). In case of doubt as to the polyunsaturated purity of an oil or shortening, ask your patient's dietitian about it.

NOTE: Petroleum or mineral oil may be prescribed as a medicinal, but normally is not used as part of a diet. *Do not give it to your patient except when ordered by the doctor.*

Acceptable vegetable oils, margarines, and shortenings are used in many ways in cooking that customarily require a "fat":

To brown lean meats, and to pan- or oven-fry fish and poultry. However, for browning meat, many cooks prefer to use nonstick pans (or a nonstick pan spray) and sear the meat without oil or shortening of any kind.

To sauté onions and other vegetables.

In cream sauces and soups made with skim milk.

In whipped and scalloped potatoes, with skim milk added.

For making bread, pie crust, cake, cookies.

For popping corn.

For making cocktail snacks.

In casseroles made with dried peas or beans.

In browning rice, and for Spanish and curried rices.

In cooking dehydrated potatoes and similar prepared foods that require fat to be added.

For pancakes, waffles, and crepes.

PANCAKES, WAFFLES. Pancakes and waffles usually are allowed in low-cholesterol diets IF they are prepared, cooked, and served with acceptable foods such as skim milk, safflower oil, egg substitutes, and so forth.

WHEAT GERM PANCAKES

237 ml./8 oz./1 cup enriched white flour
13 ml./8/10 oz./2½ tsp. baking powder
2.5 ml./1/6 oz./½ tsp. salt
15 ml./½ oz./1 tbsp. sugar
118 ml./4 oz./½ cup wheat germ, toasted with honey
296 ml./10 oz./1¼ cups skim milk
30 ml./1 oz./2 tbsp. acceptable vegetable oil
118 ml./4 oz./½ cup low-fat cottage cheese

Sift together flour, baking powder, salt, and sugar; add toasted wheat germ. Combine milk and oil, stir into dry ingredients just enough to moisten them. Add cottage cheese, mix to desired consistency. For a smooth batter, mix in a blender.

Drop batter by spoonfuls onto hot greased pan. Cook until bubbles appear on upper surface, then turn and brown other side. Makes ten 4-inch pancakes.

PASTRY, PIE. Pastries and pies have the same restrictions, as far as low-cholesterol diets are concerned, as breads and cakes (which see). Traditional flaky pie crusts and shells made with butter or most shortenings have far too much cholesterol, and if made with an acceptable margarine may not taste good to your patient. The crumb crust below has pleased many finicky eaters.

CRUMB CRUST FOR PIE

237 ml./8. oz/1 cup dry crumbs made from melba toast, graham crackers, cornflakes, or other crisp dry cereal
59 ml./2 oz./¼ cup sugar
30 ml./1 oz./2 tbsp. acceptable vegetable oil
1 ml./1/10 oz./¼ tsp. cinnamon

Preheat oven to 190°C/375°F.

Toss ingredients until they are well moistened with oil. Pack carefully into 9-inch pie pan, covering sides and bottom. Bake 10 minutes at 177°C/350°F. Fill with desired filling.

PEANUT BUTTER. Unfortunately, this popular snack and sandwich spread is not allowed in many low-cholesterol diets because of its monosaturated fat content. However, some doctors and dietitians do allow it, so if your patient wants peanut butter there is no harm in asking.

POULTRY. As they usually are prepared and cooked, chicken, duck, goose, squab, turkey, and most other wild and domesticated poultry are high in saturated fat and cholesterol. But they generally are allowed in low-cholesterol diets if the skin is first removed, either before or after cooking. There is a fairly thick layer of fat directly under the skin, but it is not absorbed by the meat; other fat deposits should not be eaten. For gravies, see Meat.

RELISHES. Many relishes such as pickles, mustards, pickle relishes, and so forth are useful in low-cholesterol diets. As a general rule, olives are not allowed. But before serving a relish, be sure that your patient is not also on a Bland or Ulcer Diet (Chapter 36).

SALAD DRESSINGS, MAYONNAISE. Many salad dressings are allowed by low-cholesterol diets. They also are commonly used, even those with a mayonnaise base, with hot and cold fish and vegetables.

Oil-and-Vinegar. For variety of taste, use different acceptable vegetable oils (see Oils) and vinegars (malt, red wine, seasoned, white distilled, and so forth) when making this traditional salad dressing. Also experiment by adding mustards, herbs, spices, and artificial seasonings.

Prepared Salad Dressings. There are many commercial salad dressings, both regular and diet types, which may be used "as is" or be changed by adding herbs, spices, pickle relish, flavored vinegar, etc. But before giving your patient a commercial salad dressing, examine the list of ingredients for forbidden items such as coconut or a hydrogenated oil.

Dry-Mix Salad Dressing Preparations. Some of these specify mixing with cream, whole milk, or whole buttermilk, which are not allowed by the average low-cholesterol diet. You usually will get good results by mixing instead with nonfat milk, nonfat buttermilk, skim milk, or reconstituted powdered skim milk or buttermilk.

Lemon Juice. Instead of a dressing, many people like to sprinkle lemon juice on salad. Try seasoning it with various herbs and spices.

Mayonnaise. Mock or imitation mayonnaise can easily be made at home, below. There also are commercial imitation mayonnaises, but before buying examine the list of ingredients for forbidden items such as coconut oil, peanut oil, hydrogenated oils, and liquid or powdered whole eggs or egg yolks.

MOCK MAYONNAISE

You may make this with a rotary beater or in a food blender.

2.5 ml./1/6 oz./¼ tsp. salt
5 ml./1/3 oz./½ tsp. dry mustard
5 ml./1/3 oz./½ tsp. sugar
Dash of red pepper or paprika
1 egg white
237 ml./8 oz./1 cup allowed vegetable oil
45 ml./3 oz./4½ tsp. vinegar.

Rotary Beater. Stir salt, mustard, sugar, and pepper together in a bowl. Add egg white, beat until foamy with rotary beater. While continuing to beat, add half the oil a little at a time; then add a third of the vinegar, then the remaining oil little by little, then the remaining vinegar.

Food Blender. Put salt, mustard, sugar, pepper, and egg white into blender, cover, and blend at medium speed for about 2 seconds. By just turning the blender on and off with each addition, blend in half the oil, 2 tbsp. at a time; stir in the last portions of oil with a long-handled rubber or plastic spatula, if necessary. Blend in 1½ tsp. vinegar, then 6 tbsp. of oil 2 tbsp. at a time. Continue blending in the remaining 3 tsp. of vinegar, then the remaining 2 tbsp. of oil.

BUTTERMILK-HERB DRESSING

237 ml./8 oz./1 cup buttermilk
15 ml./½ oz./1 tbsp. prepared mustard
5 ml./1/3 oz./1 tsp. minced onion
1 ml./1/25 oz./⅛ tsp. each dried dillweed, salt
10 ml./2/3 oz./2 tsp. finely chopped fresh parsley or 5 ml./1/3 oz./1 tsp. dried parsley
Dash of black pepper

Combine all ingredients in a covered jar, shake well to blend. Chill overnight or several hours before serving. Can be stored in refrigerator for 1 week.

YOGURT DRESSING

10 ml./2/3 oz./2 tsp. lemon juice
15 ml./½ oz./1 tbsp. acceptable vegetable oil
118 ml./4 oz./½ cup plain yogurt from skim milk
3 ml./1/6 oz./½ tsp. each paprika, salt
1 ml./1/25 oz./⅛ tsp. garlic powder
Dash of Tabasco sauce

Mix all ingredients in blender for 5 minutes at medium speed.

SAUCES. Most modern cookbooks have recipes for sauces for low-cholesterol diets; however, be sure that all the ingredients are allowed your patient. Or you may wish to change a forbidden sauce to one suitable for your patient; often this can be done by substituting a few ingredients, such as safflower for coconut, peanut, or olive oil, and using egg white or egg substitute (see Eggs) instead of whole eggs or egg yolks.

To avoid food monotony, you may change or add acceptable ingredients to the following sauces.

ALL-PURPOSE SAUCE FOR MEAT, FISH, POULTRY

44 ml./1½ oz./3 tbsp. acceptable vegetable oil
30 ml./1 oz./2 tbsp. each chopped onion and chopped green pepper
118 ml./4 oz./½ cup sliced fresh or canned mushrooms
473 ml./16 oz./2 cups stewed or fresh tomatoes
3 ml./1/6 oz./½ tsp. salt
Dash of pepper
Optional: Few drops of Tabasco sauce. 3 ml./1/6 oz./½ tsp. basil

Cook onion, green pepper, and mushrooms in oil over low heat for about 5 minutes. Add tomatoes, seasonings, and simmer until sauce is thick, usually about 30 minutes.

Here are three suggested recipes using this All-Purpose Sauce:

Meat Casserole: Cut lean veal or other meat into bite-size cubes, and brown in pan on top of stove or under the broiler. Combine with All-Purpose Sauce, cover, and cook gently or simmer on top of stove, or bake in 177°C/350°F oven, for about 1 hour.

Fish: Add cooked fish to All-Purpose Sauce, heat thoroughly, and serve on rice. Or pour heated sauce on broiled or baked fish.

Poultry: Cut poultry into bite-size pieces, brown in vegetable oil; add All-Purpose Sauce, cover, cook slowly or simmer until poultry is tender. Or place raw poultry pieces and sauce in a baking dish and bake in 177°C/350°F oven until tender, basting occasionally.

NOTE: To get the full flavor of the sauce into the poultry meat, remove skin before cooking.

HERB SAUCE

59 ml./2 oz./¼ cup/½ stick margarine
3 ml./⅛ oz./⅙ tsp. each thyme and crushed rosemary leaves

Melt margarine in a small saucepan, stir in herbs.

Serve Herb Sauce on cooked peas, green beans, zucchini, and other vegetables.

Herbs other than thyme and rosemary may, of course, be used. This is an excellent sauce for experimenting—but be careful! Mixed herbs can produce odors and tastes that are not always popular.

SEASONINGS, HERBS, AND SEASONED SALTS. Herbs and nearly all seasonings except chocolate and coconut are allowed in low-cholesterol diets. Some commercial seasonings may contain coconut or peanut oil or other forbidden ingredients; examine carefully the listed contents on each label. Also, be sure that your patient is not on a Bland or Ulcer Diet (Chapter 36) that may forbid certain seasonings.

SHORTENING, see Oil.

SNACKS. Any food allowed by a low-cholesterol diet is suitable for a snack. However, snacks generally should not be large enough to constitute a meal, nor should there be so many between-meal snacks as to spoil your patient's normal mealtime appetite. However, snacks can be important nutritional aids for people who are small, finicky, fussy eaters.

SPREADS. Conventional spreads such as strained honey, jam, jelly, margarine, and so forth for breads are welcome in most low-cholesterol diets, as they can do so much to make food attractive to bed-weary patients. Cinnamon or nutmeg mixed with granulated sugar (about 1 part spice to 5 parts sugar) liberally sprinkled on margarine may make it more acceptable to people who do not like the taste of margarine.

SWEETENERS. Honey (raw or processed), sugar (brown, white, granulated, powdered), and most other natural sweeteners (corn syrup, maple sugar and syrup, etc.) are allowed in low-cholesterol diets, but generally should be used in moderation.

> NOTE: Commercial artificial sweeteners may or may not be allowed, depending on their contents and your patient's condition. Before serving any, be sure to consult your patient's doctor.

THICKENERS. Arrowroot, cornstarch, rice flour, wheat flour, and other foods that do not contain saturated fat or cholesterol may be used for thickening sauces, gravies, soups, and so forth in most low-cholesterol diets.

VEGETABLES. All vegetables generally are allowed in low-cholesterol diets, provided they are not prepared or served with forbidden foods such as butter, lard, cream, whole milk, cheese (except uncreamed cottage cheese), ham, pork, coconut or peanut oil, hydrogenated oil, whole eggs, egg yolks, and so on. Vegetables that you serve hot for one meal may be used in a salad a few meals later. Low-cholesterol sauces can be colored and flavored to go well with vegetables. Herbs and spices can do much to change the taste of vegetables and make them more attractive to fussy eaters. Here are several popular combinations of herbs and vegetables:

Rosemary with peas, cauliflower, squash
Oregano with zucchini
Dill with green beans, carrots
Marjoram with Brussels sprouts, carrots, spinach
Basil or dill with tomatoes

Chopped parsley and chives, sprinkled on just before serving, enhances the flavor and appearance of many vegetables.

Cooking Vegetables: Boil, steam, or pressure cook vegetables. With suitable utensils, cook in a microwave oven.

SAMPLE 7-DAY MENU FOR LOW-CHOLESTEROL DIETS

Most of the foods suggested here usually are prepared with one or more items that are not allowed in low-cholesterol diets. Suitable substitutions are easily made (egg whites for whole eggs, liquid or powdered skim milk instead of whole milk, margarine for butter, etc.), and as a rule there will be no appreciable change in taste or appearance. However, some changes in seasoning or amounts of ingredients may be needed, and this can be a trial-and-error experiment; for best results, tell your patient what changes you have made and ask for suggestions. Bookstores and public libraries usually have or will get for you cookbooks that are primarily for medical diets or have worthwhile sections devoted to them. Also, booklets regarding low-cholesterol diet foods generally are available free or at very low cost through your visiting nurse, Public Health Department, or American Heart Association.

Recommended amounts of food usually are given in a low-cholesterol diet prescribed by a doctor. Amounts are, of course, based on a patient's age, sex, physical build, activity, and general condition.

Remember that the foods listed in the following menus are only suggestions, based on a balanced diet (Chapter 30). Change the meals to satisfy your patient's likes and dislikes, but maintain a proper balance of foods. You should also ask your visiting nurse for menu suggestions based on the meat, produce, etc., that are available in your shopping area. AND—when buying any packaged food examine the list of ingredients carefully to make sure that they are allowed your low-cholesterol-diet patient!

DAY No. 1

BREAKFAST

Orange or tomato juice
French toast, made with egg substitute and acceptable oil
Powdered skim milk drink, or
Coffee, tea with liquid or powdered skim milk, sugar to taste

MIDMORNING

Fruit or berries

LUNCH

Uncreamed cottage cheese vegetable salad
Toast with margarine, jam, or jelly
Fruit, canned or fresh peaches
Juice drink, or
Coffee, tea with skim milk, sugar to taste

MIDAFTERNOON

Fruit juice and crackers (saltine or graham)

DINNER

Broiled hamburger patties
Whipped/mashed potatoes, green peas
Tossed green salad, vinegar-and-oil dressing
Bread or toast, whole wheat
Sherbet
Skim milk, or
Coffee, tea with skim milk, sugar to taste

BEDTIME

Cornstarch or rice pudding, skim milk

DAY No. 2

BREAKFAST

Fruit juice
Applesauce
Scrambled eggs (egg substitute)
Toast, margarine, jelly or jam
Skim milk, or
Coffee, tea with liquid or powdered skim milk, sugar to taste

MIDMORNING

Gelatin dessert

LUNCH

Uncreamed cottage cheese and fruit salad
English muffin or toast, margarine
Skim milk, flavored, or
Coffee, tea with liquid or powdered skim
milk, sugar to taste

MIDAFTERNOON

Apple or banana

DINNER

Vegetable soup
Steak, lean, broiled
Baked potato, carrots
Angel food cake
Coffee, tea with liquid or powdered skim milk, sugar to taste

BEDTIME

Fruit juice

DAY No. 3

BREAKFAST

Fruit juice
Half grapefruit
Cereal
Toast, jam
Skim milk, or
Coffee, tea with liquid or powdered skim milk, sugar to taste

MIDMORNING

Bread pudding, made from approved bread

LUNCH

Creole rice with mushrooms
Vegetable, lettuce salad with acceptable dressing
Sliced fruit
Skim milk, flavored, or
Coffee, tea with liquid or powdered skim milk, sugar to taste
Bread pudding

MIDAFTERNOON

Fruit slush

DINNER

Lean meat and vegetable stew
Whole-wheat bread
Tossed green salad
Fruit pie, crumb crust (see Pastry, Pie)
Skim milk, or
Coffee, tea with skim milk, sugar to taste

BEDTIME

Angel food cake

DAY No. 4

BREAKFAST

Fruit juice
Stewed apricots
Oatmeal or dry cereal, skim milk, sugar to taste
Cinnamon toast
Skim milk, flavored, or
Coffee, tea with liquid or powdered skim milk, sugar to taste

MIDMORNING

Fruit juice, saltine crackers

LUNCH

Roast chicken
Baked noodles with mushroom sauce
Carrots, broccoli
Fruit cocktail or compote
Juice drink, or
Coffee, tea with liquid or powdered skim milk, sugar to taste

MIDAFTERNOON

Fruit juice or dish of fresh fruit

DINNER

Broiled fish with herb sauce
Scalloped potatoes, green peas
Lettuce and tomato salad
Pudding
Coffee, tea with liquid or powdered skim milk, sugar to taste

BEDTIME

Fruit gelatin

DAY No. 5

BREAKFAST

Apple or apple juice
Scrambled eggs (egg substitute)
Cornmeal muffins, jelly, enriched margarine
Skim milk, or
Coffee, tea with liquid or powdered skim milk, sugar to taste

MIDMORNING

Orange or banana

LUNCH

Tomato soup
Sliced turkey sandwich on French bread
Grated carrot and apple salad
Coffee, tea with liquid or powdered skim milk, sugar to taste

MIDAFTERNOON

Grapefruit or other fruit juice

DINNER

Lamb or lamb chops with mint sauce or jelly
Boiled potatoes, green beans
Lettuce salad, buttermilk-herb dressing (see Salad Dressing)
Baked apple
Coffee, tea with skim milk, sugar to taste

BEDTIME

Hot cocoa made with skim milk

DAY No. 6

BREAKFAST

Grape juice
Cooked or dry cereal, skim milk, sugar to taste
Cinnamon or jelly toast
Skim milk, or
Coffee, tea with liquid or powdered skim milk, sugar to taste

MIDMORNING

Banana

LUNCH

Green pepper stuffed with rice, lean ground beef
Uncreamed cottage cheese salad with sliced tomatoes
Bread or toast
Mixed cut-up fruit (apple, banana, grapes, orange, etc.)
Skim milk, or
Coffee, tea with liquid or powdered skim milk, sugar to taste

MIDAFTERNOON

Apple or orange

DINNER

Roast chicken
Broccoli with lemon juice, mashed potatoes
Salad (shredded lettuce, carrots, chopped sweet pickles)
Pumpkin chiffon pie, graham cracker crumb crust (see Pastry, Pie)
Skim milk, or
Coffee, tea with liquid or powdered skim milk, sugar to taste

BEDTIME

Skim milk

DAY No. 7

BREAKFAST

Orange juice
Dry cereal or wheat germ pancakes (see Pancakes)
Muffin with margarine, jelly
Skim milk, flavored, or
Coffee, tea with liquid or powdered skim milk, sugar to taste

MIDMORNING

Fruit or slush

LUNCH

Beef and vegetable soup
Head of lettuce salad with lemon juice
French bread, or roll
Skim milk, or
Coffee, tea with liquid or powdered skim milk, sugar to taste

MIDAFTERNOON

Tapioca pudding

DINNER

Roast beef or lamb
Mashed/whipped potatoes, mixed vegetables
Uncreamed cottage cheese and fruit salad
Whole-wheat bread or toast, jelly
Gingerbread square, with powdered skim milk diet whipped cream
Coffee, tea with liquid or powdered skim milk, sugar to taste

BEDTIME

Gelatin dessert, fruit mix

NOTE I: Whether you make up or are given your patient's menu, change it every so often to keep from serving the same foods too often or on the same days of the week. Remember, if your patient ever says something like, "It must be Tuesday, cottage cheese salad for lunch," you have not been changing the diet sufficiently.

NOTE II: Midmorning, -afternoon, and bedtime snacks are optional. Do not overfeed your patient.

43 Low-Sodium Diets

Persons whose circulation of blood would be impaired by the retention of liquids, and others with certain heart or kidney conditions often are put on low-sodium diets. Formerly, low-sodium diets tended to be quite drastic as to the foods they forbade. But today, due to the potent diuretics available (agents that increase the excretion of body fluids), low-sodium diets usually are less restrictive; in fact, people often have very little feeling of being on a diet. Common table salt (sodium chloride) and any seasoning containing sodium are the principal forbidden items.

NOTE: Artificial "table salt" or salt substitute may be allowed. But be sure to ask the doctor or dietitian which brand is best for your patient.

Sodium-restricted diets generally are classified as:

Mild. This restricts the amount of sodium to half the normal intake, or approximately 2,500 mg. per day. Very little salt should be used during the preparation of food, and none at the table.

Moderate. A total of only 1,000 mg. of sodium is allowed in a moderate diet.

A quarter-teaspoon of salt contains about 575 mg. sodium. One shake of salt contains about 200 mg. sodium.

Strict. All foods should be prepared and eaten without salt.

NOTE: The doctor or dietitian will of course specify the amount of sodium allowed in your patient's diet.

As in the case with any medical treatment, a low-sodium diet should be used only as prescribed and directed by your patient's doctor or dietitian. You will be given all necessary instructions as to the foods and amounts allowed, how they should be prepared, the food that should not be used, and how long your patient may have to stay on the diet. Also, you probably will be given daily or weekly menus. Make sure that they include foods that are readily available where you shop. Your visiting nurse very likely can give you some good buying suggestions.

Based on sodium content and the severity of the diet in which they are allowed, food substances are graded as Mild, Moderate, and Strict. In the following lists the amount of sodium in one unit of a food is given. Information on low-sodium menus is at the end of this chapter.

NOTE: Foods for sodium-restricted diets are, of course, in the four basic food groups: Dairy Products, Meats, Fruit and Vegetables, and Breads and Cereals (Chapter 30). A low-sodium diet should be well balanced.

Generally you can substitute freely among food substances having the same sodium content per equal units. You must, however, make proper adjustment when substituting foods that have different amounts of sodium per unit. For example, if Food A has 10 mg. of sodium per unit of 227 gm./8 oz. and the same unit of Food B has 20 mg., then a half-unit (113.5 gm./4 oz.) of B has the same sodium content as, and could substitute for, a whole unit of A.

FOODS ALLOWED AND NOT ALLOWED IN A MILD (2,500 MG.) SODIUM-RESTRICTED DIET

This is the basic list of foods allowed in sodium-restricted diets. Some of these foods are forbidden in Moderate and Strict Sodium-Restricted Diets, and added to the foods not allowed in the Mild Diet. The amount of any of the allowed foods that you may serve your patient depends on the total amount of sodium allowed by the prescribed diet.

NOTE: Omit any food that seems to give your patient gas or other discomfort.

DAIRY PRODUCTS, MILD SODIUM DIET

Foods Allowed. One unit, 237 ml./8 oz./1 cup, of any of the following foods provides a negligible amount of sodium:

Evaporated whole milk, reconstituted (water added)
Nonfat buttermilk, unsalted
Nonfat powdered milk
Skim milk
Whole milk
Whole milk buttermilk, unsalted
Low-fat milk

Foods not allowed. All commercial foods made of milk:

- Butter, salted
- Chocolate milk
- Condensed milk
- Ice Cream
- Ice milk
- Malted milk
- Milk mixes
- Milkshakes
- Sherbets

MEAT (FISH, POULTRY), MEAT SUBSTITUTES, MILD SODIUM DIET

Foods Allowed. One unit is 28.3 gm./1 oz. cooked food, and contains 25 mg. of sodium:

- Meat, poultry, fresh, frozen, or canned:
- Beef
- Lamb
- Liver (beef, calf, chicken, lamb, pork)
- Pork, fresh only
- Poultry
- Rabbit
- Tongue
- Veal

Fish, fresh, frozen, or water-pack canned, all including shellfish as allowed by the doctor or dietitian.

Meat Substitutes. Each specified unit, below, contains 25 mg. of sodium:

- American cheddar cheese—28.3 gm./1 oz.
- Cottage cheese, lightly salted—56.6 gm./ 2 oz./¼ cup
- Egg—1
- Peanut butter, low-sodium (see label)—59.2 ml./2 tbsp.
- Swiss cheese—28.3 gm./1 oz.

Fats. Each specified unit, below, contains a negligible amount of sodium:

- Butter, sweet or unsalted—9.9 ml./1 tsp.
- Cooking fat, oil—9.9 ml./1 tsp.
- Cream, heavy, sweet or sour—29.6 ml./1 tbsp.
- Cream, light, sweet or sour—59.2 ml./2 tbsp.
- French dressing—29.6 ml./1 tbsp.
- Margarine, unsalted—9.9 ml./1 tsp.
- Mayonnaise—9.9 ml./1 tsp.
- Nuts, unsalted—6 small

Foods not Allowed:

- Any canned or frozen meat to which sodium has been added; study label
- Bacon, bacon fat
- Brains
- Commercial salads and dressings, unless they are a low-sodium dietetic type approved by your patient's doctor or dietitian
- Corned meat
- Dried beef
- Frankfurters, hotdogs
- Ham
- Kidneys
- Luncheon meats (cold cuts)
- Olives
- Salt pork
- Sausage
- Smoked meats
- Sweetbreads

FRUITS AND VEGETABLES, MILD SODIUM-RESTRICTED DIET

Foods Allowed Fruit: fresh, frozen, canned, cooked, or dried. Each specified unit, below, contains 2 mg. of sodium:

- Apples, blackberries, oranges, raspberries, strawberries, melons—237 ml./8 oz./1 cup
- Applesauce, banana, fruit cup or mixed fruit, grapefruit, mango, tangerine—118.3 ml./4 oz./½ cup
- Apple juice or cider, cranberry juice, pineapple juice, orange juice, grapefruit juice—76.9 ml./2.7 oz./⅓ cup
- Apricot nectar, grape juice, prune juice—59.2 ml./2 oz./¼ cup
- Apple, fig, pear, orange, peach, tangerine—1 medium-size
- Apricot—2 medium-size
- Banana—½
- Cherries—10
- Dates—2
- Grapefruit—½ medium-size
- Grapes—12
- Plums, prunes—2

NOTE: If calories are restricted, avoid glazed or sweetened fruit, and those canned in heavy syrup.

Vegetables: For simpler listing, vegetables are listed in three groups based on sodium content per unit:

Group I. One unit, 237 ml./8 oz./1 cup, of any of the following provides a negligible amount of sodium:

- Asparagus
- Bean sprouts
- Broccoli
- Brussels sprouts
- Cabbage
- Cauliflower
- Chicory
- Cucumber
- Eggplant
- Endive
- Escarole
- Green beans
- Lettuce
- Mushrooms
- Mustard greens
- Okra
- Peppers, red, green
- Radishes
- Squash, summer; yellow; zucchini
- Tomato juice, unsalted
- Tomatoes
- Turnip greens
- Wax beans

Group II. Of each of the following, one unit, 118.3 ml./4 oz./½ cup, provides 9 mg. of sodium:

- Onions
- Peas, fresh, dehydrated; no frozen
- Pumpkin
- Rutabaga
- Squash, acorn, butternut, Hubbard, winter
- Turnip, white, green

Group III. Each specified unit, below, provides 5 mg. of sodium:

- Beans, baked—59.2 ml./2 oz./¼ cup
- Beans, dry lima or navy, cooked—118.3 ml./4 oz./½ cup
- Beans, fresh or frozen lima, cooked—78.9 ml./2.7 oz./⅓ cup
- Corn—½ small ear or 78.9 ml./2.7 oz./

Cowpeas, dried split green or yellow, cooked—118.3 ml./4 oz. /½ cup
Hominy—118.3 ml./4 oz./½ cup
Lentils, dried, cooked—118.3 ml./ 4 oz./½ cup
Parsnips—157.7 ml./5.3 oz./⅔ cup
Peas, cooked—118.3 ml./4 oz./½ cup
Rice, cooked—118.3 ml./4 oz./½ cup
Sweet potato—½ small or 59.2 ml. /2 oz./¼ cup
White potato—1 small
White potato, mashed/whipped—118.3 ml./4 oz./½ cup

BREADS AND CEREALS, MILD SODIUM-RESTRICTED DIET

Foods Allowed Breads. Each specified unit, below, provides 200 mg. of sodium:

Biscuit, roll—1
Bread—1 slice
Cornbread—1 1½-in. cube
Melba toast—4 pieces 3⅓ x 1½ x 1 in.
Muffin—1 medium-size
Pancakes—2 3-in. cakes
Waffle, yeast—1 3-in. square

Cereals: cooked, slightly salted. Each 118.3 ml./4 oz./½ cup unit of the following provides 200 mg. of sodium:

Farina
Grits
Oatmeal, old-fashioned, not instant
Rolled wheat
Wheat meal

Cereals: dry. Each specified unit, below, provides 200 mg. of sodium:

Shredded wheat—⅔ large biscuit
Other dry cereals—177.4 ml./6 oz./¾ cup minimum

Miscellaneous "grain" products. Each specified unit, below, provides 200 mg. of sodium:

Barley, uncooked—44.4 ml./1½ oz./1½ tbsp.
Cornmeal—59.2 ml./2 oz./2 tbsp.
Crackers, low-sodium dietetic—5 2-in. square
Flour—73.9 ml./2½ oz./2½ tbsp.
Macaroni, cooked—118.3 ml./4 oz./½ cup
Matzo, plain—1 5-in. square
Noodles, cooked—118.3 ml./4 oz./½ cup
Popcorn, homemade, no salt; only unsalted butter, fat, or margarine—354.9 ml./12 oz. /1½ cups
Rice, brown or white, cooked—118.3 ml./4 oz./½ cup
Spaghetti, cooked—118.3 ml./4 oz./½ cup
Tapioca, uncooked—59.2 ml./2 oz./2 tbsp.

FREE FOODS FOR MILD, MODERATE, AND STRICT SODIUM-RESTRICTED DIETS

The following foods contain so little sodium that they generally are allowed in all sodium-restricted diets in reasonable amount. But because there may be a reason other than sodium control that has kept them off the list of allowables given you, be sure to ask the doctor or dietitian before serving them to your patient.

Beverages, low-calorie and carbonated, usually allowed if sweetened by calcium cyclamate, not sodium cyclamate. Examine the label.

Candy, unless your patient's caloric intake is restricted, usually is allowed in reasonable amount IF it is homemade without salt.

Coffee, coffee substitutes, tea as a rule are allowed in moderation with milk, cream, sugar to taste. Examine the labels of special mixes or preparations of these items to see if sodium has been added.

Herbs and spices are excellent for making meals more appetizing. Here are some suggestions:

- Allspice—ground meats, peaches, stews, tomatoes
- Bay leaf—meats, poultry, soup, stews, tomatoes
- Dill—pot roasts
- Ginger—chicken, fruit
- Mint—fruit, lamb, peas
- Mustard, dry—meats, salads, sauces
- Nutmeg—cottage cheese, fruit, pie crust, potatoes
- Oregano—beef, pork
- Parsley—braised meat, peas, potatoes

Honey, jam, jelly, marmalade, or syrup usually are allowed in small amounts at a meal unless your patient is on a calorie-restricted diet.

Lemon, lime juices usually are allowed in reasonable amount as flavorings.

Nuts, unsalted, usually permitted in reasonable amount.

Seasonings such as celery, garlic, onion flakes or juices to which no sodium has been added. DO NOT use any seasoned salts, including celery, garlic, and onion salt.

Sugar, unless your patient's caloric intake is restricted, usually is allowed in reasonable amount for flavoring coffee, tea.

Tomato juice, unsalted, with garlic, green pepper, or onion may be an appetizing base for your patient's chops, roast, steak, or ground meat patties.

FOODS FORBIDDEN IN SODIUM-RESTRICTED DIETS

Regardless of the severity of a sodium-restricted diet, there are some substances that are forbidden almost without exception. These foods have a high sodium content, it being used mainly as either a flavoring or a preservative:

- Bouillon soup
- Broth
- Canned, dried soups
- Catsup
- Celery salt
- Garlic salt
- Instant cereals, desserts, soups
- Meat tenderizers

Olives
Onion salt
Pickles, all kinds
Prepared mustard
Relishes
"Seasoning" salts of any kind, for any purpose
Sauces in general, especially soy sauce, meat sauce, steak sauce, etc.

FOODS ALLOWED AND NOT ALLOWED IN MODERATE AND STRICT SODIUM-RESTRICTED DIETS

The foods allowed and not allowed by the Mild Sodium-Restricted Diet are the basis of the Moderate and Strict Diets. The contents of these two diets are found by eliminating various foods allowed by the Mild Diet.

DAIRY PRODUCTS, MODERATE AND STRICT SODIUM-RESTRICTED DIETS

All dairy products allowed in the Mild Diet are allowed by the Moderate and Strict diets, except that buttermilk must be unsalted.

If your patient is on a diet of less than 2500 mg. of sodium, it is necessary to use small amounts of low-sodium milk products. Ask the doctor or dietitian which of these suitable products are available in your marketing area.

MEAT (FISH, POULTRY, MEAT SUBSTITUTES), MODERATE AND STRICT SODIUM-RESTRICTED DIETS

Foods not Allowed (Eliminated from meats allowed by the Mild Diet):

Brain
Clams
Crab
Kidney
Lobster
Scallops
Scampi
Shrimp

Restrictions on other meat foods:

Canned meat, fish, and poultry must be of a low-sodium dietetic type.
Cottage cheese should be unsalted, and all other cheese should be of a low-sodium dietetic type.
Eggs are limited to one per day.
Fish. Use only fresh or dietetically canned (unsalted) fish.

FATS: The same fat foods listed in the Mild Sodium-Restricted Diet are allowed in the Moderate and Strict Diets.

FRUIT AND VEGETABLES, MODERATE AND STRICT SODIUM-RESTRICTED DIETS

FRUIT: All fruit allowed for the Mild Diet can be served in the Moderate and Strict Sodium-Restricted Diets.

VEGETABLES: All vegetables allowed for the Mild Diet are also allowed by the Moderate and Strict Diets except:

- Beet greens
- Celery
- Chard, Swiss
- Dandelion greens
- Mustard greens
- Kale
- Lima beans, frozen
- Peas, frozen
- Spinach
- Tomato juice should be a dietetic type with a very low or no sodium content

BREADS AND CEREALS, MODERATE AND STRICT SODIUM-RESTRICTED DIETS

The foods allowed in the breads and cereals listing of the Mild Diet may be used for Moderate and Strict Sodium-Restricted Diets except:

- Bread, yeast rolls, and cooked cereals must be made without salt.
- Quick breads such as biscuits and coffee cake must be made with either sodium-free baking powder or low-sodium dietetic mixes. Read the labels on these packaged goods carefully.
- A dry cereal must have no more than 6 mg. of sodium per 100 gm. of cereal. Again, read the package label carefully.
- DO NOT USE SELF-RISING CORNMEAL, FLOUR, GRAHAM CRACKERS, SALTED POPCORN, POTATO CHIPS, AND PRETZELS!

MENUS FOR SODIUM-RESTRICTED DIETS

As a rule, you will be given a daily or weekly menu specifying the foods and amounts allowed by the sodium-restricted diet prescribed for your patient; the foods should be listed according to the Basic Food Groups, Chapter 30, for a balanced diet. If there are foods that your patient particularly likes and wants that are neither allowed nor forbidden by the diet material, ask the doctor, dietitian, or nutritionist about them.

If planning the menu is entrusted to you, be sure to follow the requirements for a balanced diet, especially as to selecting foods from each basic group (Chapter 30), but omitting the items not allowed your patient. It is not particularly difficult to plan menus for sodium-restricted diets, once you have made a list of all the foods allowed.

44 Calcium, Low-Gluten, Phosphorous, and Potassium Diets

Calcium, Low-Gluten, Phosphorous, and Potassium diets seldom are prescribed for home nursing or entrusted to inexperienced nurses. The meals are not necessarily difficult to prepare, but a patient's reaction to special diets such as these can change in a very short time. Some changes can be extremely important; only someone with the proper medical experience can tell, and know what emergency treatment may be necessary. Also, laboratory tests often must be made at frequent intervals to find out exactly how the patient is responding to a diet, and what changes should be made. Then more tests are made to determine what effect the new diet is having.

If you must undertake the care and feeding of someone on a calcium, low-gluten, phosphorous, or potassium diet, you will be given detailed instructions by the doctor or dietitian as to the foods, amounts, and methods of preparation and serving that are required, and what reactions your patient may have. Be sure to follow the instructions in every detail; a failure to do so could be very injurious to your patient. Also, expect your visiting nurse to visit more often, to give your patient and you extra help if necessary.

CALCIUM DIETS

The development of firm and rigid bones and teeth is only one of many benefits that come from having enough calcium in the body. It is also necessary for proper functioning of the heart, nerves, and muscles, and for the passage of certain secretions through membranes of the body. In addition, calcium can prevent rickets . . . is important in activating enzymes, particularly those in the digestive system . . . is essential for satisfactory lactation by nursing mothers . . . and is almost vital to the coagulation of blood, for without enough calcium in the system, blood will not clot and any kind of bleeding is extremely difficult to stop.

Useful calcium is found in so many foods that the normal, well-balanced daily diet (Chapter 30) generally has enough for the average person in good health. However, various illnesses, abuses of the body, and extraordinary demands made on it can create conditions in which calcium intake must be reduced (a Low-Calcium Diet) and increased (a High-Calcium Diet).

LOW-GLUTEN DIETS

Gluten is an albumin, a type of protein, that comes from certain grains and vegetables. Persons with various disorders in the absorption of food from the intestinal tract often are prescribed a low-gluten or even glutenfree diet. These disorders, which are due to too much gluten in the body, often take a long time to overcome.

Gluten-control diets need not be unappetizing even though they forbid many commonly popular grains and vegetables.

PHOSPHOROUS DIETS

Phosphorous, a major source of energy for muscle contraction, is important for general growth . . . maintenance of body weight and strength . . . good development of bones and teeth . . . and the prevention of rickets.

Phosphorous is in so many foods that the normal, well-balanced diet (Chapter 30) usually contains enough for the average person in good health. But due to various illnesses, abuses of the body or unusual stresses placed on it, sometimes phosphorous intake must be reduced (a Low-Phosphorous Diet) or increased (a High-Phosphorous Diet). Pregnant and lactating women frequently are put on High-Phosphorous Diets; this should be done only by the woman's doctor.

Phosphorous diets are based on specified amounts of certain proteins, fats, and carbohydrates selected to change the patient's intake of phosphorous according to a definite schedule.

POTASSIUM DIETS

Potassium, or technically the potassium *ion*, is of major importance in the proper maintenance of body cells. Together with sodium and chloride, potassium helps maintain a balance of acids and other chemicals in the body. In proper balance with calcium and magnesium ions, potassium ions are vital for normal stimulation of muscle tissue, especially those of the heart. Potassium ions also have an important part in the conducting of nerve impulses.

Diets that control the amount of potassium absorbed by the body are prescribed mostly for patients who have been fed intravenously for a fairly long time . . . diabetics, under certain conditions . . . patients having severe attacks of diarrhea . . . patients who regularly are being given diuretics.

45 Diabetic Diets

Diabetes, of which there are several kinds, is a chronic or continuing disease caused by metabolic disorder. It is, today, incurable. But the symptoms of diabetes can be made less severe (diabetics can lead a normal life) and the patient's life prolonged by modern treatment. Modern treatment of diabetes is a continuing program of controlled diet, medicine, and exercise; diet is the most important.

Keeping to a diabetic diet often is very difficult for both patient and nurse. Difficult for the patient, because the diet nearly always requires that drastic changes be made in established and enjoyable eating habits. Difficult for you, the nurse, because foods must be prepared and served exactly as prescribed by the diet, and as a rule accurate record must be kept of the patient's actual intake of food; it also may be necessary to keep track of the patient's elimination (Chapter 49). But although diabetic diets are strict in what they forbid, they do offer a wide variety of foods and allow for many substitutions.

To help in the planning of balanced meals (Chapter 30), and to be able to easily substitute foods to satisfy a patient's likes and dislikes, diabetic diet foods are classed or grouped in lists called "Exchanges." These are:

List #1—Milk Exchanges
List #2—Vegetable Exchanges
List #3—Fruit Exchanges
List #4—Bread Exchanges
List #5—Meat Exchanges: Lean Meat
Medium-Fat Meat
High-Fat Meat
List #6—Fat Exchanges

In addition, there is a group of free foods, which usually can be used in unlimited amounts in preparing and serving meals, and a group of forbidden foods.

Except for the forbidden items, foods in a listing usually may be substituted for one another, but only according to strict rules based on their amounts of carbohydrates, proteins, fats, and Calories.

Because of the importance of food intake—eating the wrong foods can put a diabetic into a fatal coma!—you must obey all the instructions of a prescribed diabetic diet. If you want to make a change, first consult your patient's doctor or dietitian; if neither of them can be contacted and it is an emergency, ask your visiting nurse.

DIABETIC FOOD EXCHANGES

To simplify all the work of preparing diets and menus for diabetics, and to provide an easy way to select foods to fit your patient's tastes, a system of "exchanges" was made for grading portions, such as 237 ml. or 1 cup, of foods.

An exchange is a unit based on certain amounts of carbohydrates, proteins, fats, and Calories; however, not all of these are in all exchanges. Exchanges are also known as choices.

A diabetic diet is based on the number of exchanges of various foods that will add up to the total daily amount of carbohydrates, proteins, and fats that a patient may have.

There are six basic lists of exchanges—Milk, Vegetable, Fruit, Bread, Meat, and Fat. Within the same list, substitutions of foods can as a rule be made on the basis of "1 exchange or portion of this for 1 exchange or portion of that." Substitutions may be made between foods in different lists; however, differences in the values of the exchanges (amounts of carbohydrates, proteins, and fats) must be taken into account, and the diet must be kept balanced (Chapter 30). Also, in some cases substitutions in one list may change the number of exchanges or portions of foods allowed in another list.

> NOTE: In the following lists of exchanges, all foods that are printed in *italic type* are *low-fat* or *nonfat*. These lists, based on the American Diabetes Association Exchange Diet, are not necessarily complete as far as your patient's doctor or dietitian is concerned; foods may be added to or taken from a list.

List #1—Milk Exchanges

This list gives the kinds and amounts or portions of milk or milk products to use for 1 Milk Exchange; low-fat and whole milks contain saturated fat (Chapter 30). 1 Milk Exchange contains 12 gm. of carbohydrates, 8 gm. protein, a trace of fat, and 80 Calories. Amounts are given in ml. (milliliters) and cups.

Nonfat Fortified Milk

Buttermilk made from skim milk	237 ml./1 cup
Canned, evaporated skim milk	118.3 ml./½ cup
Powdered (nonfat dry, before adding liquid)	118.3 ml./½ cup
Skim or nonfat milk	236.6 ml./1 cup
Yogurt made from skim milk (plain, unflavored)	236.6 ml./1 cup

Low-Fat Fortified Milk

1% fat fortified milk (omit ½ Fat Exchange)	236.6 ml./1 cup
2% fat fortified milk (omit 1 Fat Exchange)	236.6 ml./1 cup
Yogurt made from 2% fat fortified milk; plain, unflavored (omit 1 Fat Exchange)	236.6 ml./1 cup

Whole Milk (omit 2 Fat Exchanges)

Buttermilk made from whole milk	236.6 ml./1 cup
Canned, evaporated whole milk	118.3 ml./½ cup
Whole milk	236.6 ml./1 cup
Yogurt made from whole milk (plain, unflavored)	236.6 ml./1 cup

List #2—Vegetable Exchanges

This list shows the kinds and amounts or portions of vegetables used for 1 Vegetable Exchange, which contains about 5 gm. of carbohydrates, 2 gm. protein, and 25 Calories. Starchy vegetables are in List #4—Bread Exchanges.

Asparagus	118.3 ml./½ cup
Bean Sprouts	118.3 ml./½ cup
Beets	118.3 ml./½ cup
Broccoli	118.3 ml./½ cup
Brussels Sprouts	118.3 ml./½ cup
Cabbage	118.3 ml./½ cup
Carrots	118.3 ml./½ cup
Cauliflower	118.3 ml./½ cup
Celery	118.3 ml./½ cup
Cucumbers	118.3 ml./½ cup
Eggplant	118.3 ml./½ cup
Green Pepper	118.3 ml./½ cup
Greens: Beet, Chards, Collards, Dandelion, Kale, Mustard, Spinach, Turnip	118.3 ml./½ cup
Mushrooms	118.3 ml./½ cup
Okra	118.3 ml./½ cup

Onions	118.3 ml./½ cup
Rhubarb	118.3 ml./½ cup
Rutabaga	118.3 ml./½ cup
Sauerkraut	118.3 ml./½ cup
String Beans, green or yellow	118.3 ml./½ cup
Summer Squash	118.3 ml./½ cup
Tomatoes	118.3 ml./½ cup
Tomato Juice	118.3 ml./½ cup
Turnips	118.3 ml./½ cup
Vegetable Juice Cocktail	118.3 ml./½ cup
Zucchini	118.3 ml./½ cup

NOTE: Some other vegetables are listed in Free Foods.

List #3—Fruit Exchanges

Listed here are the kinds and amounts or portions of fruits equaling 1 Fruit Exchange, which is 10 gm. of carbohydrates and 25 Calories. Amounts or portions are given in size of fruit, quantity, ml. (milliliters), or cups.

Apple	1 small
Apple Juice	78.9 ml./1/3 cup
Applesauce (unsweetened)	118.3 ml./½ cup
Apricots, fresh	2 medium
Apricots, dried	4 halves
Banana	½ small
Berries: Black-, Blue-, Raspberries	118.3 ml./½ cup
Strawberries	177.5 ml./¾ cup
Cherries	10 large
Cider	78.9 ml./1/3 cup
Dates	2
Figs, fresh	1
Figs, dried	1
Grapefruit	½
Grapefruit Juice	118.3 ml./½ cup
Grapes	12
Grape Juice	59.1 ml./¼ cup
Mango	½ small
Melon: Cantaloupe	½ small
Honeydew	1/8 medium
Watermelon	236.6 ml./1 cup
Nectarine	1 small
Orange	1 small
Orange Juice	59.1 ml./¼ cup
Papaya	177.5 ml./¾ cup
Peach	1 medium
Pear	1 small
Persimmon, native	1 medium
Pineapple	118.3 ml./½ cup
Pineapple Juice	78.9 ml./1/3 cup
Plums	2 medium
Prunes	2 medium
Prune Juice	59.1 ml./¼ cup
Raisins	2 tbsp.
Tangerine	1 medium

NOTE: Cranberries may be used as desired, a Free Food, IF NO SUGAR IS ADDED.

List #4—Bread Exchanges

Here are the kinds and amounts or portions of breads, cereals, prepared foods, and starchy vegetables that are counted as 1 Bread Exchange, which contains 15 gm. of carbohydrates, 2 gm. of protein, and 70 Calories. Amounts or portions are given in size, cm. (centimeters), of item, quantity, and ml. (milliliters) and cups, or spoonfuls.

Breads, see Prepared Foods

Cereals

Barley (cooked)	118.3 ml./½ cup
Bran Flakes	118.3 ml./½ cup
Cereal (cooked)	118.3 ml./½ cup
Cornmeal (dry)	2 tbsp.
Flour	2½ tbsp.
Grits (cooked)	118.3 ml./½ cup

Pasta (cooked): Macaroni, Noodles, Spaghetti	118.3 ml./½ cup
Popcorn (popped, no fat added)	709.8 ml./3 cups
Puffed Cereal (unfrosted)	236.6 ml./1 cup
Ready-to-eat Unsweetened Cereal	177.5 ml./¾ cup
Rice (cooked)	118.3 ml./½ cup
Wheat Germ	59.1 ml./¼ cup

Crackers

Arrowroot	3
Graham, 6.25 cm./ 2½-in. square	2
Matzo, 10 x 15 cm./ 4 x 6 in.	½
Oyster	20
Pretzels, 7.8 cm./ 3⅛ in. long x .3 cm./⅛ in. diameter	25
Rye Wafers, 5 x 8.75 cm./ 2 x 3½ in.	3
Saltines	6
Soda, 6.25 cm./ 2½ in. square	4

Dried Beans, Lentils, and Peas

Baked Beans, no pork (canned)	59.1 ml./¼ cup
Beans, Lentils, Peas (dried and cooked)	118.3 ml./½ cup

Prepared Foods

Biscuit, 2-in. diameter (omit 1 Fat Exchange)	1
Bread: enriched white, pumpernickel, whole grain (omit 1 Fat Exchange)	1 slice
Bun, plain, small (omit 1 Fat Exchange)	1
Corn Chips (omit 2 Fat Exchanges)	15
Corn Muffin, 2-in. diameter (omit 1 Fat Exchange)	1
Cornbread, 2 x 2 x 1-in. cube (omit 1 Fat Exchange)	1
Crackers, round, butter-type (omit 1 Fat Exchange)	5
Muffin, plain, small (omit 1 Fat Exchange)	1
Pancake, 12.5 cm./ 5-in. diameter, 1.25 cm./ ½ in. thick (omit 1 Fat Exchange)	1
Potato Chips (omit 2 Fat Exchanges)	15
Potatoes, French Fried, 5 to 8.75 cm./ 2 to 3½ in. long (omit 1 Fat Exchange)	8
Waffle, 12.5 cm./ 5-in. square, 1.25 cm./½ in. thick (omit 1 Fat Exchange)	1

Starchy Vegetables

Corn	78.9 ml./⅓ cup
Corn on Cob	1 small ear
Lima Beans	118.3 ml./½ cup
Parsnips	157.8 ml./⅔ cup
Peas, Green (canned or frozen)	118.3 ml./½ cup

Potato, White	1 small	*Winter Squash, Acorn or Butternut*	118.3 ml./½ cup
Potatoes, mashed	118.3 ml./½ cup	*Yam*	59.1 ml./¼ cup
Pumpkin	177.5 ml./¾ cup		
Sweet Potato	59.1 ml./¼ cup		

List #5—Meat Exchanges: Lean Meat

This list gives the kinds and amounts or portions of lean meat and other protein-rich foods (fish, poultry, milk products, vegetables) that count as 1 Exchange of Lean Meat, which contains 7 gm. of protein, 3 gm. of fat, and 55 Calories. Amounts or portions are given in gm. (grams) and oz. (ounces), ml. (milliliters) and cups, or quantity.

Fish

Any, fresh or frozen Clams, Oysters, Scallops, Scampi, Shrimp	5, or 28.35 gm./1 oz.	*Canned Crab, Lobster, Mackerel, Salmon, Tuna*	59.1 ml./¼ cup
		Sardines, drained	3

Meat

Beef: Baby beef (very lean), chipped beef, chuck, flank steak, plate ribs, plate skirt steak, round (bottom, top), rump (all cuts), spare ribs, tenderloin, tripe	28.35 gm./1 oz.	*Lamb: Leg, loin (roast, chops), rib, shank, shoulder, sirloin*	28.35 gm./1 oz.
		Pork: Leg (center shank, whole rump), smoked ham (center slices)	28.35 gm./1 oz.
		Veal: Cutlets, leg, loin, rib, shank, shoulder	28.35 gm./1 oz.

Milk Products

Cheeses containing less than 5% butterfat	28.35 gm./1 oz.	*Cottage cheese, dry and 2% butterfat*	59.1 ml./¼ cup

Poultry

MEAT WITHOUT SKIN: Chicken, Cornish Hen, Guinea Hen, Pheasant, Turkey	28.35 gm./1 oz.

Vegetables

Dried beans, peas (omit 1 Bread Exchange)	118.3 ml./½ cup

List #5—Meat Exchanges: Medium-Fat Meat

This list gives the kinds and amounts or portions of medium-fat meat and other protein-rich foods (dairy products, vegetables) to use for 1 Exchange of Medium-Fat Meat, for each of which omit ½ Fat Exchange, except where a different amount is specified. Amounts or portions are given in gm. (grams) and oz. (ounces), ml. (milliliters) and cups or spoonfuls, or quantity of an item.

Dairy Products

Cheese: Farmers cheese, Mozzarella, Neuchâtel, Ricotta	28.35 gm./1 oz.
Parmesan, grated	45 ml./3 tbsp.
Cottage cheese, creamed	59.1 ml./¼ cup
Egg (high in cholesterol)	1

Meat

Beef: Corned beef (canned), ground (15% fat), rib eye, round (ground commercial)	28.35 gm./1 oz.
Organ meats (high in cholesterol): Heart, kidney, liver, sweetbreads	28.35 gm./1 oz.
Pork: Canadian bacon, boiled ham, Boston butt, loin (all cuts tenderloin), shoulder arm (picnic), shoulder blade	28.35 gm./1 oz.

Vegetable

Peanut butter (omit 2 additional Fat Exchanges)	*30 ml./2 tbsp.*

List #5—Meat Exchanges: High-Fat Meat

Here are the kinds and amounts or portions of high-fat meat and other protein-rich foods (milk products, poultry) to use for 1 Exchange of High-Fat Meat, for each of which omit 1 Fat Exchange. Amounts or portions are given in gm. (grams) and oz. (ounces), quantity of an item, or size in cm. (centimeters) and in. (inches).

Meat

Beef: Brisket, corned beef (brisket), chuck (ground commercial), ground beef (more than 20% fat), hamburger (commercial), roast (rib), steaks (club, rib)	28.35 gm./1 oz.
Lamb: Breast	28.35 gm./1 oz.
Pork: Country-style ham, deviled ham, loin (back ribs), pork (ground), spare ribs	28.35 gm./1 oz.
Veal: Breast	28.35 gm./1 oz.
Processed Meats:	
Cold Cuts, 11.25 cm./4½-in. square, .3 cm./⅛ in. thick	1 slice
Frankfurter	1 small

Milk Product

Cheese: Cheddar types	28.35 gm./1 oz.

Poultry

Capon, meat only, no skin	28.35 gm./1 oz.
Duck (domestic) meat only, no skin	28.35 gm./1 oz.
Goose, meat only, no skin	28.35 gm./1 oz.

List #6—Fat Exchanges

Here are the kinds and amounts or portions of fat-containing foods used for 1 Fat Exchange, which contains 5 gm. of fat and 45 Calories. Amounts or portions are given in ml. (milliliters) and spoonfuls (tea-, table-), quantity, or size in cm. (centimeters) and in. (inches).

Food	Amount
*Avocado, 10 cm./4-in. diameter**	⅛
*Margarine, soft, tub or stick***	5 ml./1 tsp.
*Nuts: Almonds**	10 whole
Walnuts	6 small
Peanuts, Spanish*	20 whole
Virginia	10 whole
*Others**	6 small
Oils: Corn, Cottonseed, Safflower, Soy, Sunflower	5 ml./1 tsp.
*Olive**	5 ml./1 tsp.
*Peanut**	5 ml./1 tsp.
Bacon, crisp	1 slice
Bacon fat	5 ml./1 tsp.
Butter	5 ml./1 tsp.
Cream: Light	30 ml./2 tbsp.
Sour	30 ml./2 tbsp.
Heavy	15 ml./1 tbsp.
Cream Cheese	15 ml./1 tbsp.
Lard	5 ml./1 tsp.
Margarine, regular, stick	5 ml./1 tsp.
Mayonnaise***	5 ml./1 tsp.
Salad Dressing: French***	15 ml./1 tbsp.
Italian***	15 ml./1 tbsp.
Mayonnaise-type***	10 ml./2 tsp.
Salt Pork, 1.9 cm./¾ in. cube	1

*Fat content is primarily monounsaturated (Chapter 30).
**Made with Corn, Cottonseed, Safflower, Soy, or Sunflower oil only.
***If made with Corn, Cottonseed, Safflower, Soy, or Sunflower oil, can be used on a fat-modified diet.

Free Foods

Here is a list of some foods that you can, as a rule, use in unlimited amounts in preparing and serving diabetic meals. However, since diet problems differ widely among diabetics, before using any of these foods be sure to consult your patient's doctor or dietitian:

Bouillon, without fat
Broth, clear
Coffee (black), decaffeinated, regular; grain-type coffee substitutes, such as Postum
Consommé
Cranberries without sugar
Diet, low-calorie beverages
Flavorings: Lemon, lime, mint, vanilla, etc.
Gelatin, unsweetened
Pickles, unsweetened
Seasonings: Celery salt, chili powder, chives, horseradish, garlic, mustard, onion salt or powder, paprika, parsley, pepper, red pepper, seasoned salts, salt, etc.
Spices: Cinnamon, nutmeg, etc.
Tea (plain)
Sweeteners, artificial (sugar substitutes)
Vinegar

Forbidden Foods

The following foods usually are not allowed in diabetic diets. However, since dietary conditions differ among diabetics, you may wish to ask your patient's doctor or dietitian about forbidden foods.

- Cake
- Candy
- Chewing gum
- Condensed milk
- Cookies
- Honey
- Jam
- Jelly
- Pie
- Soft drinks, except diet (see Free Foods)
- Sugar
- Syrup

DIABETIC DIETS

Diabetic diet plans must be designed to meet the needs of the individual person. They are based on the person's age, activity level, present weight in relation to that person's ideal weight, and other medical conditions that may exist.

The American Diabetes Association bases the number of Calories required on the patient's ideal body weight, as measured in kg. (kilograms), and level of physical activity, as follows:

20 Calories per kg. ideal body weight = Caloric intake for weight loss

25 Calories per kg. ideal body weight = Caloric intake for maintaining present weight

30 Calories per kg. ideal body weight = Caloric intake for an increase of activity or for weight gain

Of the total number of Calories needed, 50 percent should be from carbohydrates, 20 percent from proteins, and 30 percent from fats. This is, of course, only a general guide, and the doctor, dietitian, or nutritionist will adjust the balance to meet the special needs of your patient.

Feeding Your Patient The diet prescribed for your patient will specify the number of Exchanges or portions of each food to be taken daily. At what time of day they are to be taken may or may not be important. If it is important, the diet will specify the food and the number of portions to be taken in the morning, noon, and evening meals, and for between-meal snacks if allowed.

It is advisable to plan your patient's meals several days at a time. It will help prevent food boredom; no matter how well a person likes a food, being given it too often, at too many meals in a row, can easily change like to dislike. Also, planning meals for several days at a time usually will simplify your shopping.

Many sick people like and really need between-meal and bedtime snacks. These usually are allowed, but must be counted into the day's total food intake of carbohydrates, proteins, fats, and Calories.

Sick people often are not hungry at a mealtime. If your patient does not eat all of a food at a meal, the uneaten portion may be served later, or you may add the amount of uneaten food to the appropriate Exchange at the next meal. For example:

If only half the hamburger bun is eaten at lunch, for dinner you could serve your patient 177.5 ml./¾ cup of macaroni or spaghetti instead of 118.3 ml./½ cup.

SAMPLE DIABETIC DIETS

Diabetic menus are based on providing a patient with a certain number of Calories per day as contained in the allowable foods selected to make a balanced diet (Chapter 30). Below are sample 1-day menus for 1,000-Calorie and 1,500-Calorie diabetic diets, given in terms of Exchanges followed by a suggested food; Free Foods may, of course, be added as desired.

1,000-Calorie Sample Diabetic Menu

BREAKFAST

1 Meat Exchange—1 egg
1 Bread Exchange—1 slice enriched white bread
1 Fat Exchange—5 ml./1 tsp. butter
1 Milk Exchange—236.6 ml./1 cup skim milk

LUNCH

2 Meat Exchanges—56.7 gms./2 oz. fish
2 Vegetable Exchanges—236.6 ml./1 cup carrots
½ Bread Exchange—59.1 ml./¼ cup noodles
½ Fat Exchange—5 pecans
1 Milk Exchange—236.6 ml./1 cup buttermilk made from skim milk
1 Fruit Exchange—1 small apple

DINNER

3 Meat Exchanges—85 gm./3 oz. top ground beef
2 Vegetable Exchanges—118.3 ml./½ cup each of beets, zucchini
½ Bread Exchange—½ slice enriched whole-wheat bread
½ Fat Exchange—2.5 ml./½ tsp. enriched margarine
1 Milk Exchange—236.6 ml./ 1 cup yogurt, plain, unflavored, made from skim milk.

1,500-Calorie Sample Diabetic Menu

BREAKFAST

1 Meat Exchange—1 egg
2 Bread Exchanges—236.6 ml./1 cup cooked rice
1 Fat Exchange—5 ml./1 tsp. enriched margarine
1 Milk Exchange—236.6 ml./1 cup whole milk
1 Fruit Exchange—118.3 ml./½ cup applesauce

LUNCH

3 Meat Exchanges—85 gm./3 oz. beef
1 Vegetable Exchange—118.3 ml./½ cup beets
2 Bread Exchanges—118.3 ml./½ cup spaghetti and ½ slice enriched whole-wheat toast
1 Fat Exchange—5 ml./1 tsp. margarine
1 Milk Exchange—236.6 ml./1 cup whole milk
1 Fruit Exchange—118.3 ml./½ cup raspberries

DINNER

3 Meat Exchanges—85 gm./3 oz. chicken meat
2 Vegetable Exchanges—118.3 ml./½ cup each of carrots, celery
1 Bread Exchange—118.3 ml./½ cup mashed potatoes
1 Fat Exchange—5 ml./1 tsp. enriched margarine
1 Milk Exchange—236.6 ml./1 cup whole milk

46 Tube-Feeding Diets

Tube feeding is done when a patient cannot take food by mouth. Feedings commonly are given through a pliable tube passing through the patient's nose and down into the stomach. It may be kept in place for a fairly long period of time. All the carbohydrates, fats, proteins, minerals, vitamins, and water needed by a patient can be supplied by tube feeding. However:

DO NOT ATTEMPT TO GIVE A TUBE FEEDING UNTIL YOU HAVE BEEN THOROUGHLY INSTRUCTED, SUPERVISED IN ALL PHASES OF THE PROCEDURE, AND APPROVED TO DO IT BY AN EXPERIENCED NURSE OR DOCTOR!

TUBE FEEDINGS

Homemade tube feedings, or the formulae to be given, are excellent breeding and growing grounds for bacteria. For this reason, you may be advised to use a sterile, commercially prepared product. In either case, mix only enough for 24 hours' use at most, and keep it tightly covered in the refrigerator. Whenever possible, mix the necessary amount for each feeding as needed.

Your patient's doctor or dietitian will prescribe the amount of formula to be given during a 24-hour period, and the frequency of feedings.

A sample tube-feeding formula is at the end of this chapter, not necessarily for you to follow but to show the ingredients that may be used. The formula for your patient will depend on the doctor's diagnosis and the physical requirements and nutritional needs of your patient. You may be given the formula as a more or less conventional recipe; or it may be given in amounts of carbohydrates, proteins, fats, vitamins, minerals, and water. In this case, the hospital dietitian or your visiting nurse probably can give you a proper recipe; if not, insist that your patient's doctor give you one.

It is most important to follow formula instructions exactly, especially when measuring ingredients.

EQUIPMENT NEEDED

Tube feeding requires a combination of highly specialized and commonplace equipment. The commonplace are the usual measuring spoons and cups, dishes and pans, funnels and pouring cups that you would need for any cooking that must be done with accurately measured and prepared ingredients.

The specialized equipment for tube feeding is selected by the doctor according to the size and type of tube that your patient can tolerate, the size container that will hold enough but not too much formula for a feeding, controls for regulating the rate of flow, and so forth. You also need equipment, usually adhesive tape, to hold the tube to your patient's head in an acceptable position. An adequate stand to hold the formula container may be required; a commercial hospital stand is best for this, although if necessary you can safely use the substitute stands suggested for an enema or irrigation/douche (Chapters 25, 26).

TUBE FEEDING

Although tube feeding should not be attempted without the positive approval of an experienced nurse, there are certain phases of it that you should know in advance:

1. *Before beginning to tube feed a patient,* make certain that the tube is in the stomach and is not clogged. To test, hold the free end of the tube in a glass of water;
   a. If a few bubbles come from the tube then cease, the tube is in the stomach and the air has been expelled.
   b. If bubbles come from the tube rhythmically or periodically, the tube is not in the stomach.
2. *Begin a feeding* by pouring into the tube a small amount of water, 30 ml./1 oz., very slowly. Then pour in the formula, allowing it to run down the side of the syringe or funnel to let any trapped air escape before you completely fill the syringe or funnel.
3. *Do not force* the formula down the tube; let it run in slowly, by gravity.
4. *When the prescribed amount of formula has been given,* rinse the tube, to clean it and keep it from clogging, by running 60 ml./2 oz. of water through it. Do not remove tube from patient unless you are ordered to.
5. *After a feeding,* the upper or free end of the tube usually is covered and fastened by adhesive tape to the patient's forehead to keep it out of the way.
6. *Sometimes a doctor may order* small amounts of formula, 45–60 ml./1½–2 oz., to be given hourly. However, it is more usual to feed 200 ml./6¾ oz. at 2–4-hour intervals.
7. *If given a totally balanced formula* containing all the daily requirements of carbohydrates, proteins, fats, vitamins, minerals, and water, a tube-fed patient can be kept in a nutritionally healthy state.

SAMPLE TUBE-FEEDING FORMULA

A variety of commercial preparations are available for easy mixing with water or milk for tube-feeding formulae. Two products in particular are very satisfactory for a low-calorie formula: Sustagen, a protein supplement, and Lonalac, a low-sodium product. However, for higher calorie requirements it is better to use a planned formula of ingredients, as in this sample tube-feeding formula. It provides 3,000 calories with a balanced ratio of 165 gm./5.8 oz. of protein, 106 gm./3.75 oz. of fat, and 346 gm./12.2 oz. carbohydrate:

.95 l./1 qt. homogenized whole milk
3 eggs
400 ml./14.1 oz. canned, frozen apple juice
30 ml./1 oz. vegetable oil
118.3 ml./4 oz. or ½ cup containers of strained baby foods:

Beef liver	4 containers
Beets	2 containers
Peaches	2 containers

354.9 ml./12 oz. or 1½ cups Sustagen or approved substitute.
Water as needed to make of total of 2,500 ml./88.25 oz. or 2.76 qt. of formula

47 Feeding Your Patient

No matter how carefully and cleverly you select, prepare, and serve the foods your patient may have (Chapters 31, 46), there often is the problem of getting it eaten, of feeding your patient. As a rule, sick people are poor eaters, usually for reasons that to them are good and sufficient. Perhaps a physical handicap or condition makes eating difficult or even painful. Perhaps your patient simply does not want to eat at that time. Or perhaps because eating is difficult or painful, your patient has become discouraged and unwilling to eat. But no matter what the problem is, or why, you must solve it. Somehow you must get the food where it belongs—in your patient!

Tricks and guile, subtle promises and outright bribes are seldom effective in getting a handicapped or an unwilling patient to eat. Sometimes a direct challenge, such as "You know you need food in order to get well—it's up to you to eat—no one can do it for you!" will work. But the most effective, and difficult, course is patience. Keep after your patient to eat, but do not nag or scold or threaten (signs of impatience). Do not let your patient dawdle or dillydally unnecessarily, but do not try to rush or force matters (signs of impatience). Explain why certain foods may be necessary or are not allowed, but do not be sarcastic about it (a sign of impatience).

HANDICAPPED PATIENTS

Handicaps that most commonly hinder a patient's ability to eat are lack of sight, poorly fitting dentures, disorders of the mouth or throat, and anything that prevents normal use of fingers, hands, or arms. The last two types of handicaps often are combined in stroke patients.

More than anything else, a handicapped patient needs encouragement. You can give hidden or secret encouragement by selecting and preparing foods that will minimize the effects of your patient's handicap; the easier it is to eat, the more your patient will want and try to eat in spite of the handicap. You give open encouragement by congratulating your patient for a successful attempt to eat or, in event of failure, by pointing out how this attempt was better and came closer to success than the previous one. But be careful not to overdo the congratulations; a mature person often resents lavish praise, especially for doing something that should not be difficult. Also, do not lie about how close your patient came to overcoming a handicap; you do not have to be caught telling many lies in order to lose your patient's trust and confidence.

Selecting and Preparing Foods When there is a choice of foods, as there is in most diets, select those that you know your patient can deal with, if self-feeding, and chew and swallow. This is particularly important at the beginning of an ailment, when every possible effort must be made to restore a patient's self-confidence. Knowing the condition of your patient, you can avoid foods that may be difficult to chew and swallow; a ground meat patty that crumbles easily may be much better for your patient than tender, juicy slices of steak. Be careful of foods that may be hard in some parts, soft in others; the flowery part of broccoli usually is quite tender, but the stalk can be tough and stringy. On the other hand, as a rule it is not good to keep a patient on foods that are too easy to chew and swallow, foods that do not offer a challenge. Tender, crumbly ground meat may be excellent at the start, but as a patient's condition improves, there should be a gradual change to more solid food in order to build the patient's self-confidence. The best encouragement a sick person gets from eating is knowing that normal, everyday foods are now a regular part of the diet.

How you serve food is especially important for the self-feeding patient who has disabled fingers, hands, or arms. To encourage self-feeding, make the food easy to be managed by knife, fork, or spoon. Prepare the cutlery with special assists or holders if necessary (Chapter 16, Handicap Aids). For the patient who will cut food, provide a sharp knife; it cuts with less effort than a dull knife, and is less apt to slip.

Prepare foods so that they are easy to cut, or serve the food already cut in bite-size pieces. This is particularly important for the patient able to use one hand only. Serve hard-to-pick-up foods, such as firm green peas, in a bowl instead of on a flat plate. Or, if the diet permits, serve an elusive food, such as green peas, with a moderately thick cheese or cream sauce; you could mash the peas slightly, but this calls more attention to the patient's difficulty in self-feeding.

The Self-Feeding Patient Before serving foods, make sure that the self-feeding patient is in a safe and comfortable position for eating. If the patient is in bed, set the bed, if adjustable, and the pillows to give dependable, comfortable support to the upper body. Assist, if necessary, putting the patient's legs in comfortable positions. If the patient will eat from a bedside table, set it in place over the bed and adjust it to a comfortable height for your patient. If a patient eats from a bedtray, clear a space for setting it on the bed.

When serving a meal, do not put it down haphazardly. Place each item—dishes, cups, glasses, cutlery, seasonings, napkin—within easy reach of the patient. However, items, such as a bowl of dessert, that will not be wanted until after most of the other foods are eaten, may be put in a slightly out-of-the-way place or taken away until wanted. Butter bread if necessary. As foods are finished, their dishes may be removed.

Many handicapped persons are too "ambitious"; that is, they try to do more self-feeding than they are able to. Failures can be so frustrating sometimes that tempers are lost and food, dishes, and cutlery may go flying across the room. Ignore it to the best of your ability, as almost any remark will further discourage your patient. Do not in any way imply that your patient has failed time and time again, and should quit trying. Keep in mind that many failures often come before achievement. To reduce the possibilities of failure, give your patient tasks that you feel certain can be done; only after regular success with simple tasks should a disabled person be allowed to tackle more complicated ones.

Whether to stay in the room or leave it while a self-feeding patient eats may be a problem. As a rule, you should not stay if in any way a patient seems embarrassed to eat in front of you. It may be that the patient is uncomfortably aware of being awkward in using knife, fork, or spoon; or of an unavoidably unusual way of chewing or swallowing. Or perhaps the patient will talk less and eat better if you are out of the room.

On the other hand, if your patient has difficulty managing some foods, the fact that you are present and ready to help often brings on the little extra effort that gets a job done. Also, eating is a social activity, and having someone to talk to while eating may stimulate a patient to eat better than if left alone to eat.

If you stay in the room while your patient eats, be unobtrusively ready to help at all times, but never offer help unless it is necessary. As a rule, it is better to let a patient try and fail than not try at all. Do not help a patient become discouraged by either preventing or unnecessarily helping an attempt at self-feeding. If discouragement does set in, your handicapped patient may become an unwilling patient, below.

Stroke Patients Among the handicapped, self-feeding usually is most difficult, especially at the start, for stroke patients. The normal use of both hands has suddenly stopped; only one hand works, and it may not be the one that the patient used the most. So on top of an overall clumsiness due to the general weakness that usually accompanies a stroke, the patient must learn to function with only one hand, possibly the one that was less skillful. To learn firsthand how this is, try transferring, without spilling, a heaping teaspoon of sugar from a bowl to a cup with your "wrong" hand (left, if you are right-handed).

In addition to the sharply limited use of hands, a stroke patient may have difficulty chewing and swallowing. Depending on how severe the stroke is, it may be almost impossible for a patient to keep a solid or liquid on the side of the mouth that still has sensation. Also, swallowing, if it does not cause a choking sensation, can be very difficult at first. Do not leave a stroke patient with these problems alone while eating.

Regardless of handicaps, make every effort to get a stroke patient on a self-feeding program as soon as possible. This is necessary primarily because of the unexpectedness and suddenness of the sickness. Usually a person is healthy one minute, has lost control of half the body the next minute. Fortunately, in time patients may regain many of their former abilities. However, it requires a great deal of determination and work by the patient. The way you help is by encouraging your patient in every way to be self-sufficient. Self-feeding is a major step toward self-sufficiency.

Of course, it does not always happen, but stroke patients often become short of temper and may have a personality change. It is especially common when they fail at some simple task that they have done thousands of times, such as raising a fork of food without spilling. Whatever you do, do not scold or complain about it. If necessary, and it well may be at the start and later on, repeat what the doctor said about strokes and how regaining the use of nerves and muscles is the result of trying, trying, trying—and trying some more. Or ask your visiting nurse to explain the facts of strokes to your patient.

Elderly Patients Elderly persons often have many of the eating handicaps experienced by stroke patients. As much as possible, work with them the same as with stroke victims. However, often elderly persons' handicaps become greater instead of improving, and as they lose physical ability you must give more help in self-feeding. But as long as a patient can do any self-feeding, encourage it.

Children As a rule, there is little difficulty in putting a child on a self-feeding program. Most children are optimistic, willing and wanting to try almost anything, and usually see a series of failures as a bigger and bigger challenge. Once a child passes the initial stage of an illness or injury, generally the problem is one of preventing physical acts that could be harmful. But be careful not to discourage a child. Often the best way to prevent an act that might be harmful, yet not discourage a child patient, is to say, "Let's ask our visiting nurse first!" Children seem to have more confidence in the visiting nurse than in their regular one (or mother), probably because they do not see the visiting nurse as often. As a general rule, a child's physical state will limit activities without prodding by parents, nurses, or others. It is easier to rely on this than to keep a child quiet.

Patients Who Must Be Fed Aside from the actual eating, everything about selecting, preparing, and serving food for self-feeding patients applies to most patients who must be fed, except those without sight.

The main rule covering patients who must be fed is: Do not rush them! To keep hot food from getting cold, keep your patient eating as steadily as possible. Do this by filling the fork or spoon while the patient is chewing and swallowing, and be ready with the next mouthful as soon as the present one is swallowed. But until your patient is ready for it, hold the filled fork or spoon down near the plate or bowl. Also, do not put too much food into your patient's mouth. To people not accustomed to it, being fed by someone creates a helpless feeling, which can be greatly increased by being given too large a mouthful of food or being fed too fast. Moreover, most people find it less tiring to chew and swallow several small mouthfuls of food than a few large ones. Give your patient a short rest occasionally or a drink of liquid between bites.

Patients Without Sight When feeding persons who cannot see, either temporarily or permanently, name and describe each food item when serving a meal. There usually is no need to go into much detail, just a simple listing will do, such as "cream tomato soup today . . . a nice green salad . . . hamburger patty . . . baked potato . . . carrots . . . orange gelatin with cookies . . . and tea." If there is a food new to your patient, describe it in some detail and perhaps hold it up close to be smelled. If your patient seems uninterested in food, use a little salesmanship in naming the items. For example, instead of saying just, "a nice green salad," go into detail, such as "a salad with bright green, crispy fresh lettuce, luscious sliced tomato, some of those green peas you like so much, and an herb dressing that really makes your mouth water." Remember what the owner of a very successful eating establishment is supposed to have said, "We sell the sizzle, not the steak." Incidentally, with many people the expression *mouth-watering* really does stimulate the flow of saliva and thereby help increase a desire for food.

When actually feeding a sightless person, name each food just before bringing it to the mouth. With children you may make a game of it, guessing what the food is before you name it.

Sightless people should be given every opportunity and encouragement to feed themselves. Describe clearly where each food is located on the plate or tray, and guide your patient's hand to it. Protect your patient and bed or clothing from spills with a large towel or bib. Do not scold if your patient makes a mess.

UNWILLING EATERS

The main problem that inexperienced nurses often have with people who are able but unwilling to eat is self-control. The nurse's self-control, not the patient's. After the work of selecting, preparing, and serving food that you know your patient can and should eat, it is extremely annoying to see it pushed aside or left untouched until it becomes unappetizing. Appearing to lose your temper to some extent may sometimes get a patient to eat. But it is better to find out why the patient will not eat properly, and remove that cause. In somewhat rare cases, a patient may refuse food because of a so-called death wish; if you suspect this to be the case, notify the doctor or your visiting nurse immediately. Most other times when a sick or injured adult will not eat, it is due to the diet prescribed, to really being "just not interested" in food, or to wanting to do something else at the time. Remember, too, that during illness nothing may taste good or as it tasted before.

Children usually present somewhat different problems and need different treatment from adults who are unwilling to eat.

Distasteful Diet A common saying about diets is, "List all the foods you like—and don't eat them!" Unfortunately, many diets seem to be exactly that. Patients are suddenly denied the foods, seasonings, kinds of cooking, and amounts that they have enjoyed, perhaps too lavishly, for many years. Now they get foods that simply do not taste right, that are unappetizing. They may accept such foods for a few days out of a sense of duty; but then they lose interest and do not care to eat. After nibbling a little of this and a smidgen of that, they really do not want any more. Aside from ordering a patient to eat, which seldom works, here are some ways of coping with the problem of a distasteful diet:

1. Make foods more attractive to a patient by radically changing the kind and/or amount of seasoning. Try different herbs with vegetables, such as dill on buttered cooked carrots, and fresh ground nutmeg on spinach.
2. Ask the doctor or dietitian to remove some restrictions from the diet to bribe your patient to eat. However, patients who win this kind of appeasement once usually will try it time and time again. Also, there are practical limits to such appeasement; if carried too far, the patient will be off the diet.
3. Ask the doctor or dietitian if you can make a deal whereby your patient follows a diet faithfully for a week or 10 days, and then has a "real meal" of just about anything. As a rule, there must be some restrictions, but most patients will accept a few restrictions in order to savor forbidden foods. Do not be surprised if after a few of these so-called real meals your patient loses interest in them and is willing to follow the prescribed diet. It commonly happens, especially if any distress or discomfort follows the "real meal."
4. With a mature and rational patient, the best way to combat a distasteful diet may be for you or your visiting nurse to explain exactly why the diet was prescribed . . . what it can do . . . and how long it must be used if followed strictly or loosely. Use all details necessary to convince your patient of the need of the diet; how this part of the body must get special nourishment, how the strain that was put on those organs must be reduced, and so forth. Spell out in plain, simple language what can and probably will happen if the diet is not followed. Many adults reject a diet simply because they do not fully understand it.

Just Not Interested in Food To some people eating is only a necessary chore. They may not actively dislike it; but they eat mainly because they believe it will keep body and soul together. They prefer some foods to others, but do not really care what they have. They are in the habit of three or more meals a day; they would be just as happy, or happier, with only one or two. They would be delighted if a pill a day would replace all meals. Although such a person probably is truthful about food's not being important and saying that anything you serve will be satisfactory, as a rule you should try to arouse some interest in eating. Your patient's ailment may be the necessary leverage to do it.

Due to a sickness or injury, a person's likes and dislikes often change. A person who was not interested in food when healthy may now take real interest in it if it is presented with much the same kind of salesmanship that often is necessary when feeding Patients Without Sight, above. If this approach works with your patient, usually it is wise to ask for suggestions for making foods more tasty; people who do not care for food for themselves often are excellent cooks and meal planners for others.

It also often happens that people's attitudes toward food change when they are sick or injured. Actually, they may not care more for food now than when they were healthy, but now they are willing to eat properly because of their physical need. Explain the purposes of food as you would to a patient on a Distasteful Diet, above.

When no kind of persuasion works with an unwilling eater, then the only solution usually is to come right out and say that no one else will benefit, no one else will be harmed by the patient's action.

Patients Who Would Rather Do Something Else Than Eat In many cases what these patients would rather do than eat is talk. This commonly happens to sick people who are left alone for fairly long periods of time. They accumulate many things to discuss with you, their nurse. If the only time you are with them is during meals and they want to talk, they will, and you cannot stop them.

The only prevention for this is to give them ample time to talk with you before mealtime. Delay serving if necessary.

Children Children who can but simply refuse to eat can be extremely annoying. Scolding them seldom works. In most cases they see nothing wrong or unreasonable in refusing to eat; their parents gave in when they refused a food just because they thought they would not like it.

Because most children are basically fair, or curious, at heart, one of the best ways to overcome the I-don't-believe-I'll-like-it objection to food is the "no thank you" helping. You agree not to force a food on the child, and the child agrees to try at least three regular-size bites of everything you serve.

Depending on the maturity of a child, you may have to play games in order to get food eaten. Games such as "this bite for you . . . this for your mother . . . this for your father . . . this for me . . ." and so on through the whole roster of relatives, friends, and pets. You can adapt this type of game to the child's ailment, such as "this bite for the bone above the break . . . this for the bone below the break," and so on.

If an unwilling-to-eat child is mature enough to understand, then you and your visiting nurse may explain why the foods are needed the same as you would to an adult patient on a Distasteful Diet.

48 Meals Can Be Fun

The little extras you do in preparing and serving meals can get your patient to eat better. That will save you work, because the better a patient enjoys meals the less time you must spend "persuading" and, often, rewarming foods to make them more palatable. The suggestions in this chapter are not difficult to follow or time consuming. And no one by itself probably will be very effective. But when you do several of these extras, the results for your patient and you can be well worthwhile.

In addition to preparing and serving meals to make them attractive, you may make them more fun for your patient by inviting some guests.

PREPARING MEALS

Foods Plan meals according to your patient's diet, while selecting foods for the greatest eye, nose, mouth, and personal appeals (Chapter 30).

Prepare and serve meals so that hot items will be hot, cold ones cold. Usually this is a simple matter of heating or chilling plates, bowls, cups, or glasses. The safest way to heat them is by soaking them in hot water for several minutes. Oven warming may make them too hot to handle, or warp or even break them. You may fast-chill dishes by soaking them in a basin of water and ice cubes. But when time permits, chilling in the freezing compartment of a refrigerator usually is more satisfactory.

> NOTE: For very slow eaters, you may need to serve foods in thermal or "heat-holding" dishes, such as one with a bottom container for hot or cold water.

Table Service Table service means the setting (plates, bowls, etc.), silver- or flatware, serving tray, placemat, napkin, and decorations or specialty.

If you use chinaware and similar place settings, use the "Sunday best" for your patient whenever practical—when there is little chance of breakage. These dishes usually are the nicest, and will make your patient feel important, like someone special who is getting the best that the home has.

If you use paper or other disposable dishes, instead of buying a large supply of one color, design, or shape, get as many different styles as you can. The variety will do much to lessen the monotony common to many ailments. It will also give you better opportunity to increase the eye appeal of meals by selecting dishes that go well with the colors of the foods.

The cutlery also should be the best that the home has. If your patient needs handicap aids for cutlery (Chapter 16), place them on the utensils before serving a meal so as to call the least attention to them. If foods are to be knife-cut by your patient, be sure that the blade is sharp. A dull knife often is difficult to handle, is apt to slip and spill foods, and can be very discouraging to a handicapped person.

If serving on a bedtray instead of a bedside or overbed table (Chapter 8), use only a sturdy one. A flimsy, wobbly tray usually makes a patient worry about spilling, especially liquids. Do not get a bedtray that is too large or heavy for your patient to move. Also, it should be high enough not to rest on your patient's legs or abdomen.

Placemats and paper napkins are made in a wide variety of colors, designs, and sizes. Get as many different styles as possible in order to give your patient a greater variety of things to see.

The decoration or specialty suggestion for adding interest to a meal can be just about anything that will fit on the patient's tray or table and is not a food item. A flower bud or bloom. An unusual leaf, a small sprig of leaves. A get-well or best-wishes card. A small toy or coloring book for a child. In short, anything that is not part and parcel of the meal, anything novel or colorful that will amuse or interest your patient during a meal and, hopefully, for a while after it.

BEFORE SERVING YOUR PATIENT

As close as possible to the planned mealtime, get your patient ready for it.

Provide items for washing, or you wash your patient's hands, and face if wanted. Except for the first meal of a day, when a more complete washing may be in order, as a rule a damp soaped washcloth, a rinse washcloth, and a towel are sufficient.

Prop your patient up in bed, or in a chair, or assist to the table if the meal will be eaten there. Make your patient warm and comfortable with a blanket, shawl, or other wrap.

If a meal will be served on a bedside or overbed table, put it in place and set it with the placemat, napkin, and cutlery.

SERVING YOUR PATIENT

When your patient is ready for a meal, serve it as soon as you can. If a person is not truly interested in eating, often the case with disabled people, an unnecessary wait between being made ready for a meal and getting it can cause further loss of appetite.

> NOTE: If your patient cannot see, name and describe each food and drink that is being served. As a rule, you should bring each item close enough for your patient to smell it distinctly and separately.

Whether to serve all the foods at once or present them in "courses," such as soup, salad, main dish, etc., may be a problem. Serving all at once usually is less work for you, but seeing so much to eat may frighten your patient. Also, by serving in courses, hot foods more easily can be kept hot, and cold foods cold. However, the best solution to the problem is what your patient is accustomed to and prefers.

GUESTS

Whether bedfast or up and around, sick people who are confined to home for more than a week or 10 days tend to become bored with their meals. Often this happens because the average nurse, experienced or not, usually serves essentially the same dishes time and time again. Diet permitting, as a rule they are foods that the patient likes. But after so many meals, too much is too much. Also, even when a good variety of food is served, too often the same or similar seasonings and ways of preparation are used—making all foods taste much alike. Fortunately, even if your patient is on a fairly strict diet, meal boredom frequently can be prevented—by brown-bag lunches and potluck dinners.

> NOTE: Brown-bag lunches and potluck dinners may involve several of the problems of visitors (Chapter 52), and therefore should not be planned without first consulting the doctor, your visiting nurse, and your patient.

Brown-Bag Lunch For simple brown-bag lunches invite some of your patient's friends, associates, or fellow employees to come and eat their lunches with your patient. You may furnish the beverage. Prepare a regular lunch for your patient or, diet permitting, make it like a brown-bag lunch with sandwiches, a boiled egg, cookies, fruit, and so forth—served in a brown bag!

For a brown-bag lunch that may have greater appeal to your patient, and reduce your work for at least one meal, suggest to each guest what to bring that your patient can eat. If your patient's diet is too restricted, ask guests to bring a novelty, perhaps an inexpensive game or puzzle, that your patient can enjoy after the lunch.

Potluck Dinner This is the same as the typical church, school, or club potluck dinner, except that each guest is told what foods are not allowed your patient. Also stress restrictions as to seasonings (highly spiced foods may be forbidden) and method of cooking (fried foods usually are not recommended). For the sake of variety in foods and flavors, ask potluck guests not to bring any dishes that you usually serve.

From a practical standpoint, a major advantage of the potluck dinner is that there usually are enough leftovers to give your patient "different" foods for the next few dinners.

Surprise! Surprise! Surprising a patient with a brown-bag lunch or potluck dinner may not be advisable. Some sick people do not care to be seen by anyone except very close friends or relatives. Others do not like brown-bag lunches or potluck dinners. Still others do not like surprises; they want to know in advance and prepare for guests. Also, looking forward to a special event may be just as beneficial to a patient as the event itself.

Sometimes it is best to mention, in a casual way, the possibility of a brown-bag lunch or potluck dinner. If your patient seems to favor it, then plan it as a surprise if you think it wise. However, keep in mind that letting your patient help in planning the event may add a world of joyous anticipation to an otherwise humdrum day.

As with so many things connected with a sick person's likes and dislikes, there is no hard and fast rule either for or against brown-bag lunches and potluck dinners. Do what the doctor allows and what you believe your patient will enjoy—but do not be surprised, or get hurt feelings, if your patient does not like it.

49 Keeping Track of Food Intake and Waste Output

If you must record your patient's food intake and/or waste output (urine, feces), it is extremely important to be accurate—accurate in your measurements, accurate in your observations, accurate in recording them. The life of a diabetic patient, for example, can depend on records of food intake, since to great extent medication is based on them. And possible internal disorders, injuries, aftereffects of surgery, and phases of an illness can be indicated by a patient's urine and/or feces.

In a record of food intake, keep track only of the amounts actually consumed, not the amounts served. As to waste output, specimens of urine or feces from a home patient seldom are required. But if they are needed, the doctor or your visiting nurse will explain how to collect them. Usually it will be your responsibility to get specimens to the laboratory.

EQUIPMENT

Little special equipment is needed for measuring a patient's food intake or waste output.

Food Intake Solid foods may be measured by *weight* with an ordinary kitchen food scale that is graduated or marked in grams/ounces, or by *volume* with a container graduated in cc. (cubic centimeters)/oz. (ounces)/cups.

Liquid foods and beverages usually are measured by *volume* by the same container used for solid foods.

Sweeteners, coffee cream or milk, and other flavorings that may be used in small quantity generally are measured in terms of level, rounded, and heaping tea- or tablespoonfuls. Seasonings such as pepper, salt, etc., seldom are measured unless used in appreciably more than the conventional "dash."

Eggs, oranges, apples, and other foods that may be considered units in themselves could be measured in terms of weight or volume, but as a rule are measured and recorded by size as small, medium, large, and extra-large or jumbo.

Waste Output For measuring urine, a liter- or quart-size or larger plastic container graduated in cc./oz. generally is satisfactory; discard it when no longer needed. For a male patient, the graduated urinal as in Fig. 8–24*a* is practical.

Feces seldom is weighed. A statement of its color, texture, and estimated amount usually is adequate for the record.

If urine or feces specimens are needed, prepared containers and instructions for filling and storing or delivering them to the laboratory should be supplied by the doctor or your visiting nurse.

FOOD INTAKE

Prior To Serving When measuring a food or beverage by weight, use *net weight*, the difference between the weight of the container empty and when it holds the food or beverage. No such adjustment is needed when measuring a food or beverage by volume.

Unless a truly accurate method is wanted for determining the amount of a food or beverage actually consumed, form a mental picture of the amount or volume of each item served in relation to its weight or volume when measured. For example, a 57-gm./2-oz. serving of chopped vegetable might make a mound so high and so wide and long; or 1183 cc./4 oz. of milk might fill a drinking glass about halfway. When your patient has finished eating or drinking, estimate the amount consumed, such as about half of the mound of chopped vegetable or half the amount of milk served.

If a second helping of a food or beverage is wanted, add its net weight or volume to that of the original serving. To prevent confusion as to the total net weight or volume served, do not serve the second helping until the first one has been completely consumed.

Actual Food Consumption In most cases, the simple method of estimating the amount of food or beverage consumed, above, is satisfactory. If not, then measure the net weight or volume of each item left by the patient and subtract them from the total amounts served.

> NOTE: If your patient has a contagious disease, you probably should sterilize containers that have been used for measuring leftover foods or beverages. Ask your visiting nurse.

Recording Food Intake Make a separate record of food intake for each 24-hour period; it usually covers the time from breakfast to breakfast, but any consistent

May 10th

Breakfast – 7:30 A.M.	
Orange juice - 200 c.c.	
4 stewed prunes	
1 egg	
2 pieces toast with butter	
Coffee – 150 c.c.	
	Snack – 10:00 A.M.
	Milk - 200 c.c.
Lunch – 12:15 P.M.	
Tuna sandwich	
Lettuce and sliced tomato	
Tea - 150 c.c.	
	Snack – 3:00 P.M.
	Orange juice 300 c.c.

Fig. 49-1 *Partially filled form for recording Food Intake*

time span is satisfactory. A simple but adequate food intake record is shown in Fig. 49–1. Date each record to assure that changes in your patient's food intake can be kept in proper sequence. For convenience, meal records usually are at the left side of the record, and between-meal snacks and beverages at the right. As a rule, the time of starting a meal or between-meal snack or beverage is noted in order to establish a pattern or sequence of the patient's intake to compare with that of the waste output. The method of preparing food often must be recorded, because how it is prepared can affect a patient's urine and/or feces. Unexpected strong changes in a patient's attitude toward foods, seasonings, etc., also should as a rule be noted on a food intake record.

Despite the many factors, above, that could be entered in a food intake record, in most cases only a few actually are required. Your patient's doctor or dietitian will provide a list of the entries that are needed, including observations of yours that may be helpful.

WASTE OUTPUT

In reporting a patient's urine and/or feces, color generally is a major factor since it may indicate the presence of, or changes in, many internal conditions. But color alone does not necessarily indicate that a patient is getting better or worse:

The color of feces can be due entirely to food pigments. A greenish feces may be the result of having eaten spinach, and the eating of large amounts of fresh fruit, such as peaches and apricots, can cause a light-color feces.

The color of urine normally will vary from pale straw to amber. Color may be affected by medicines and some foods. For example, rhubarb commonly makes urine either brown or orange in color.

Another important factor in waste output is patient discomfort during urination or a bowel movement. Unusual stress, prolonged stress, pain, or strain in either of these functions should be noted on the record. If severe, report them to the doctor or your visiting nurse as soon as possible.

To simplify your work and consolidate data for the doctor or your visiting nurse, waste output records, as in Fig. 49–2, usually are written on the back of the food intake record.

Urine If reports of your patient's urine are required, flush out the urinal with clean water and empty it before use. Do not leave any water in it! Pour the urine into the measuring container, or take the reading direct from a graduated male urinal (Fig. 8–24*a*), and record the amount in cc./oz.

Record the color of the urine. Usually it is a combination of colors instead of a pure one—greenish instead of a strong green, brown-red instead of a true brown or a true red, and so forth. Describe the color as accurately as possible, using as many terms as you feel necessary, such as *light* or *dark* . . . *yellow, greenish, brown-red* . . . *clear* or *cloudy*, etc.

You also may be required to record the odor of urine. Fresh, normal urine is generally considered as having a not particularly unpleasant odor; it may be faintly aromatic. Under certain conditions it may have a strong, easily identifiable

Urination	B. M.
7:00 A.M. – 300 c.c.	
	8:30 A.M. – copious amt, tarry black
10:30 A.M. – 200 c.c.	
2:15 P.M. – 250 c.c.	
	6:15 P.M. – moderate amt, soft formed, brown
7:00 P.M. – 200 c.c.	
	11:00 P.M. – moderate amt, liquid

Fig. 49–2 *Partially filled form for recording Waste Output*

odor, such as that of ammonia. However, urine's odor is significant only in a fresh specimen.

If a patient has a bowel movement and urinates in the bedpan at the same time, generally you cannot measure the amount of urine or determine its color or odor accurately. Make this notation on the record.

Feces Reports of a patient's feces usually describe its color, texture, and odor, and give a rough estimate of the amount. Exact weight and specimens seldom are required.

As with urine, feces usually is a combination of colors, ranging from a clayish white to tarry black, and should be reported with as many descriptive terms as you feel are necessary. Normal color of feces ranges from light brown to dark brown.

The texture of feces usually is described as firm, semisoft, or liquid. Firm feces may further be described as very firm or hard, in small pellets, rough, and so forth.

The normal odor of feces is generally considered as not being very disagreeable nor particularly strong. Although changes in odor often are due entirely to changes in a patient's diet, they should be reported. So also should a particularly foul odor of feces.

Usually the amount of feces is adequately described as copious, moderate, or small.

Recording Waste Output When the back of a food intake record, Fig. 49–1, is used for recording waste output, you need to fill in only the times of urination and bowel movements and pertinent data, as in Fig. 49–2. Because there usually are more urinations than bowel movements in a 24-hour period, urine reports customarily are at the left side of the record.

When recording liquid intake and waste outut, total it for each 24 hours. For example, a patient may have taken in 2,000 cc./2 l./67.6 U.S. Fl. oz./21 U.S. Fl.

qt. of liquid, and excreted 1,800 cc./1.8 l./60.9 U.S. Fl. oz./ 1.9 U.S. Fl. qt. of urine. It can be listed in any of the following ways:

	Cubic Centimeters	*Liters*	*U.S. Fluid*	
	cc.	l.	oz.	qt.
Intake	2,000	2	67.6	2.1
Output	1,800	1.8	60.9	1.9

IN GENERAL...

As a rule, food intake and waste output will not be identical, but the amounts should be fairly close. When they are not:

If intake is much greater, more than about 15 percent, than waste output, be sure to report it to the doctor or your visiting nurse. Of course, part of the difference between intake and output usually is due to the loss of body fluids by perspiration and respiration.

When waste output is greater than food intake, the patient may be suffering dehydration; this can be serious and should be reported to the doctor immediately. Two dehydrating actions that usually do not need to be measured before reporting to the doctor are vomiting and diarrhea.

50 Suggestions for the Working Nurse

Despite objections that many people have to "routine" living, it is the only practical way of making sure that your patient will receive proper care. Unless there is a schedule for serving meals, cleaning and dressing your patient, making the bed and freshening the room, giving medicine, and so forth, important services may be overlooked. Also, most sick people prefer an established daily life. They look forward to meals, baths, a back rub, exercise, etc., at set times, and tend to fret if a service is late and become annoyed if it occurs before they are ready for it. To sick people in general, time passes slowly. If two welcome breaks in a day, such as a meal and a back rub, occur closer together than usual, it merely means that there will be a longer wait for the next break.

Most experienced nurses want a routine because it enables them to do their work the best way without overtaxing their strength or losing needed rest. This is especially important in the case of someone who is nursing at home and working full-time at an outside job.

As a rule, the most practical routine for both nurse and patient is one based on the work, play, and rest schedule in effect when the patient was well. If, for example, you and your patient had your main meal in the middle of the day and a light one at night, there usually is no need to change that habit simply because of your patient's ailment.

Aside from being more practical, keeping to an established way of living usually is better for a patient's frame of mind. An abrupt change, obviously due to the patient's condition, stresses its real or imagined seriousness; and the real or imagined extra work it makes for you and the family may give your patient a strong feeling of guilt or of being a burden. Keeping to the accustomed way of living gives the average sick person a sense of security, a feeling that "things aren't so bad." And it often prevents the confusion as to where they are and with whom that so often afflicts elderly sick people.

If, however, you are employed full-time outside the home, changing an established way of living may be essential. Usually the easiest way to make this change is to plan the new schedule in detail before presenting it, with explanations when necessary, to your patient and the rest of the family. If there are objections, listen to them patiently, but keep in mind that the purpose of the new schedule is to enable you to give your patient the best possible care. In order to get your plan more readily accepted, you may have to make some changes that will, at worst, be only minor inconveniences; if you think that this may be necessary, plan them in advance and give in only after sufficient discussion with all persons involved.

SUGGESTED SCHEDULINGS

Any scheduling of nursing care depends on the condition of your patient. One who is confined to home but can be up and around most of the time usually needs much less care than one who can be out of bed for only very short periods; these situations are covered in detail in Chapter 51. For general care, here are some changes in routine living to consider.

BATH. Normally a patient is bathed (bed, shower, or tub) between breakfast and the noon meal. Instead, schedule it for shortly before or after the evening meal. It may, of course, be given just before a patient's bedtime. But since the bed usually is made at bathtime and the back rub given at bedtime, bathing then can make this time unnecessarily busy and tiring for you and your patient. If your patient is not confined to bed, a daily bath may not be necessary; one every other day may be adequate.

BED. The bed usually is made during a patient's bath. This is almost essential when giving a bed bath (Chapter 23), but may be changed to any convenient time for the average shower or tub bath patient.

BACK RUB. A back rub usually is given just before a patient's bedtime to encourage sleep. Additional rubs may be given at any time you and your patient feel it necessary.

EXERCISE. Depending on the condition of your patient, prescribed exercise may be given during a bath (Chapter 28), or at any other time of day or night.

MEALS. For most people not engaged in hard manual labor, breakfast is a light meal, and either the noon or the evening meal is light and the other the main one. Some people are accustomed to two, four, or five instead of three meals a day. Eating habits are among the most difficult to change; but for most nurses who work full-time outside the home and must also prepare the meals, having the main one after work usually is the practical solution.

VISITING. Every day you should spend some time simply visiting with your patient, being a good listener. If between outside working and nursing at home your day seems too short for a listening session, try dressing or undressing in your patient's room—let your patient talk while you are busy.

WORKING. If you work full-time outside the home, it may be necessary to have someone—a neighbor, relative, or friend—drop in during the day to see if your patient needs anything. If you cannot get home at noon to prepare luncheon, you may have to do it before going to work. Many communities have Meals-On-Wheels service available. A well-balanced meal is brought to the home at the noon hour. If a special diet is necessary, it can be arranged. Check your community services or ask your visiting nurse for this service.

51 Planning the Care of Your Patient

Whether your patient is confined to home but otherwise leads an almost normal life, or is bedfast and unable to move, planning the proper care involves protection as well as the more physical nursing services such as bathing, feeding, giving medicines and so forth.

PROTECTION

In addition to guarding against disease and infection, protect your patient against:

- Accidents
- Overexertion
- Visitors
- Boredom
- Despondency

Accidents Only patients who are physically, mentally, and emotionally able and willing to care for themselves in an emergency should ever be left alone at home for even a short time, and that is not recommended. If your patient does not have full control of all faculties and you must leave the home for even a few minutes, get someone to replace you. It can be anyone, adult or child, who at least can and will summon help in an emergency. If, however, your patient has been asking for food, beverage, medicine, activity, etc., that is restricted or forbidden, warn your replacement against giving in to your patient's pleas; better, get someone you know will not give in.

Regardless of how much or how little nursing care sick or injured people need, keep in mind that they are disabled and that they:

1. *May be confused* at times as to where they are, the seriousness of their condition, and what they should or should not do. This often occurs to sick

elderly people, to persons with recent head injuries, to patients having certain fevers or infections, and to persons who have had certain kinds of surgery. Patients showing any signs of confusion or disorientation must never be left at home alone or with people who cannot control them. To prevent injuring anyone, keep especially close watch on a patient who has or has had any period of confusion or disorientation and must use a sharp or pointed article such as a knife, fork, pen, pencil, scissors, etc.

2. *May not safely* be able to go up or down stairs, get in or out of bed or a chair, take a shower or a tub bath, or go to the toilet. Do not leave such patients alone at home ever, unless you are absolutely certain that they will not attempt an unsafe action.

3. *May need safe floors.* If your patient uses crutches, a walker, cane, or wheelchair, remove all scatter or throw rugs, mats, or small carpets. They can cause serious falls, and make it difficult to operate a wheelchair.

NOTE: Crutches, canes, and walkers without wheels should always be equipped with safety caps to prevent sliding on slippery surfaces such as hardwood, linoleum, and cement floors.

4. *May fall out of bed.* Except for patients having the mildest disabilities, such as a light cold or a broken finger, the bed should be equipped with guardrails (Chapter 8), which should be locked in the protective position whenever the patient is left alone. This is particularly important for the protection of sick elderly people, stroke patients, persons in casts, people who have had recent surgery or had an injury-accident, persons with certain fevers or infections, patients who are in any way confused or disoriented. If your patient objects to guardrails, ask your visiting nurse to explain why and when they are necessary.

Overexertion Regardless of their kind or stage of disability, many sick or injured people want to try an exercise or activity that they believe will help them even though it has not been approved by, or even discussed with, the doctor. This often is done to show you how well they are—thanks to your care and work! But they do not realize what can happen if an exercise is too strenuous or they fall. Improper or too much exercise can open a nearly healed wound; a fall can easily break bones. If you even suspect that your patient is too eager, then you or your visiting nurse should explain exactly what can result from unapproved activity. Explain in plain, simple, blunt words and do not try to spare your patient's feelings. If you believe it is necessary to say, "Only a fool would do that," say it! The important thing is your patient's health and safety. In some cases (but consult the doctor first), the best solution is to let a patient try a nonprescribed exercise while you are there to help if necessary; let the patient learn the hard way what can and cannot be done. If your patient does it safely and with no adverse side effects, you both will be pleased.

NOTE: As a general rule, too-eager patients should not be left alone at home. However, just knowing that someone is present, even a child only old enough to tattle, will deter them. Tell the child what things the patient should not do. Children usually respond well to this kind of responsibility.

Exercise is, of course, essential to everyone's welfare (Chapter 28), and you must encourage your patient to do all that the doctor or therapist prescribed. But too much of a prescribed exercise can be as harmful as one that is basically too strenuous for your patient or does not give certain parts of your patient's body proper muscular activity.

Visitors Regardless of how well they know and like one another, visitors (Chapter 52) nearly always tire sick and injured people. Experienced nurses know this, which is why they so often "look in" on a patient who has visitors. If you see or even suspect that visitors are tiring your patient, suggest that it is time for them to leave; insist on it in no uncertain terms when necessary. As a rule, only two or three visitors at a time should be allowed to see a patient.

Protecting your patient against long-staying visitors can be a difficult task, particularly when patient and visitors unite against the common enemy—you!

Boredom Persons who were moderately to very active before becoming sick or injured often suffer from boredom, especially when their condition is improving. The healthier they feel, the more they tend to "forget" why they are confined to home or to bed. They obey orders, often simply because they feel that they are paying for the doctor's advice and must get their money's worth. They regard any rest period as something to suffer through. They encourage themselves to become "bored" with any and every thing . . . books, radio, TV, puzzles, games, visitors, special foods—nothing holds interest for them.

A patient's boredom can become a serious problem. However, there are several practical ways to stop it, or at least to keep a patient from wallowing in it. It may be that a frank discussion of the reasons for the enforced rest or confinement will help a patient accept it. Or a patient may accept it if the doctor gives an approximate length of time that it must be endured.

To get some patients out of their boredom a sort of shock treatment may be needed. It may be a sharp scolding. Or a threat to quit nursing—although a threat that you obviously cannot keep is worse than useless. Ask your visiting nurse, who probably has had much experience with "bored" patients, to help solve the problem.

Despondency The older sick and injured persons are and the less able they are to care for themselves, the more likely they are to become despondent, feel unwanted, neglected. It often leads to dangerous self-pity, ranging from dark mutterings such as, "If it wasn't for me, you could . . ." to threats of deliberately wasting away or even committing suicide. Always keep close watch on patients who threaten or frequently talk about self-destruction; they are more likely to try it than other persons are.

Not all patients suffer despondency, and how severe such spells are may greatly depend on how long a patient will be confined. Those who will be laid up for a fairly short time often become irritable, but not necessarily despondent. Mild attacks of despondency often do not last very long; your visiting nurse may be quite helpful in stopping them and advising how you may prevent future ones. In the case of deep despondency, or long-lasting or frequent mild attacks, consult your patient's doctor.

PLANNING THE NURSING CARE

The number of nursing services that you must give your patient and the schedule of providing them are equally as important. Failure to follow a schedule can result in a number of harmful things, ranging from mildly disturbing or upsetting your patient to causing painful bedsores (Chapter 15) and some or all of the many disuse disabilities due to lack of exercise (Chapter 28).

To help you plan the care of your patient, here is a list of common nursing services that are needed, and practical suggestions for providing them. To ease your workload, schedule your nursing work to fit in with other demands made on your time. It may simplify making up a schedule and keeping to it if you mark each service with a reminder of when it should be done, such as *M* for Morning, *A* for Afternoon, *E* for Evening, *D* for Daily, *EOD* for Every Other Day, *W* for Weekly, and so on.

☐ BACK RUB (Chapter 18). Most patients learn to enjoy back rubs very much in very short time. There is no harm in giving your patient one anytime, but there are certain times when one should be given. It depends on the condition of your patient:

1. Patients who are up and around for most of the time usually do not require back rubs unless they have real difficulty in going to sleep at bedtime.
2. For crutch, cane, walker, and wheelchair patients who are fairly active in moving themselves around, the back rub is excellent for relaxing tense and tired muscles. For less active persons, back rubs can help keep muscles limber and stimulate circulation of the blood.
3. Patients who are confined to bed for most of the time generally need a back rub as an aid to going to sleep at normal bedtime.

NOTE: Whenever giving your patient a back rub, examine the bony prominences for signs of pressure, which could become bedsores (Chapter 15).

☐ BATH (Chapter 23). Because sick and injured people often are not as strong, agile, and capable as they think they are, let them take a shower or a tub bath only when you or another competent person is nearby to give immediate help if needed. How often bathing should be done depends on the condition of your patient:

1. Unless the patient is receiving external medication, a daily bath usually is not as important for patients who are up and around most of the time as for those who are less active.
2. Crutch, cane, walker, and wheelchair patients generally should be bathed daily; however, it is more important for the inactive patient, especially

one who must be given a bed bath, than for one who can have a shower or a tub bath.

3. Patients who are confined to bed for most of the time should be bathed daily. If other factors permit it, patients who are allowed out of bed for sufficient time should have a shower or a tub bath, or even a sponge bath. Give other patients a bed bath, with them in bed or sitting on the side of it. Encourage your patient to do as much of the work of bathing as possible.

NOTE: Use the bathtime to inspect your patient for signs of potential bedsores. This is also an excellent time for your patient's exercise (Chapter 28).

☐ BED (Chapter 13). How often you should remake the bed with fresh linen depends on the condition of your patient. You should, of course, keep the bedding smooth and free of wrinkles.

1. Unless a patient who is up and around most of the time is being given external medication, as a rule you need not change bed linen more often than you would for a healthy person.

2. Bed linen for crutch, cane, walker, and wheelchair patients who must be given a bed bath is generally changed daily. But unless such patients who can be tub, shower, or sponge bathed are receiving external medication, usually there is no need to change bed linen more often than you would for a healthy person.

3. Linen for patients who are bedfast for most of the time and must be given a bed bath generally is changed daily. But for patients who can shower, tub, or sponge bathe . . . spend most of the day "in bed" resting on a cot, daybed, etc. . . . and are not receiving external medication, usually there is no need to change bed linen more often than for a healthy person.

4. Make the bed daily, with a change of linen, for patients who are allowed out of bed for only limited time. After the bed bath is a good time for your patient's first out-of-bed period. It also is a good time for you to remake the bed, and a good opportunity for you to observe your patient's reaction to being out of bed.

NOTE: When your patient gets out of bed, if you are not going to change the linen, pull the top sheet and bedding down over the foot of the bed to air; it should air for at least an hour if possible.

5. Change bed linen daily for bedfast patients. Encourage your patient to help as much as possible, even if only by moving from one side of the bed to the other. Be sure to keep the regular and draw sheets free of wrinkles. Whether or not your patient feels them, wrinkles can irritate the skin and cause pressure points that could become bedsores.

☐ BEDSORES (Chapter 15). Patients who are up and around most of the time and lead fairly normal lives seldom develop bedsores. All others, including those confined to wheelchairs, should be examined for potential bedsores several times a day. Two particularly good times to do it are at morning bath time and before a patient goes to sleep at night.

☐ CLEANING THE ROOM. How much thorough room cleaning and daily tidying up you should do depends on the condition of your patient.

1. Except for appearance sake, as a rule the only thorough room cleaning and daily "lick and a promise" necessary for patients who are out of their real beds for most of the time is the same as for a healthy person. Use your own good judgment, but excessive cleaning usually is not necessary.
2. Rooms for patients who are confined to their real beds for most of the time usually should be thoroughly cleaned twice a week, especially in dusty regions, and tidied up daily. If your patient's time out of bed is long enough, it may be the practical time for cleaning.

NOTE: Immobile patients often are more aware of and troubled by the real or imagined lack of cleanliness of their rooms than other patients.

☐ DRESSING PATIENTS. The extent of dressing and how much aid you should give depend on the condition of your patient. Patients should, when practical, wear clothes that they like, including underwear as well as outer garments.

1. Patients who are up and around most of the time, even if using crutches, or a cane, walker, or wheelchair, usually can dress themselves in whole or in part. Encourage them, even if it does take considerably more time than if you dressed them, as it provides excellent exercise. Dressing usually is done before a patient gets into a wheelchair, unless dressing in the chair is more convenient.
2. Patients who are out of their real beds most of the day, but confined to daybeds or couches, may be treated the same as those who are up and around most of the time, 1 above, or who are confined to bed, 3 below. Relatively active patients, and those who can and will keep themselves covered by a light blanket or afghan to prevent chilling, may be dressed in clothes of their choice. Less active patients, and those unwilling or unable to keep themselves adequately covered for warmth, usually are treated as bedfast patients, following.
3. Patients who are confined to their real beds for most of the time commonly wear pajamas (often just the tops) or nightgowns, with or without a bedjacket or sweater. The patient gown, hospital-type (Chapter 8) or substitute, is extremely practical for immobile patients, as it is the easiest of all to put on or remove from a helpless person. Change pajamas or gowns at least daily; two or more times a day in hot or humid weather, and for patients who perspire somewhat freely. When out of bed, patients should wear dressing gowns or bathrobes that will keep them comfortably warm and

prevent chills. Bedroom slippers or mules also should be worn, or heavy socks if a patient prefers them.

NOTE: When getting patients out of bed who have been bedfast for more than 2 weeks, always put shoes on them to support the arches of the feet.

☐ EXERCISE (Chapter 28). Give, assist with, or supervise all exercises exactly as prescribed by the doctor or therapist. Keep close watch on lazy and too-eager patients, as too little and too much or too strenuous exercise can be harmful.

GETTING IN AND OUT OF BED (Chapter 14). Give only the aid that is absolutely necessary to help your patient in and out of bed, as these actions usually provide good exercise.

1. Moving a patient directly from bed to a wheelchair, or from chair to bed, must never be done unless the wheels are locked. Patients who are expert in moving between wheelchair and bed may be allowed to do it unaided, but you should be nearby to give emergency help.
2. Patients in the early stages of recovery from severe sickness, injury, or surgery, and those who have been confined to bed for about 10 days or more, usually are much physically weaker than in their normal condition. Have your patient sit on the edge of the bed with feet dangling for 5 to 10 minutes before getting off it. This allows the patient's equilibrium and blood pressure to adjust before standing; without such adjustment, the patient is apt to have a dizzy spell or, in extreme cases, a blackout.

☐ HANDICAP AIDS (Chapter 16). Use all the handicap aids available to make your patient comfortable and more self-sufficient.

☐ MEALS (Chapter 30). As well as being important nutritionally, meals can give patients mental and emotional stimulation by making them feel that they are improving, and that they are wanted by their friends and relatives.

1. As a rule, patients who can be out of bed for any time, other than for just going to the toilet, should eat with the family. The meal that the patient is most likely to have to prepare is the midday one; the more of this work that the patient does, the better. If a patient is unwilling or unable to prepare meals in keeping with a diet, you should plan meals that can be served with minimum effort, such as heat-holding containers of soup and the main dish, salad in the refrigerator, etc. When a patient regularly must be left alone for a meal, make it a definite part of the day's schedule.
2. Patients who are allowed out of bed for very brief times usually have all meals in bed. They may occasionally have the main meal with the family. Ask the doctor. The pleasure a patient gets from eating with the family may outweigh possible harm caused by being out of bed longer than usual.

3. Encourage patients who are more or less immobile to do all self-feeding possible, regardless of how it may prolong a meal. Meals often are a major interest for these patients; make every effort to prepare tasty, attractive foods that your patient likes and are allowed by the diet.

☐ RADIO, RECORDERS, TELEPHONE, TELEVISION (Chapter 16). For patients who can use and want them, place the telephone, radio, record player or tape recorder, and television sets (or remote controls for them) within easy reach.

☐ SHIFTING POSITION IN CHAIR. To help prevent bedsores (Chapter 15), patients who spend most of their time in regular chairs or wheelchairs should shift their weight every 30 minutes. Those who can should push down on the armrests to lift themselves off the seat, and stay there for about 30 seconds. Patients who cannot lift themselves should shift weight by raising one buttock, then the other, off the seat for about 30 seconds each.

☐ TOILET. For the sake of exercise (Chapter 28) and to protect your patient's sensibilities, give your patient the least assistance in all phases of going to the toilet.

1. Patients who are up and around most of the time, unaided or with crutches, cane, or walker, and wheelchair patients who can move themselves directly between bed and chair usually need only the same assistance as for Getting in and out of Bed, above. It may also be necessary to help them on and off the toilet.

2. Wheelchair patients who should be moved in and out of their chairs as little as possible and those who cannot move themselves safely in or out of their chairs and must be left alone at home should be given a urinal or a bedpan (Chapter 8) as needed. If you must leave the home and your patient can use a urinal or a bedpan without assistance, leave it with your patient to spare possible embarrassment of having to ask for it; cover it with a towel.

3. Bedfast patients who are allowed out of bed for only very brief periods usually prefer to go to the toilet, especially for bowel movement, than have a bedpan or urinal in bed. Ask the doctor if trips to the toilet are included in your patient's allowed time out of bed.

4. If your patient may not get out of bed to go to the toilet, encourage the use of urinal and bedpan at regular times, such as on awakening in the morning, at bathtime, before lunch and dinner, and at normal bedtime. If you must leave the home for a while, plan such trips for soon after your patient has had a bowel movement or urinated. If this cannot be done, leave a bedpan and a urinal, each covered by a towel, within easy reach of a patient who can use it with little or no assistance. The person who is watching out for your patient while you are gone probably could give the bedpan or urinal; but sick people often dislike receiving these items from people they do not know well.

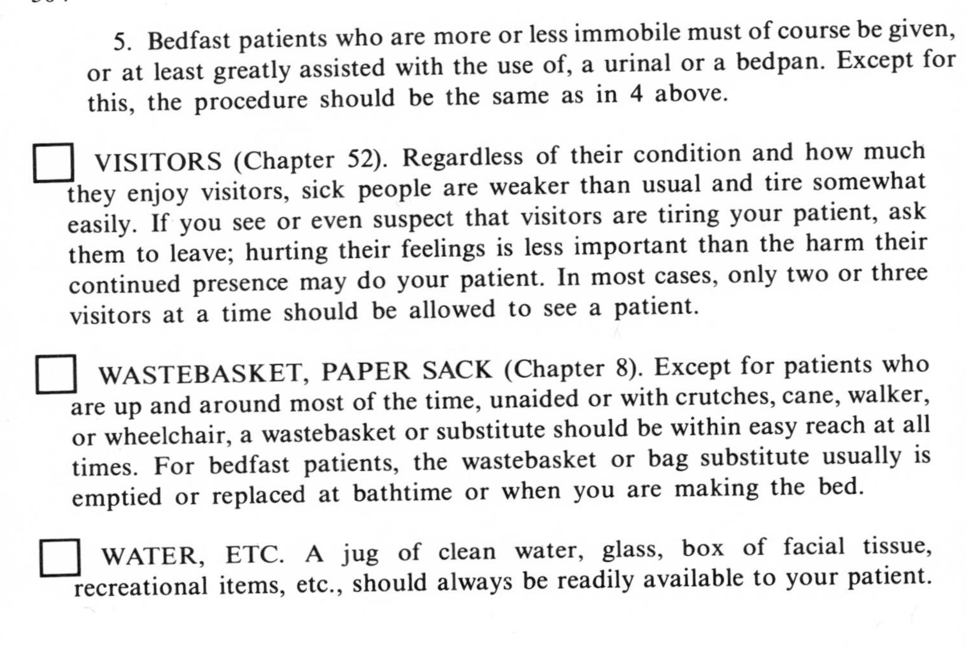

5. Bedfast patients who are more or less immobile must of course be given, or at least greatly assisted with the use of, a urinal or a bedpan. Except for this, the procedure should be the same as in 4 above.

☐ VISITORS (Chapter 52). Regardless of their condition and how much they enjoy visitors, sick people are weaker than usual and tire somewhat easily. If you see or even suspect that visitors are tiring your patient, ask them to leave; hurting their feelings is less important than the harm their continued presence may do your patient. In most cases, only two or three visitors at a time should be allowed to see a patient.

☐ WASTEBASKET, PAPER SACK (Chapter 8). Except for patients who are up and around most of the time, unaided or with crutches, cane, walker, or wheelchair, a wastebasket or substitute should be within easy reach at all times. For bedfast patients, the wastebasket or bag substitute usually is emptied or replaced at bathtime or when you are making the bed.

☐ WATER, ETC. A jug of clean water, glass, box of facial tissue, recreational items, etc., should always be readily available to your patient.

52 Visitors

As well as being the best thing that can happen to patients, a visitor can be the worst. Visitors can fill patients with the strongest reasons for getting well, and they can drive patients to utmost exhaustion.

One of the more difficult problems confronting the average inexperienced nurse is visitors and what to do about them. Who should be allowed to see your patient, who should not. How long should visitors be allowed to stay. How to get rid of visitors, without hurting their feelings if possible. What to do with gifts, especially candy and other eatables.

There is only one answer for all problems about visitors: do whatever is best for your patient. Be polite, be firm, tell what little white lies may be necessary—but do what is best for your patient!

VISITING HOURS

Although a major reason for caring for a patient at home is to get away from the regimentation of a hospital, establishing visiting hours for your patient may be the only way that will enable you to do your work and get necessary rest. Of course, it depends to great extent on the condition of your patient; the less you must do for your patient, the less visitors can get in the way. However, in order to give yourself time to get certain basic work done as well as assure your patient of some rest periods, you should set aside certain times as visiting hours.

WHEN VISITORS ARRIVE

Always ask your patient's permission before admitting a visitor!

Whether your patient is suffering from a physical, emotional, or mental illness or from an injury, remember that sick people tire easily and, often, unexpectedly. By the time a visitor who had phoned just a short time before arrives, your patient may really have gotten too tired to want to see anyone. Take your patient's word for it, and explain it to the visitor.

Never take it for granted that a patient wants to see relatives who come to visit. Relatives and in-laws often believe that "their" sick people just naturally want to see them any and every time they care to visit; some feel that sick people are obliged to receive relatives and in-laws. But there may be several reasons why relatives and in-laws are the people a patient does not want to see. Relatives and in-laws are not necessarily friends, and often have nothing in common with the patient to talk about. Relatives and in-laws frequently are self-appointed bearers of bad news. Because they have decided that the patient should know, they repeat fact or fiction about how a business is doing . . . a competitor they think has been promoted . . . trouble they understand children have gotten into . . . an "affair" the patient's spouse is supposed to be having, and so on. Also, relatives and in-laws frequently feel that a patient will benefit from hearing how someone with a similar ailment died but could have been saved by a different doctor (not your patient's) and different treatment (not your patient's). So before ushering in relatives or in-laws for a visit, ask your patient.

Never take it for granted that a patient wants to see friends, fellow employees, or business associates who come to visit. Bonds that hold people together when all are healthy often break when one of them is sick or injured, and a sickroom visit may be embarrassing for all. Also, for purely personal reasons, many patients do not care to be seen by people outside the immediate family. So again, be sure to ask your patient before bringing in visitors.

When your patient does not want a visitor, remember that sick people often have sudden and unexplainable changes of mood, and some other time may welcome that visitor warmly. Therefore, try not to hurt the presently unwanted visitor's feelings. Give a plausible excuse for your patient's being unavailable. There are many things that you can say and that a reasonable visitor will accept . . . patient is sleeping . . . doctor is very strict about visiting hours . . . too many visitors the last few days . . . patient had a poor night/morning/afternoon and simply does not feel up to having visitors now. Follow your excuse with a suggestion that the visitor come back again, but should telephone first.

What if a visitor will not accept an excuse and insists on seeing your patient? In most cases a person like this deserves no consideration, so simply say that your patient is not now having visitors—and put the visitor out.

Sometimes a member of the patient's family will object to your turning away of visitors, and object on the grounds that the patient should be allowed to entertain guests. Simply state that your patient is not an entertainer, at least not at the moment, and that your patient's sickness or injury is not a sideshow or nightclub act.

THE WELCOME VISITOR

Before admitting a visitor, it may be advisable to briefly describe your patient's condition; but in doing this be very careful not to give out information that your patient does not have. Most visitors are naturally curious about sickness and injury. Your "official" account (after all, you *are* the nurse) should satisfy the visitor's curiosity and prevent questions and remarks that are better left unsaid. Describing your patient's condition also gives you an ideal opportunity to tell a visitor how long to stay, something that can be of utmost importance, below.

There is, of course, the argument that by describing your patient's condition you take away your patient's pleasure of doing it. Possibly true—unless you warn the visitor to simply listen to your patient and ask reasonable questions.

GIFTS

If your patient is on a diet, candy, pastries, ice cream, certain beverages and other goodies may not be allowed. If they are brought as gifts, thank the donor and explain why your patient may not have them.

Books and magazines are, in general, safe gifts for sick people. However, some people have very strong likes and dislikes of reading material.

Recorded or taped music often is a very welcome gift, particularly when the music is the type the patient likes best. In self-defense, however, you may have to put a limit on how loudly and how often it is played.

Clothing such as bed jackets, nightgowns, bathrobes, shawls, slippers, and so forth usually are practical and welcome gifts. If appropriate, tell the donor in advance what style, color, size, etc., your patient prefers.

Flowers and potted plants are, of course, reliably safe gifts for almost all sick or injured people who are not allergic to certain pollens.

HOW LONG SHOULD A VISITOR STAY

Regardless of a patient's condition, and of the warmth of feeling between patient and visitor, you should get rid of a visitor as soon as your patient shows any sign of being tired. (You would be amazed by how often hospitalized patients must be given sedatives to offset the exhaustion caused by too many visitors or visitors who have stayed too long.)

Because of your close contact as the nurse, probably you will sense oncoming tiredness before your patient does. The minute you do, say something to the effect that visiting time is ended, or say to the patient, "You look as if you are getting tired." If after a few minutes the visitor or visitors show no sign of leaving, say clearly and with authority that your patient is tired and needs rest. If that does not produce results, go stand beside the open doorway as if waiting to usher the visitors out. Remember that when visitors do not have sense enough to leave when first told to, you must take positive action. The good of your patient is far more important than a visitor's hurt feelings.

There is no hard and fast rule regarding length of visits since so much depends on the kind of illness, a patient's general physical and emotional condition, and wishes. In some cases a five-minute visit may be ample. On the other hand, a patient may enjoy a long, relaxed visit with certain people. Experienced nurses often arrange some sort of signaling whereby a patient can indicate when a visit should end.

Remember, the "right" visitor can give your patient's spirits a tremendous lift and provide enjoyment from the memory of the visit in days ahead. But even the "right" visitor must not be allowed to stay too long.

PART TWO

You—the Patient

What you can do and should not do in order to be a good and well-liked patient as far as the doctor, your nurse and visiting nurse, family and friends are concerned.

53 So You're Going Home

If you are like most sick or injured people, you are all eagerness to get out of the hospital or similar institution and go home. But for your own good, do not be in too much of a rush. Take time enough for you and your home nurse to get the instructions and equipment and supplies needed for your proper care. Take a little more time to thank the people who have been caring for you.

THE INSTRUCTIONS YOU'LL NEED

Before leaving the hospital or other treatment center, have your home nurse meet with your doctor and you regarding the care you must have when you are home. Particularly if your nurse is inexperienced, this meeting may prevent most of the worry that the three of you otherwise probably would have about your getting the proper nursing care.

Even though the doctor and attending professional nurses and technicians may have told you what care you will need at home, ask the doctor to repeat the instructions in detail while your home nurse is present. You, if at all possible, and your home nurse should write down the instructions in detail—rest periods, bathing, meals, medication, limitations on activities, kind and amount of exercises, everything about the care you need. Before the doctor leaves, compare your written notes with your nurse's. Remember that most people do not "hear" instructions exactly the same way. Also, most people write in detail the parts of instructions that they think are most important, and for the others simply jot down some reminder words. So for your own good, be sure that your set of written instructions and your nurse's are the same. They can also save a lot of arguments between you and your nurse as to what you should or should not have, should or should not do.

If your home care will involve a complicated diet or cooking, or special exercises or other therapy, the doctor usually will ask the dietitian or therapist to meet with you and your home nurse. Whether or not they have *M.D.s* behind their names, they are experts in their fields and deserve the same respect as your doctor. And they should be able and willing to explain their instructions clearly.

While receiving instructions from the doctor, dietitian, or therapist and reviewing them with your home nurse, be sure that you understand them thoroughly. If there is anything that you are not sure of, no matter how small and unimportant it may seem—ask for an explanation. Keep asking until you do fully understand; many medical terms sound alike and are confusing to nonprofessionals.

HELP KEEP THE WELCOME MAT OUT

Particularly if you have been there for more than just a few days, before checking out of a hospital or similar institution, make it a point to thank personally the people who have cared for you. Hospital personnel from the doctor to the cleaning people are accustomed to gripes and complaints from patients and patient's friends and relatives, but seldom do they get a "Thank you for all you have done."

Be practical. Not only will the thanking make you feel better, it usually will be remembered and get you better service if and when you must return. Help keep the welcome mat out for yourself—just in case.

Hospitals generally have a form that may be filled out asking for honest criticism and helpful suggestions. Do not be afraid to tell your unpleasant experiences, if any. But keep in mind that deserved bouquets are also appreciated.

54 So You're Home Now

You're home now—things will be different! No more being told what to eat, when to eat, when to sleep, when to wake up! No more do this, do that! No more "We feel better now, don't we!" You know how well you feel. You know what you can do, what you want to do, what you will do! You're home now—you'll have it your way!

Perhaps.

But in most cases, no.

Unfortunately, most people coming home from a hospital, convalescent home, or other treatment center bring with them a false sense of strength. No matter how serious or severe their sickness or injury, they commonly believe that just the act of coming home is proof positive that they are getting better, and that further recovery depends chiefly on how hard they work at it. Even patients who must be carried in and put to bed immediately tend to feel that they now should do more than they could in the other place. Patients who were allowed out of bed for limited times often firmly believe that now, at home, they should and can be up and around all they want . . . that the more they do the better it will be for everyone . . . and that most of being an invalid is, for them at least, a state of mind!

Frequently, however, the simple truth is that going home was considered as being less harmful than keeping a patient under full-time professional care in a qualified institution. Some of the practical reasons for this decision are the cost of institutional care and the patient's genuine need of it, patient homesickness, and TLC—the Tender Loving Care that can be given by a patient's family and friends.

WHAT ABOUT YOU?

Of course, in *your* case the doctor may have realized that you no longer really needed professional care, that you understood and would do what you should do, and that you could be relied on to give your home nurse all necessary instructions and directions.

Fine!

But for your own good and regardless of what the doctor said about your going home, promise yourself not to do too much now that you are home, and promise not to try to be boss. Chances are you will discover that these promises, like good intentions, are easier made than kept. But keep in mind this rule of thumb:

If you follow your doctor's and visiting nurse's instructions carefully you will have an easier time of it than if you force yourself to do what you think you ought to be able to do.

ABOUT OVERDOING

Especially during the first few days after coming home, convalescing patients tend to do more than they should. Some feel that they should be more active than they are allowed to be, that they should stop babying themselves, and that too much exercise is better than not enough. Others are so much happier for coming home that they believe themselves stronger than they are. Other patients overdo because they feel ashamed of appearing weak and in need of help. And others do more than they should in order to keep their home nurse from having to do so much work.

But what usually happens when artificial or forced strength gives out? Even if you are lucky and collapse safely onto a convenient bed or soft chair, there will be frantic calls to your doctor or the visiting nurse, perhaps a return to the institution you were so glad to leave, and a completely unnecessary load of worry and extra work for your home nurse.

So when you come home as a patient, instead of showing how strong and healthy and eager you are, be smart and follow your doctor's instructions. If you believe that they should be changed, decide what you think the changes should be. But before making any changes, ask your doctor or visiting nurse. Do not try to wheedle or browbeat permission from your home nurse—nursing you as you are probably is tedious enough without having another worry added to the load.

YOUR STATUS

If you return as a more or less dependent invalid to the home that you used to "rule," simple day-to-day living in it can become quite irritating for you. And for your home nurse. And for your family in general. Unfortunately for you, whether or not home life becomes almost unbearable for everyone in it depends mainly on you.

Face it. Your sickness or injury made an important change in your home. Others now have to do the work that you did, make the decisions that you made. Just as you did things your way, "they" do things their way. Usually they are not acutely aware of doing things differently from the way you would, but to you it is very obvious. And annoying. Naturally. Especially since you know from your own experience that your ways are the proper, practical ways. However, remember that "they" are now in command and that you have to get along with them and their ways. Here are some patient-proven *don't*'s and *do*'s for you that should help:

Don't try to be boss!

Do wait until your opinion is asked for, even if it is a very long wait.

Don't volunteer instructions for doing tasks . . . what tools and materials to use . . . where to start . . . how to work—right to left, left to right, top to bottom, bottom to top, outward from the middle, inward from the edges, or any other way that you know is best.

Do let whoever is doing a job do it her/his way even though you would do it differently.

Don't say or look, "If you had done it my way," when she/he falls flat on her/his face trying to do something her/his way.

Do be thankful that (as you no doubt will learn in fairly short time) "they" can get things done and made good decisions without your guidance.

Don't fuss and fret that you have nothing to do because no one wants you to do anything. This will change as "they" learn more about your limits and abilities, so enjoy it while you can! Relax—and help everyone!!

Do the tasks that "they" allow you and try to do them the way "they" suggest—at least, for as long as "they" are there to watch you. Keeping everyone happy should be part of your job.

Don't give in to doing it "their" way when you know, and possibly learned the hard way, a better way of doing it. For example, if someone insists that you get in or out of a bed or chair a certain way, and you have learned a method that is more practical for you, tell "them" so. After all, you are only protecting yourself.

Do, if you are consulted on how to perform certain tasks, respond cheerfully, and give instructions as clearly and simply as you can. Sometimes this is quite difficult, and it would be much easier for you to do the job rather than teach someone. But make the most of the opportunity to pass some of your knowledge and skill on to other members of the family.

Observe the above few *do*'s and *don't*'s and you probably will be the easy-to-care-for kind of patient that nurses, even inexperienced ones, like to help. At least, you will not be the kind of sick person whose nurse, family, and friends can hardly wait to be rid of.

55 On Suffering in Silence

First—be careful!

Suffering in silence or without complaint can be the best or the worst thing you can do to your nurse and to yourself. Whether "smiling despite the agony" or "biting the bullet" is wise or foolish depends on the nature of your suffering, on the effect your behavior may have on your nurse (especially if inexperienced), and on the effect it may have on you. The reasons for and against suffering in silence may change from day to day, even from minute to minute. However, with some careful thought you probably can decide wisely whether silent suffering can make you a wonderful patient or an extra worry to everyone concerned.

The most important factor in deciding whether to suffer in silence is honesty. Total, all-out honesty. Honesty in the questions you ask yourself, honesty in your answers. If you cannot give a definite answer to a question, be *honest enough* to say, "I don't know," and *smart enough* to consult your doctor or visiting nurse. There are three basic questions to ask yourself:

First, what is the nature of your suffering?

Second, what effect will your suffering in silence have on your nurse? and,

Third, what effect will it have on you?

All questions are equally important. Cheat on any answer if you wish—you will be the one to suffer the most.

NORMAL AND ABNORMAL PAIN

Almost all surgery and injuries, many medical treatments and some diseases produce pain. The severity, acuteness, and length of pain periods usually change as a disability progresses, and so does the patient's reactions to them. When a pain period becomes more severe, more intense, and lasts longer, most patients fear relapse and deterioration. When pain lessens, patients usually tend to thrill with thoughts of recovery. Unfortunately, both increases and decreases of pain can be misleading; they may be normal or abnormal, depending on the patient and the disability.

Since changes in pain may be normal and a good sign in your case, always ask the doctor in advance what to expect in the way of pain, when, and for how long. *Have your home nurse, especially if inexperienced, present when getting this information from your doctor.*

Ask what kind of pain to expect. Try to identify it in your own words, such as a sharp, stabbing sensation . . . a hot tingle . . . cramping . . . a deep ache . . . hot flashes . . . severe itching . . . painful joints, and so forth. Keep asking until you know exactly what to expect—what pain will be normal and natural for your condition, approximately when it should start, how long it may last. Of course, pain periods seldom start and stop exactly on schedule, and often the actual pain is different from what you have expected. But as long as they are reasonably close to the doctor's prediction, as a rule you can safely consider a pain period to be normal and not worth worrying about unduly. Admittedly, "reasonably close" is vague; however, if a pain period was supposed to start on the third day, usually any time from late in the second day to early in the fourth would be reasonably close.

If there are serious differences between actual and predicted pain, it may be abnormal and your doctor or your visiting nurse should be consulted immediately. There are many factors that may indicate abnormal pain—it starts appreciably sooner or later than predicted ... it is much greater than predicted ... the character or kind of pain changed. What nearly always marks a change of pain as being abnormal is how quickly it occurs—a *sudden* increase or a *sudden* decrease or total stoppage of pain, or pain *suddenly* appearing in a new location. In any of these cases, notify your doctor or nurse immediately, and do not even consider "suffering in silence."

SHOULD YOU SUFFER IN SILENCE?

Regardless of whether your pain periods are normal or abnormal, sooner or later you probably will face the problem of whether or not you should suffer in silence. Of course, you will notify your doctor at once of abnormal pain; you are not being brave, just extremely foolish, if you do not. You also should tell the visiting nurse, particularly if you cannot contact the doctor.

But what about your "private" nurse, especially if inexperienced, and your family and friends? Do you tell them, or should you suffer in silence? There is no rule of thumb except, perhaps, that you should give utmost consideration to its possible effects on your nurse and on you, the two most important people involved. Here are some points to consider for and against suffering in silence. Be honest in judging how they may affect your nurse and you.

How It May Affect Your Nurse Probably your nurse, especially if inexperienced or a spouse, relative, or friend, is more concerned and worried about you than you are, and for two good reasons:

1. An experienced nurse may have had many patients with your problems and knows what to expect almost from hour to hour, and therefore does not worry unduly as long as everything is normal. But without this background, the inexperienced nurse usually is not aware of the differences between normal and abnormal pain, and tends to worry excessively about the care you are getting. The worry usually is greater when there is a close personal relationship between nurse and patient.

2. You may have been disabled for so long a time, or possibly your present condition is so much less painful than it was a while ago, that you are not fully aware of normal or abnormal changes in it. As a result, you may worry less about yourself and your disability than an inexperienced nurse will.

Keeping in mind the two main reasons why an inexperienced nurse may worry more about you than you do, try to decide whether your "suffering in silence" will increase or decrease that worry.

Possibly the most difficult question to answer honestly is, Do you feel that you really can "suffer in silence," really can conceal your pain and worry? If you try and fail, your nurse most likely will think that your reason for trying to deceive is much greater than it actually is. Also, once you are caught fibbing about your condition, your nurse is sure to doubt you the next time you say that everything is all right. Of course, there is more than one way to "suffer in silence" successfully. Some patients actually can keep all sign of tension due to pain from showing in face, speech, or action. Others admit to more than usual pain, but insist that it is so mild that it really is not important. Still others may try to make a joke of it: "It hurts, but not nearly as much as I'd hurt me if I was the pain." Some persons try to minimize their pain on the basis that holy people of their knowledge have suffered more and gained spiritually by it. And then there are those who try to bluff their nurses by boasting that their pain is much greater than it is—"Why, this is the worst kind of pain anyone ever had! It's driving me crazy! It's been this way for the past six months!" If you are determined to conceal your pain from your nurse, try any means that you feel you can make work.

Now assume that you can successfully "suffer in silence" and deceive your nurse. With lessened worry about you, or at least no increase of worry, an inexperienced nurse may tend to lessen the care that you should receive. No intentional slackening of care, but a natural easing off based on the feeling, "My patient is so much better now that we can relax a little." No omission nor neglect of things that seem very important, but only of apparently minor matters, such as allowing forbidden goodies into your diet, giving medicine at irregular times and perhaps missing a dosage now and then, admitting too many visitors, interrupting your rest periods, and so forth. No one of these may be harmful, but many of them put together may cause a relapse.

Another possible reaction by an inexperienced nurse to your successful suffering in silence is a feeling or expectation that you should now improve quickly. Without either of you being aware of it, and without your doctor's permission, your nurse may urge you to get "up and around" sooner than you should, and you may force yourself to do it. The possible result—a relapse due to overexertion.

Also, your successful suffering in silence may lead an inexperienced nurse to feel unwanted and unneeded before you are safely able to care for yourself. This can cause neglect; unintentional, but harmful. Or, again unintentionally and unaware of it, your nurse may experience a certain resentment at your apparent rapid recovery; possibly there will be a feeling that it is now time for the weary nurse to become the patient and the ex-patient to do some nursing. These reactions are not due to dislike or bitterness, and often do not occur; but they can happen as the result of a sudden, probably completely unexpected removal of the pressure caused by worrying about you. Remember that parents who have spent hours searching and praying for a lost child often want to spank it hard when the little darling is found quietly playing at home.

If it seems that "suffering in silence" is noble and heroic and that not to do it is being very selfish, done to assure you better nursing care, keep in mind that as a patient your prime job is to improve as quickly as possible. The sooner you do, the sooner you can pay back some of the tender loving care that you received.

How Suffering in Silence May Affect You When disabled in any way, almost all of us are torn between the desire to get special attention and the wish to show everyone, especially ourselves, that we do not need it. This makes "suffering in silence" a unique and frustrating problem. If we are completely successful and no one knows that we are suffering, no one knows what we are achieving—we win the blue ribbon, so to speak, but cannot claim it or we automatically lose it.

Fortunately, there is a more practical side to suffering in silence. First, assume that it will not lessen the nursing care that you need. Then decide which will really make you feel better mentally and emotionally: talking about your suffering, or not mentioning it. As a rule, the better you feel mentally and emotionally, the better you feel physically.

Suppose you decide, and have good cause, to talk about your suffering:

1. Do not talk about it so often that your nurse and everyone else wants to avoid you—soon you may have no audience.
2. Do not go into such great detail that you lose your audience. Your abdominal surgical wound may fascinate you and your doctor, but make other people queasy.
3. Listen to accounts of debilities that have occurred to other people, no matter how boring they may be. They may take your mind off your own trouble for a few minutes, and you may even learn something useful.
4. If you discuss your condition calmly, intelligently, and without demand for sympathy, you may find that it eases your tensions and fears. The simple act of admitting to discomfort or pain often makes it easier to bear. Also, as a rule you will be admired by your listeners—admiration is one of the nicest tributes to receive.

Now suppose that you decide not to talk about your suffering:

1. You may or may not have more visitors than otherwise. Many people who visit obviously sick persons seem to forget those who appear to be well on the road to recovery.
2. You will have to keep your pain and suffering in the past tense—"It really hurt back then, when I was so sick"—and lose about 90 percent of the sympathy you may be entitled to.
3. You must be careful not to show any trace of the discomfort you may feel—or all your efforts to suffer in silence will go for nothing.

On the other hand, if you can get away with it, if no one except your doctor and the visiting nurse suspects that you do not feel as well as you pretend, there can be intense, deep satisfaction that gives a wonderful feeling of achievement. This takes many sick people a long way on Recovery Road.

56 Smile—It Could Be Worse

Smile, and the world smiles with you—complain, and you're left alone, especially if you complain for the sake of complaining.

You may know sick people who really try to make the most of their illness. Their conversation jumps from one ache and pain to another. You mention the weather—they might like it if they felt better. You hope they will enjoy the little gift you brought—you should know that they are too sick to enjoy anything. You are thankful that they have such a good doctor—they swear it is a wonder that they are still alive. They are so fortunate to have such a competent nurse—you have no idea of all the necessities that are not done! Their voices are weak. Not so weak that you will miss any words, but weak enough to stress the horrors of their ailments. Finally there is nothing more you can think of to say, and between you and the patient settles a silence broken by dramatically spaced-out sighs of painful exhaustion.

Does this seem at all familiar, as if it just might have occurred during your present disability? Have you fewer and fewer visitors? Are their visits shorter? Does your nurse spend less nonworking time with you?

Due to the difficulties that you are going through, you may have forgotten that healthy people have troubles, too. Also, you may have forgotten that healthy people often are embarrassed by, or slightly ashamed of, their good health when in the presence of disabled people. And, you may have been complaining too much.

Of course, no one expects you to bubble with laughter, joy, and merriment when you are disabled. Especially not soon after coming down with a sickness or shortly after surgery or an injury. But after the initial stage has passed, or when you have accepted the fact that you must put up with an affliction, you usually begin to feel better.

As soon as you begin to feel better in any way at all, show it! Do not keep it secret from anyone, especially not from your nurse, relatives, and friends. Those who were with you during the worst times have a right to know that you really do feel better. But in many cases just *saying* that you feel better will not work. No matter how strongly you say it, chances are that several of the people close to you will be convinced that you do not feel better, that you are simply putting on an act to mislead them. So you must *show* and *keep showing* them that you feel better.

How you can show them depends, obviously, on your condition. But no matter how it restricts your actions, if you really want to show that you feel better you probably can find a way. It may take a lot of original thinking. For example, if you cannot smile with your lips, or it could not be seen because of bandages on the lower part of your face, try smiling with your eyes; usually just the thought that you want to smile will bring a happy expression to your eyes. Or, wink in a friendly, even lascivious way. Or, waggle your eyebrows. Or, roll your eyes suggestively. It need not be much, just something to show that the time is gone when all you wanted was for everyone to know and sympathize with your every ache and pain.

LIVE IT UP!

If your condition permits it, a very good way to show that you feel better is to return as much as possible to your normal behavior. Go all out, even though some of your relatives and friends, even your nurse, may not approve of the way you dressed and behaved. It may be that their disapproval without being willing to stop you (remember, you still are sick and require some indulging) will add a bit of beneficial spice to your life:

—If you used cosmetics before, use them now if you want. If you cannot apply them as you like, ask your nurse or an empathetic relative or friend to do it for you.

—If you wore your hair long and "they" cut it short, let it grow if you want. But do not let a love of long hair interfere with proper treatment of your ailment.

—If you cherished clothing bright with psychedelics, and you still find it comfortable, wear it.

—If your life-style depends on subtle or on strong perfume, cologne, or deodorant, apply it or them as conservatively or as liberally as makes you content.

—If your culture opposes frequent baths, clean faces and hands, try to persuade the doctor, nurse, family, and friends that cleanliness is not for you. You may win. Or they may refuse to attend to your needs. Not only do they have their rights, they are in a better position to get them than you are. Console yourself with a bit of practical advice: if you can't lick 'em, join 'em!

No matter how you go about it, when you feel better let your nurse, your family and friends know it. Be positive in ways that count. Stop whispering your needs—speak up. Stop asking someone to fetch the things that you can get—get them yourself. Stop being picky-picky about your food—eat it and be thankful that you can. Stop feeling sorry for yourself—or no one else will. And most of all, whenever you can—

SMILE!—IT COULD BE WORSE! You know that for a fact. It was worse, until you got to feeling better.

57 Give Your Nurse a Hand

Whether or not they are paying for services, there is a tendency among sick people to expect the nurse to do all the work. Not just the bathing, feeding, dressing, soothing, and entertaining of sick people, but all the other work as well.

Generally this is not done intentionally. Without meaning to, however, sick people often fall into a habit of thoughts such as "The nurse is healthy and wants to help me" . . . "I'm weak—let the nurse do it" . . . "I'd like to help, but even simple little tasks tire me so" . . . "The doctor said I must rest" . . . "It's the nurse's responsibility to do the work" . . . "It's so hard for me to move around and get what I want—and so much easier if the nurse moves me or fetches what I want" . . . "Whatever must be done of a professional nature, the nurse has been shown the correct way and can do it much more easily without my help."

If you are like so many people who have been disabled by sickness, surgery, or an injury, perhaps you can think of several more good reasons why you should let your nurse do all the work.

Too often, you get away with it.

Of course, no one wants you to do anything that is beyond your capabilities or could harm you. The doctor probably told you and your nurse what activities you should not do. Other than avoiding such activities, you should do as much for yourself as you possibly can. This is one very important step in regaining your strength.

IF THE NURSE DOES TOO MUCH FOR YOU . . .

Occasionally an inexperienced nurse tends to do too much for a patient. Instead of accepting the patient's disability for what it really is, the inexperienced nurse may believe it is worse. Even though the doctor said that the patient should be encouraged to move about without assistance, the inexperienced nurse often first hovers by like a mother hen, then slips a supporting arm around the patient. Or, instead of letting the patient reach for an item, the inexperienced nurse rushes to fetch and deliver it.

What if this happens to you?

One result is that you, the patient, may not get the beneficial movement, the normal exercise that you need. Instead of helping you overcome or learn how to cope with your disability, your nurse makes it an even greater obstacle.

Another result is what often happens to your nurse. When starting to take care of you, all the unnecessary extra assistance and fetching usually seems advisable. After all, if you need nursing care you must be in a very weakened condition, almost helpless. But as the novelty of being a nurse wears off (it may be replaced by a resentment of the seemingly endless extra work, and the aches of tired hands and feet and back) the unnecessary extras that you have been getting become too much of a burden.

The relationship between your nurse and you may become somewhat tense. Your nurse feels that waiting on you hand and foot when you do not really need it is too much—it is high time for you to make an effort to do more for yourself! Possibly you blame your nurse for not letting you do enough things for yourself. Unless both of you are careful, this situation easily can flare into a rapid fire of "I did's" and "I didn't's."

GIVE YOUR NURSE A HAND

No matter how obliging your nurse is, the more you do for yourself the better your nurse and you are likely to get along with each other and, even more important, the sooner you will recover from your disability or learn how to live with it. As a rule, coping with a disability is the most difficult, physically, at the onset of an illness or shortly after surgery or an injury. But the sooner you start trying to cope with it, by doing whatever you can for yourself, the better for you.

The so-called size of the first self-nursing task that you attempt is not important. To build confidence in yourself, and in your nurse, select a task that you feel certain of being able to do. Once you have mastered it, tackle another one. Advance yourself to increasingly difficult tasks as your strength and ability improve. However, until you have mastered several tasks, as a rule it is best to avoid any that you think you may not be able to do. The more successes you have, the less likely you are to be badly discouraged by attempting a task that is too much for you.

While taking over as many self-nursing tasks as you can for your own benefit, try where possible to do those that your nurse dislikes or finds the hardest to do for you. Certainly, sometimes your efforts undoubtedly will be more hindrance than help. Perhaps you are slow and hold up other work. But your nurse will be so pleased with your effort that a slight inconvenience will not matter.

58 Mealtime

Whether or not food and eating are particularly interesting or important to you, feeding you probably is one of your nurse's more troublesome day-in day-out problems. What to serve you? Which foods allowed by your diet do you like very much? Which are all right, but you would rather not have? Which do you positively dislike? Also, how much food should you have, and how much do you really want? These are simple questions that you could easily answer and thereby save your nurse much worry and extra work.

However, if you are like so many of the sick people who are being cared for by inexperienced nurses, in order to spare yours worry and work you probably take what is served. Each meal may consist of your favorite foods prepared just as you like; but the same dishes served several times often become tiresome and tasteless. Or meals may be foods your nurse likes and believes that "everyone" likes, but that you eat only to be polite. Or, the foods served you may be those that nutritionists say are the best for mankind, but that almost make you gag to swallow. Still, rather than put your nurse to extra work preparing other foods, and rather than hurt your nurse's feelings by saying that you do not like the food, either you force yourself to eat or insist that you do not feel well enough to eat.

Claiming that you do not feel well enough to eat is quite likely to worry your nurse into making a needless call to the doctor or your visiting nurse. Especially is this likely if you feel it necessary to give forth the groans and other signs of pain or discomfort needed to prove your claim of not feeling well enough to eat.

Forcing yourself to eat food that you do not like will get the nutrients into your body, but they probably will do little real good. Moreover, forcing yourself to swallow food that is repulsive to you can give you severe indigestion or even make you vomit. However, there may be some specific foods that are vitally important for you to have. In this case, try eating very small portions at first, and gradually increase them as you become accustomed to the taste. This will require self-discipline and positive thinking on your part. It will not be easy, but it can be done, especially if your health depends on it.

EAT WHAT YOU LIKE

To make things simpler for your nurse (and to pamper yourself in a healthy manner, if you care to see it that way), study your diet carefully and list the allowable foods in the order of "I like very much," "all right, but not my favorite," and "no thanks!" If more than one way of cooking or other food preparation is allowed, list them in order of preference, too. If your diet is limited, you also should indicate which foods you would prefer to have most often and which the least often.

Discuss the list with your nurse, and if you have suggestions as to how you like certain foods prepared or served, say so. Do not limit this to the main dishes, but also discuss the kinds and amounts of seasonings, relishes, dressings, and condiments that you like and dislike. Your dislikes are just as important as your likes, and the more you specify what you want to eat, the easier you make the job of feeding you.

However, keep in mind that sick people's taste for food frequently changes. Sooner or later you may find that something you really enjoyed while healthy seems to have lost its appeal. This is perfectly natural, so do not hesitate to tell your nurse that you do not want a certain food anymore.

Of course, in specifying what foods you want and how they should be prepared, you should be practical. Do not insist on dishes that are beyond your nurse's ability to prepare as you want; for example, not all good cooks can make light, fluffy soufflès. Nor should you request foods that take a long time to prepare and need constant watching, especially if your nurse is employed outside the home. You should also take into account the season of the year and the family food budget. This practical approach to meals will simplify your nurse's work and do much to eliminate any worry that you are not getting enough variety of food.

TRY SOMETHING NEW

With most people, foods tend to be habit forming. For example, you may have the habit of eating beef and chicken, and seldom have turkey, pork, or lamb. You may regularly have green peas and carrots, and only rarely eat squash, zucchini, cabbage, string beans, rice, potatoes, and so forth. You may be in the habit of having your vegetables simply boiled, drained, sprinkled with salt and pepper.

Try breaking away from your habit foods as much as your diet and other considerations allow—and you may have many pleasant surprises! Try different cuts of meat, different seasonings, different vegetables and ways of preparing them, different salads and dressings, fruit and desserts, hot and cold beverages. You may believe you will not like something you have never tasted, this often happens; but do not firmly make up your mind in advance not to like it. And if at times you suspect your nurse of serving dishes that you have not had before, be polite enough to try them graciously. You may be glad you did.

HOW MUCH FOOD YOU WANT

Under normal circumstances, sick people should neither stuff nor starve. They should not eat too much for comfort at a meal, nor should they feel uncomfortably hungry after one. If either condition persists for more than three or four consecutive meals, consult your doctor, nutritionist, or visiting nurse. Even with so-called starvation diets for essential quick loss of weight, as a rule steps are taken to suppress excessive pangs of hunger; if not, the patient suffers needlessly and frequently will get extra food by whatever means possible.

> NOTE: In order to keep you from "stuffing" or "starving," it may be necessary to give you more and smaller meals each day, or it may require smaller servings. Although you may have been taught to "eat everything on your plate," if this will cause you distress and discomfort, don't do it. Forget your upbringing and leave what you cannot eat. If you find that you cannot eat as much as you should, ask for more frequent meals and smaller servings. Sometimes the sight of a large amount of food on a plate destroys the appetite.

In most diets, the amount of food prescribed for a meal is based on what the "average" patient should eat comfortably. Of course, if you are not "average," you may want more or less. If there is only a small difference between the amount served you and the amount that you want to eat, tell your nurse. Do not secretly dispose of excess food, and do not sneak the extra food you may want. Simply ask for smaller or larger servings.

> NOTE: Under certain conditions, especially with diabetes, it is extremely important that accurate records be kept of the food consumed. If you secretly dispose of food or sneak additional, you will falsify the records and possibly harm yourself seriously.

GETTING READY TO EAT

Preparing and serving meals is not always a simple task for a nurse, particularly for one who is in a strange kitchen or is not experienced in cooking and food handling. Help with meals by getting ready for them as much as you can.

If you are not confined to bed and can carry things about, set your tray or set your and your nurse's places at the table. Clear away any clutter on the table; it can be unappetizing. Breakfast and dining tables often are messy catchalls for books, magazines, mail, newspapers, clothing, and so forth.

If you are confined to bed, do what you can toward putting yourself in position to eat, and clear the bed to make room for the meal tray. If the bedside table is within convenient reach, clear space on it for the glass or cup of beverage that may be brought with your meal; it usually is easier to clean up a spill on a table than on the bed.

And finally, make up your mind to eat, without word or sign of complaint, the meal your nurse brings you. True, there may be some food that you do not like, and you may have mentioned it before. But now is not the time to complain. Wait until your nurse is not tired from preparing *your* meal. Then, when your annoyance and your nurse's fatigue have diminished, mention the food you did not like, and why.

59 Use Those Muscles!

For many patients-at-home, just the usual moving around and helping with the tasks of normal family life provide sufficient daily exercise. If you need more exercise or should do specialized or therapeutic-type exercises, undoubtedly your doctor or therapist has given you and your nurse adequate instructions. (For basic information on exercising, see Chapter 28).

Whether your program consists of just normal daily living exercise or conventional calisthenics, or highly specialized exercises prescribed by the physician, two things you must be careful to avoid are babying yourself and overworking yourself. Others can suspect, but only you can know for sure when you are babying or overworking yourself. Both can seriously retard, or even prevent, your recovery.

WHY BABY YOURSELF?

Because of your disability, or possibly due to the length of time you have been disabled, you may tire easily from nearly any kind of exercise, and some of them really may be painful to do. Naturally you tend to avoid them, and you should—until you have discussed them, particularly those that cause pain, with your doctor or therapist. If the answer is that you should do those exercises, then do them with a reasonable amount of moderation at the start. But do not baby yourself.

Patients who baby themselves about exercising are those who quit too soon, and usually refuse to try it again. For example, the instant a muscle feels the least bit used or tired, or the instant there is a twinge of pain, even one hardly worth the weakest kind of an "ouch," they stop. They have had it. No more exercising today, tomorrow, next day. It hurts, it is much too strenuous for a weakened condition, and no matter what the doctor says, no more of it. Anyhow, the doctor is not here to see how agonizingly painful, how positively exhausting it is. Certainly, exercise is necessary—for most other people.

Moderation is the intelligent approach to all exercises. Here are some practical ways to be moderate in your exercising:

1. Exercise at the start for a limited time, possibly 5 minutes, then stop, regardless of not being tired or feeling pain. Exercise again when you feel up to it, but this time do it for, say, 10 minutes, then stop. Next time exercise for 15 minutes, then for 20. Of course, if at any time you feel too tired or have severe pain, you should stop immediately. The next time exercise for a shorter period; after that lengthen them by fewer minutes, say, 2 instead of by 5 minutes.
2. Instead of basing your exercising program on time, as in 1 above, base it on a certain number of exercises, such as flexing your hands. So many complete flexes the first time, so many more the next, and so forth. Again, if you reach a stage where it is too tiring or painful, stop; and when you renew your exercising, increase it by a fewer number each time, or do the same number of exercises for several days.
3. Do not exercise to the point of exhaustion. Instead, exercise only to the point where you feel that you could do it a few more times without injury but would rather stop for a few minutes' rest. If pain is your warning sign, stop exercising after it is a slight twinge but before it hurts badly.

The greatest benefit from exercising in moderation comes from keeping to a practical schedule of increase until you reach the desired regular amount. If you try to advance faster on some days than on others, you are likely to become discouraged on days when you cannot advance as quickly; also, you may harm yourself by overworking.

WHY OVERWORK YOURSELF?

Most disabled people who overwork themselves in exercising are simply victims of their own pride. They want to show themselves and everyone else that they can do more exercise than the doctor or the therapist recommended. They want to prove that because they do more they will recover in shorter time. Exercising in moderation is all right for weaklings, for those who baby themselves through life, but not for them.

As a rule, it does not take much time for these patients to overwork themselves into a state of exhaustion; the body will take so much abuse, and then just quit working. Also, excessive exercise after surgery and other wounds can weaken the healing process. Admittedly, overexercising does not necessarily produce drastic results, but it can. As a rule, it does give a warning in advance; but people who deliberately overexercise generally consider this as just another sign that hard work, tiredness, and pain usually go hand in hand. Moreover, a person who overexercises and is not injured at the start tends to keep overexercising until there is damage.

60 Join the Family!

After the first few days of a person's sickness-at-home, family life tends to zigzag back to normal. Unfortunately, this surprises many sick people. Still more unfortunately, many of them try to delay the return to normal family life; they probably rank high among the people of whom it has been said, "They enjoy poor health."

Two of the more popular ways of trying to prevent the return of normal family life are:

1. Retire from it as obviously as you can. Make everyone fully aware of the fact that you no longer are able to be an active member of the family. Deny all responsibility. Speak only when spoken to. Become a hermit at home as far as your family and friends are concerned.
2. Take over complete management by self-appointment. Insist that you be consulted, always, for everything. Let it be known that your decisions and opinions are final and binding. Make yourself the center of family attention and activities.

If you succeed in either of these efforts, you undoubtedly will delay if not totally prevent the return of normal family life in your home. You also will make caring for you, in both meanings of the term, extremely difficult for everyone, especially your nurse. Moreover, you are very likely to bring down upon yourself every discomfort that your disability allows. Aside from all that, in most cases just being sick is not sufficient reason for anyone to become a hermit, or to expect to become the center of family affairs.

ON BEING A HERMIT

When you are sick at home, as a rule there are very few reasons why a doctor would want to keep you away from your family and friends. They are easy-to-understand reasons. Your sickness is in a dangerously contagious stage, people should not needlessly be exposed to it . . . you are in a weakened state and easily might catch another sickness, such as a cold . . . your disability may be such that you must be shielded from the excitement, noise, and clatter of visitors in your sickroom . . . certain people should be kept away from you simply because they antagonize you, make you nervous. Of course, there could be other reasons why your doctor would want to isolate you at home, reasons that would be explained to you and your nurse.

Given a valid medical reason for your being isolated from family and friends, most of them will think of you frequently with sympathy and hope for your betterment. You are still with them in spirit at least, and they look forward to when you can get together again in the flesh. Meanwhile, and to help take your mind off your troubles: Get-well cards . . . flowers . . . books . . . various other remembrance gifts. And, often, offers of practical help such as getting your medicines . . . bringing prepared meals to your home . . . running errands and doing other services that can lessen your nurse's workload.

But if you voluntarily choose to shut yourself away from everyone, more and more of your relatives and friends will, as time goes by, forget you. Naturally. You keep yourself out of sight too long—and the "out of mind" naturally follows. Also, each person is apt to feel singled out as someone that you do not care to see—so naturally each one does not care to see you. Making yourself a hermit without good cause usually is done to get sympathy and attention, and usually has the exact opposite effect.

There is, of course, a seemingly valid reason why people want to avoid family and friends after getting certain diseases or following an injury or surgery. They are disfigured. They are in some way shamed. They do not wish to be seen. They fear the forced, expressionless faces of their relatives and friends. They dread questions they know are based on morbid curiosity. They will hide in isolation until they are accustomed to themselves, and then they will face and defy their family and friends, challenge them to say the wrong thing, to look the wrong way! But with most people, the longer they put it off, the harder it becomes to confront a nondisfigured public—and, they reason, since they have waited this long, it will not hurt to wait a while longer.

But there are several important factors that many disfigured people seem to overlook at the onset of their affliction. If you are one of them, remember:

1. Whatever happened to you, it appears to be more repulsive or crippling to you than to anyone else.
2. It is natural for your family and friends to be curious about what happened to you; it would be unfriendly if they were not. Answer their questions, but avoid details that you prefer not to talk about at that time. If they persist, simply tell them that you would rather not talk about the details.
3. Unless you keep making an issue of it, chances are that the people you live and work with will soon stop making unnecessary and embarrassing special arrangements for you.
4. Most mature people that you now meet for the first time probably will think of your affliction as being "normal" for you, and not make anything of it one way or another.
5. The sooner you start and the faster you learn to live with your affliction—and join the family!—the sooner you, your family, and your friends will accept you for what you are and what you can do.

ON BEING THE CENTER OF ATTENTION

If you are sick or disabled at home and are not being a hermit about it, you probably will, at the start, receive more flattering attention than you did when healthy. This is natural. But unless you know how to cope with it, the special attention can become a disaster for you and your family.

In order to help you build confidence in yourself, and to assure you that you do have an important role in family life and activities, it is fairly common for members of the family to ask your opinion on various matters. You were never before considered by the family to be an expert on public affairs, but now what do you think of the latest political mess? Who's to blame in the current popular scandal? Is now a good time to buy or sell? Is it getting better or worse? Do you really think this will look good? Your experience, your expertise, is not at issue. Qualified or not, your opinion, your judgment on this, that, and the other thing suddenly is in demand. It is ridiculous, if you mentally stand off and look at it, but it is flattering. It does make you feel sort of good all over. And it does give you the opportunity to air some opinions you have long wanted to.

But if you, like people who believe their own publicity, take it the wrong way instead of accepting it for what it is worth, you and your family and friends may be headed for serious trouble.

With many people, suddenly becoming the center of attention makes them believe that they deserve it. Thanks to their disability, they now have time to think about the important things, whatever they may be. Thanks also to their disability, those people who have different opinions will not disagree too strongly for fear of causing a relapse. So opinions are freely offered first whenever asked for, then whenever anyone else has an opinion, and finally when there really is no need for an opinion.

It does not take much of this to antagonize your family and friends to the point of leaving you alone if at all possible. If they cannot get away from you and you persist in settling their affairs for them, sooner or later the time will come when tempers break and you are told in no uncertain terms to mind your own business. This usually is followed by apologies for having hurt your feelings, but the damage has been done. There is now a wall of mutual ill will between you, with you feeling that most of your family and friends are on the other side. Chances are that you, in self-defense, still feel qualified to render an opinion or make a decision; but now there is no demand for them, no attention paid them. Naturally you and everyone else involved feel hurt and want to avoid one another.

And it all could have been prevented so easily if, at the start, you had admitted to yourself that your opinions about things you did not know had been asked only in an attempt to make you feel important.

SO JOIN THE FAMILY!

So do not be a hermit unless the doctor orders it, and do not attempt to take over the thinking for the family, but fit yourself in where you can, considering your condition.

Join in family discussions, but do not try to dominate or trade on your disability.

Join in the planning of family activities even if you know you cannot participate in them. But be careful not to inject yourself so deeply into an impossible-for-you activity that your being unable to participate will spoil it for the others.

Make a real effort to share the enjoyment of what happened to others through their telling it to you. This may be hard for you to pretend at first, but after a while you probably will learn to get real pleasure out of the pleasures of others.

And if you suffer from a permanent disability, ask your family to help you, from the start, by not making special concessions to it that are not absolutely necessary. Keep in mind that most blinded people soon learn to say, "I'll see you," without wincing, and that many permanent wheelchair patients say, "I'll run over," without giving it a second thought. But regardless of how you plan to behave and how strong your determination, if your disability is permanent it is almost certain that you will need the total support and cooperation of your family and friends. You in turn must cooperate and participate in their efforts to help you.

Join your family instead of hiding from it or attempting to boss it, and you will be surprised by what they can and will do for you.

Glossary

Abrasion the rubbing or scraping off of skin, or of mucous membrane, from the body; often called skinned, as in skinned elbow.

Abscess a localized collection of pus in any part of the body; caused by disintegration or displacement of tissue.

Acute sharp, severe, sudden, rapid onset (of a disease) with severe symptoms and a short course; often dangerous. Opposed to **chronic.** An acute hospital is one for the immediate and, usually, short confinement for sickness or injury, as opposed to a convalescent hospital or home.

Allergy (allergic reaction) oversensitive or excessive reaction by a person to something (an allergen) that most people do not react to at all. Common allergens are bacteria, drugs, food, house dust, pollens.

Antibiotics natural and synthetic substances that stop the growth of or destroy harmful bacteria in the body. Do not confuse with **antibody.**

Antibody obscure but important protein substances produced in and by the body to protect it against an antigen or foreign substance, usually a disease-producing agent, that has entered the body. Do not confuse with **antibiotics.**

Antiseptics substances that slow or inhibit the growth of disease-producing microorganisms; weaker than **disinfectants.**

Asepsis sterile condition due to freedom from germs, infection, any form of life; excluding germs rather than attempting to destroy them. See **antiseptics.**

Atrophy a wasting away of any part of the body (flesh, organ, tissue cell), usually due to lack of proper nutrients or exercise.

Autoclave apparatus for sterilizing surgical instruments, dressings, etc., by applying heat (steam) under pressure. See **asepsis.**

Blister a collection of clear, watery fluid under the skin; may be caused by disease (fever), burn, counterirritant, irritating chemical, or by pressure on and chafing of the skin.

Bruise (contusion) an injury, usually a fall or a blow, that breaks the capillaries under the skin but not the skin.

Catarrh an old-fashioned term for the discharge from an inflamed mucous membrane. Do not confuse with **cathartic.**

Cathartic **laxative,** purgative. Do not confuse with **catarrh.**

Chronic long-continued, -term, -duration; persistent, prolonged, repeated. Opposed to **acute.**

Concussion (of the brain, cerebral) often due to a blow on the head, or a fall on the end of the spine, strong enough to cause either temporary or prolonged unconsciousness; the skull may or may not be fractured. A mild concussion may cause no more than slight dizziness and a headache of short duration.

Contusion a **bruise.**

Convulsion uncontrollable, often violent, spasms or contractions of muscles usually alternating with relaxation of muscles; often called **fits, seizures.**

Cyanosis blue-grayish color in the skin (especially of the face, hands, feet) due to lack of oxygen in the arterial blood.

Debridement surgical removal of dead or damaged tissue, or of foreign material, often necessary in treating neglected bedsores.

Disinfectants substances that kill bacteria outside the body. There are many disinfectants; all should be used only as directed by the doctor, pharmacist, or manufacturer. Disinfectants are stronger than **antiseptics.**

Disoriented mentally confused; unable to estimate direction, location, time, or to recognize persons, places, things.

Eruption a breaking out, as in a skin **rash.**

Fits see **convulsions.**

Fracture a break in, or the breaking of, a bone. A break of cartilage may be called a fracture.

Gamma globulin a special protein in human blood; contains disease-fighting **antibodies.**

Hallucination perception (feeling, hearing, seeing, smelling) of things that have no reality.

Hemiplegia paralysis of only one side of the body, usually due to a **stroke** or to injury of blood vessels in the brain.

Hemorrhage bleeding; abnormal, but not necessarily copious, discharge or escape of blood internally or externally from an artery, vein, or capillary.

Laceration cut or wound, usually with irregular edges; a tear.

Laxative a mild **cathartic;** generally should be taken only on doctor's advice, as self-dosage is more apt to cause than to cure constipation.

Malaise a general feeling of being ill or unwell; may or may not be accompanied by headache or nausea.

Narcotic a drug that causes sleep or stupor (near-unconsciousness, numbness, somnolence, stunned condition, stupefaction) while relieving pain; can also stimulate and exhilarate; easily habit forming. Addiction to narcotics much easier to get than to get rid of.

Nausea feeling sick to the stomach and about to vomit; biliousness; queasiness; also called air-, motion-, sea-, travel-sickness.

Obsession an overwhelming idea, or emotion, such as fear, that persists in one's consciousness in spite of attempts to forget it. However, the difference between obsession and "having faith" in an idea or an emotion often is difficult to distinguish; many great people seem to have been obsessed.

Pain threshold the point at which a stimulus, such as heat or pressure, first makes an impression on a person's consciousness or arouses a response. Pain thresholds are not constant; they vary with the same person at various times, and with various people.

Paralysis complete or partial loss of function, particularly loss of sensation or of voluntary motion; temporary or permanent loss; caused by injury to the brain, nervous system, or to a muscular mechanism.

Paraplegia (paraplegic) **paralysis** of both legs; usually accompanied by paralysis of bowel and bladder, making the paraplegic incontinent.

Pica strong craving for strange or unusual foods, or for nonfood substances such as clay, plaster.

Plasma the liquid part of blood, in which the blood cells and **platelets** float. Do not confuse with blood serum, which is the clear liquid that separates from blood when it clots.

Platelets in circulating blood of vertebrates, the small colorless disks that aid in clotting of blood.

Prone (position) lying horizontally, face downward.

Quadriplegia (quadriplegic) **paralysis** of both arms and both legs; see **paraplegia.**

Range of motion area over which, or limits to which, a joint may move.

Rash superficial eruption of the skin, usually temporary; reddish color, the color varying with the cause of the rash.

Seizures see **convulsions.**

Sensory perception recognition of a person, place, thing, or action caused by stimulation of one or more of the senses (hearing, sight, smell, taste, touch).

Serum, blood see **plasma.**

Shock in general, upset body functions due to inadequate amounts of blood carrying oxygen to the tissues and return of blood to the heart. Usually associated with injury, but may be caused by many conditions including drug reaction, dehydration, hemorrhage, infection, poisoning. See also **trauma.**

Sordes foul, brownish-black scales or crusts that accumulate on teeth and lips from secretions of the mouth during continued, low fevers; dirt, filth.

Spasm sudden, involuntary, uncontrollable muscular contraction.

Stress emotional or intellectual force, strain, or tension that tends to upset a person.

Stroke sudden paralysis caused by injury to the brain or to the spinal cord; also called apoplectic fit, apoplexy, brain hemorrhage, paralytic stroke.

Supine (position) lying horizontally on the back, face upward.

Symptom any observable change in bodily functions or mental behavior indicating the presence or kind or phase of disease, especially when regarded as an aid to diagnosis.

Trauma an injury; physical, emotional, or psychological.

Wound damage to the soft parts of the body structure in which the skin is cut or torn. Incised wound is one caused by a cutting instrument; puncture wound is made by a pointed instrument. The great risk in a wound is infection.

General Index

Also see Foods and Feeding Your Patient Index, pages 341–44

Page numbers in italics refer to illustrations

Abdominal respiration, 134
Accidents, protecting patient against, 296–97
Accuracy in dealings with the doctor, 8–9
Age, bedsores and, 92
Airborne transmission of disease, 67
Air deodorant and freshener, 55
Air mattress, 94
Alcohol, denatured or rubbing, 56, 58
Altitude, respiration and, 133
Animate vectors, 64
Ankle protectors (doughnuts), 107–8, *107*
Ankles, exercises for, 112
Anxiety. *See also* Fears; Worries
  reporting to doctor, 11–12
Arm, paralyzed, 194
Aspirin for fever reduction, 119
Atrophies, 189–90
Attention, being the center of, 328–29
Axillary temperature, 126
Auxiliary bed padding, 26–27

Baby powder, 56
Bacilli, 63
Back rub, 113–16, *115*
  giving a, 114–16
  lotions or alcohol for, 56
  planning, 299
  as preparation for sleep, 183
  scheduling, 295
Bacteria, 62–63. *See also* Microorganisms
Baking soda enema, 167
Bandaged patients, bathing, 147
Base, 198
Basins
  bath, 22, *22*
  emesis. *See* Emesis basin
  sitz bath, 160, *160*
Bath basins, 22, *22*
Bath blanket, 23, 79
  for enemas, 164
  for irrigations, 173
  for vaginal douches, 178
Bath-Ease safety seat, *148*, 149
Bathing. *See* Baths
Bathlifts, 88, *89*
Bath oils, 142
Baths (bathing)
  bed, 145, 155–57
  equipment for, 144–45
  while making the bed, 71, 79
  planning, 299–300
  ring cushions for, 39, *39*
  scheduling, 295
  shower. *See* Shower baths
  sitz, 159–61, *160*
  as sleeping aid, 184
  sponge, 145, 154–55
  temperature of water for, 145–46, 150, 160–61
  therapeutic, 143–44
  time of day for, 144
  tub. *See* Tub baths
Bath safety guard- or grabrails, 149–50, *149*
Bath salts, 142
Bath seats, *148*, 148–49
Bathtub. *See also* Tub baths
  getting a shower bath patient in and out of a, 151–52
  getting a tub bath patient in and out of, 153
  guardrails and grabrails for, 149–50, *149*
  irrigating in a, 175–76
  safety strips or mats for, *147*, 147–48
  sitz baths in a, 160, 161
  vaginal douche in a, 179–80, *179*
Bathtub transfer seat, 148–49, *148*
Bed, 23, *24*
  getting in and out of, 302
  guardrails for. *See* Bed guardrails
  hospital, 23, *24*
  irrigating in, 176
  making the. *See* Making the bed
  moving patient between chair and, 87, 302
  moving patient in, 85–86
  preparing patient for sleep and, 183
  protecting patient from falling out of, 297
  vaginal douche in, 179–80, *179*
Bed assists, 101–2, *102*. *See also* Trapeze bars
Bed baths, 145, 155–57
Bedboards, 29–30, 43
Bed cleanliness, bedsores and, 93
Bedding, 70. *See also specific bedding items*
  envelope corners for, 77–78, *78*
  fan-folding, 78, *78*
  folding, 72, *72*
  holding, 71
  loosening, 78
  sequence of, 72
Bedding frames (or cradles), 30–31, *30, 31*
  with foot support strip, 109, *109*

for toe protection, 108
Bedfast patients
bathing, 155–57
bedsores and, 92
irrigations for, 173, 176
shampooing hair of, 158–59
toilet assistance for, 303
Bed guardrails, 23, *24*, 297
remaking the occupied bed and, 80
Bedlamp, 31
Bed linen. *See also* Bedding; Making the bed; *and specific items*
frequency of change of, 300
washing, 68
Bed mattresses. *See* Mattresses
Bed padding, 23, *25*, 25–27, 94
Bedpan(s), 31–33, *31, 32*, 303
emergency (newspaper), 32–33, *32*
for enemas, 163
giving a, 32
transmission of disease and, 69
for vaginal douches, 178
Bedridden patients. *See* Bedfast patients
Bed rinse/shampoo tray, 27, *27*
Bed sheets. *See* Sheets
Bedside aid kits, 33
Bedside tables, 33, *33*
Bedsores, 90–95, *90*, 191
bed padding for prevention of, 23, 26, 94
causes of, 92–93
cushions for prevention of, 38–39, *39*, 94
early detection of, 91
light massage for, 116
prevention of, 93–94
preventive treatment of, 91–92, 103–4
treatment of, 95
when to examine patient for, 300–1
Bedspread, 34. *See also* Bedding
folding, 72
installing, 77
Bed springs, 29
Bedtray, over-the-lap, 33
Bed wedge pillows, 23, 29, *29*
Behavioral changes, 4
Bell, 34
Benzoin, for bedsore prevention, 92
Bidet
irrigating on a, 175
vaginal douche on a, 179
Bite, transmission of disease by, 69
Bladder stones, lack of exercise and, 190
Blankets, 34. *See also* Bedding
bath. *See* Bath blanket
installing, 77
rolled, to prevent foot rotation, 111
Blanket support, 30, *30*, 31, *31*
Bleeding: reporting to doctor, 12
Blood clots, 191
Blood pressure, 135–42. *See also* Sphygmomanometers
auscultatory measurement of, 138, 141–42
definition of, 136
diastolic, 137
direct measurement of, 138
indirect measurement of, 138
lack of exercise and rapid fall in, 190–91
palpatory measurement of, 138
recording, 137–38
systolic, 136–37
taking, 138–42
variations of, 137
Blood pressure cuffs, 35, 140
Body deodorant, 56
Body lotions, 56, 145
for body rubs, 114
Body mechanics, 81–84
Body powder, 56
for body rubs, 114
Body rub. *See also* Back rub
lotion and powder for, 114
massage distinguished from, 113
Body temperature, 117–28. *See also* Chills; Fever; Thermometers
abnormal or excessive changes in, 119–20
axillary, 126
Celsius and Fahrenheit degrees for measuring, 117
Celsius (centigrade)-Fahrenheit conversions, 127–28
dangerous extremes of, 120
environmental temperature and, 119
fluctuations in, 118
normal, 118
oral, 126
pulse and respiration changes and, 117–18, 133
recording, 120–22, *120, 121*
rectal, 125–27, *127*
reporting to doctor, 14–15
taking, 125–27, *127*
times of taking, 120
Books, 102
Boredom, 298
Bottom sheet, 72. *See also* Sheets
fitted, 74
installing, 74–76, *75, 76*, 80
tightening a, 75–76, *76*
Bowel movement. *See also* Constipation; Feces; Incontinence
reporting to doctor, 13
washing patient after, 142
Breakfast tray, over-the-lap, 33
Breathing (breath). *See also* Respiration
Cheyne-Stokes, 134
difficulty in, 12, 13
shortness of, 12, 13
Buttermilk-herb dressing, 252

Call system, electric, 34
Calluses on feet, 112
Canadian cane, 36, *36*

Canadian crutches, 38, *39*
Canes, 35–37, *35–37*, 297
Carafe, 37
Castile enema soap, liquid, 162
Casts
  bathing patient in, 147
  bedsores and, 93, 94
Celsius (centigrade) degrees, 117
Celsius (centigrade)-Fahrenheit conversions, 127–28
Chair. *See also* Wheelchairs
  commode, 38, *38*
  moving patient between bed and, 87
  shifting position in, 303
Change of position
  in chair, 303
  preventing disuse disabilities and, 191, 192
Chec medical bathlift, 88, *89*
Cheyne-Stokes breathing, 134
Children. *See also* Infants
  carrying, 83
  pulse rate of, 129
  rectal temperature of, 127
  retention enemas for, 168
  soap enemas for, 162, 163, *163*, 166–67
  wheelchairs for, 54, *54*
Chills, 119
  reporting to doctor, 13
Chlorophyll ointment for bedsores, 95
Chronic disease, bedsores and, 92
Circulatory disturbances, lack of exercise and, 190–91
Cleaning. *See* House cleaning; Room cleaning
Cleansing enemas, 161–67. *See also* Soap enemas
Clock, 37
Cocci, 63
Comfort, patient's, 7–8
Commode, 37, *38*
Commode chair, 38, *38*
Communicable diseases. *See also* Transmission of disease
  reporting of, 66
Complaining by patient, 319
Confusion (disorientation), 296–97
Consciousness, loss of, 13
Constipation, lack of exercise and, 190
Contagious diseases. *See* Communicable diseases; Transmission of disease
Contractures, joint, 190–92
Control of limbs, loss of, 13
Convulsions, 13
Cooking utensils, washing, 65
Cornstarch as body powder, 56, 114
Cotton, 56–57
Cotton swabs, 57, 58. *See also* Q-Tips
Coughing, transmission of disease by, 67
Crutches, 38, *39*, 297
  tips for, 36
Cups, 40
Cushions, seat, 38–39, *39*
Cuts and scratches, transmission of disease and, 65, 67–68

Decubitus ulcers. *See* Bedsores
Denervation atrophy, 190
Dental floss, 57
Dentifrice, 57, 59
Dentures, 184
Deodorant
  body, 56
  room, 55
Despondency, 298–99
Diastolic blood pressure, 137
Diets, 205–80
Diplococci, 63
Discussions of family affairs, 5
Disease. *See also* Microorganisms
  definition of, 62
  infectious, 62
  transmission of. *See* Transmission of disease
Disorientation (confusion), 296–97
Disuse atrophy, 190
Disuse disabilities, 189–92
Doctor
  accuracy in dealings with, 8–9
  getting all the facts from, 9–10
  home nurse as go-between for patient and, 8
  house calls by, 15–16
  instructions of, 10, 17–18, 311, 313
  telling doctor that you are to be nurse, 9
  visits to or by, 15–17
  when to call the, 11–15
  writing down instructions from, 10, 17–18
Douche. *See* Vaginal douche
Douche bag for irrigations, 172, *172*
Drainage from a wound or sore, 14
Draw sheets, 40, *40*
  installing, 76, 80
  moving a patient with, 85–86
Dressing patients, 301–2
Drinking glass, 40
Drinking straws, 40
Drinking water. *See* Water
Dust, diseases transmitted by, 64, 65
Dusting powders, 56
Dust mop, 65
Dyspnea, 134

Eggcrate® bed padding, 25, *25*, 26
Eggcrate® cushion (or pad), 38–39, *39*
Eggs, low-cholesterol diet and, 247
Elderly patients, feeding, 283
Electric blankets, 34
Electric shavers, 45
Electric sheets, 28
Emesis basin (kidney basin), 40–41, *41*
  for enemas, 164
Endocrine glands, 198, 199
Enemas, 161–70
  baking soda, 167

cleansing, 161–67
equipment for, 162–64, *163*
high, 166
retention, 168–70
saline/salt, 167
soap. *See* Soap enemas
Entertainment, 102
Envelope corners, 77–78, *78*
Eruptions, 14
Exchanges. *See* Diabetic Food exchanges
Excretion, 199
Exercise, 189–95, 302, 325–26
active, 193
for ankles, 112
disuse disabilities due to lack of, 189–91
excessive, 189, 297–98, 326
feet, 112–13
general, 193
objections of patients to, 192
passive, 193–94
patients who baby themselves about, 325–26
preventing disuse disabilities and, 191, 192
scheduling, 295
therapeutic, 193
for toes, 112
with trapeze bar, 194–95
Eye-tiring activity, as sleeping aid, 184

Face, washing, 142–43
Facial tissue, paper, 57–58
Family affairs, discussions of, 5
Family life, 327–30
Family room, moving your patient to, 6–8
Fan-folding bedding, 78, *78*
Fears, 4. *See also* Anxiety
pain and, 196
of sick people, 9
Fecal-and-oral transmission of disease, 69
Feces, reporting, 290, 292, 293
Feet. *See also* Foot care; *and entries starting with* Foot
bedsore preventive devices, 94, 104–8, *104, 105, 107, 108*
bedsores on, 94, 103–4
exercises for, 112–13
loosening bedding for the, 78
lubrication of, 113
washing, in bed, 156–57, *156*
Fever. *See also* Body temperature
aspirin used to reduce, 119
Floors, safe, 297
Flotation pads. *See* Water pads
Folding bedding, 72, *72*
fan-folding, 78, *78*
Fomites, 64
Foot calluses, 112
Foot care, 107–13. *See also* Feet; *and other entries starting with* Foot
bedsore preventive treatment, 103–4
exercises, 112–13
lubrication, 113
soaking and washing, 103
toenails, 112, *112*
Foot cradle, 30, *30*, 108
Foot drop, 108–10
Foot guard, 108, *108*, 109, 111
Foot rotation, 111–12
Foot support band, 30
Foot support boards, 109–10, *110*
Forearm cane, 36, *36*
Fork holders, 98–99
Fracture pans (slipper bedpans), 31, *31*
Furniture, dusting, 65
Furniture arrangements, changes in, 5, 6

Gas, Harris flush for expelling, 167
Genitals. *See also* Vaginal douche
irrigations of, 171, 173–76
Gifts from visitors, 306
Glass, drinking, 40
Gloves, 41, 65, 68
for irrigations, 173
for sitz baths, 160
for vaginal douches, 178
Gown
hospital (patient), 42
nurse's, 70
Grabrails, bath, 149–50, *149*
Guardrails, bath, 149–50, *149*
Guardrails, bed, 23, *24*, 297
remaking the occupied bed and, 80

Hair
blow-drying, 158
long, 159
shampooing and care of, 146, 157–59
Handbell, 34
Handicap aids, 95–102, 302
bed assists, 101–2, *102*
reaching aids, 100–1, *100*
reading aids, 100, *100*
telephone, 96
writing aids, 99, *99*
Hand lotion, 56
Hands, washing, 65, 69, 142–43
Harris flush, 167
Heat lamp for bedsores, 95
Heel cups, 104–7, *105*
Heel protectors, 104–7, *104, 105*
Hemoglobin, 200
Hermit, being a, 327–28
Home environment, 6–8
Home Health Aides, 19
Homemakers, 20
Hormones, 199, 200
Hospital bed, 23, *24*
Hospital gown, 42
House calls by doctors, 15–16
House cleaning, 65. *See also* Room cleaning
Hoyer patient lifts, 88, *88, 89*

Hypodermic needles, 68
Hypostatic pneumonia, 191

Immobility. *See also* Bedfast patients
  bedsores and, 92
Inanimate vectors, 64–65
Incontinence, 192
  bedsores and, 93
Infants. *See also* Children
  soap enemas for, 162, 163, *163*, 167
Infection of bedsores, 95
Infectious disease, 62. *See also* communicable diseases; Microorganisms; Transmission of disease
Ingrown nails, 112
Inner-lip plate, *97*, 98
Insects, transmission of disease by, 64, 68
Intercom, 34, 42
Intravenous feeding, 200
Invacare bath chair lifts, 88, *89*
Irrigations, 170–76
  in a bathtub, 175–76
  in bed, 176
  on a bidet, 175
  drying patient after, 173
  equipment for, 172–73, *172*
  of genitals and perineal/rectal areas, 173–76
  pressures of, 172, 175
  "Scotch," 171
  temperature of, 171
  on a toilet, 173–75
  types of flows, 172
Irrigation solutions, 171

Joint contractures, 190–92

Kidney basin (emesis basin), 40–41, *41*
  for enemas, 164
Kidney stones, lack of exercise and, 190
Knives, for handicapped patients, 97, *97*

Lamp, bed, 31
Lifeguard bathtub rail, *149*, 150
Lifting a patient, 81–84, *82*. *See also* Mechanical lifts
Lights (lighting), 184. *See also* Lamp, bed
  changes in, 5
Living room, moving your patient to, 6–8
Lubricants, 59
  for enemas, 164
  for feet, 113
Lubricating retention enemas, 168–70

Magazines, 102
Making the bed, 70–81
  general preparation for, 70–71
  handling the bedding, 71–72
  occupied bed, 79–81, *80*
  planning, 300
  scheduling, 295
  unoccupied bed, 73–79, *73, 75, 76, 78*
Malnutrition, bedsores and, 92
Massage. *See also* Back rub; Body rub
  for bedsores, 91, 116
  light, 116
  with portable shower heads, 154
  shower baths as, 150
Matey Bantam holder, 100, *100*
Mats, safety tub, 147–48
Mattress cover, 43. *See also* Bedding
  installing, 80
Mattresses, 42–43
  bedsores and, 94
  polyfoam or foam, 42, 43
  turning, 43
Mattress pads, 43. *See also* Bedding
  installing, 73–74, *73*, 80
Measuring cups, pitchers, and spoons, 43
Measuring medicines, 61
Mechanical lifts, 81–82, 87–88, *88, 89*
Mechanically soft diet, 225–26
Medicaid, 18
Medical records, 10–11, 16
Medicare, 18
Medicinal retention enemas, 170
Medicines. *See also* Pain pills; Sleeping pills
  do's and don't's, 61
  patent, 60
  prescription, 59–60
Metabolic disturbances, lack of exercise and, 190
Metabolism, 200
  basal, 198
Microbes, 62
Microorganisms, 62–66. *See also* Transmission of disease
  portal of entry of, 63
  preventing spread of disease-producing, 65
  transmitting agents (vectors) of, 64–65
  virulence of, 63–64
Mouthwash, 57
Moving a patient, 79–89
  in bed, 85–86, 94
  bedsores and, 94
  between bed and chair, 87
  body mechanics and, 81–84
  carrying a patient, 83–84
  help from patient, 84–85, *84*, 87
  in and out of bed, 302
  lifting a patient, 81–84
  mechanical lifts for, 87–88, *88, 89*
  for remaking a bed, 79–81, *80*
  shower bath patients, 151–52
  sliding board for, 45, *45*, 87
  tub bath patients, 153
Muscular atrophy, 189–90
Music. *See also* Stereo system
  as sleeping aid, 184

Nails
  ingrown, 112

trimming, 143
washing, 143
Newspapers, 102
Nightingale, 41
Noise, 4–5, 185
NREM sleep, 181
Numbness in the extremities, reporting to doctor, 14
Nurse's gown, 70
Nutrition, 197–206
Nutritional retention enema, 170

Oil retention enemas, 168–70
Ointments for bedsores, 95
Oral temperature, taking, 126
Ortho canes, 35, *35*, 36, *36*
Ortho forearm crutches, 38, *39*
Osteoporosis, lack of exercise and, 190
Overexertion, protecting patient from, 297–98
Oxygen, 201

Padding. *See also* Cushions
bed, 23, *25*, 25–27, 94
for foot support boards, 110
for vaginal douches, 178
Pads
mattress. *See* Mattress pads
water, 51, 94
Page turner, 100, *100*
Pain, 195–96, 315–18
Pain medication, 195–96
bedsores and, 92
Paper facial tissue, 57–58
Paper towels, 58
for enemas, 164
Paralyzed arm, 194
Patent medicines, 60
Pathogenicity, 64
Patients
family life and, 327–30
giving your nurse a hand, 320–22
instructions from doctor, dietitian, or therapist, 311
overdoing by, 313
status of, 313–14
suffering in silence by, 315–18
thanking hospital personnel, 312
Pen or pencil holders, 99, *99*
Peri bottle, 172, *172*
Perineal areas
sitz baths for, 159–61, *160*
washing, in bed, 157
Perineal/rectal area, 171
irrigations of, 173–76
Peristalsis, 201
Perspiration
bedsores and, 93
pillowcases and pillow tickings and, 44
Petroleum jelly, 59
Pillowcases, 44. *See also* Bedding
installing, 79
Pillows, 44
bed wedge, 23, 29, *29*
encasing, 79
for foot rotation prevention, 112
plumping up, 44, 79
Pillow tickings, 44
Pitcher, 37
measuring, 43
Planning the care of your patient, 296–304
nursing care, 299–304
protection, 296–99
Plumping up pillows, 44, 79
Pneumonia, hypostatic, 191
Portal of entry of microorganisms, 63
Posey foot guard, 108, *108*, 109, 111
Posey ventilated heel protector, 104, *104*
Position, change of
in chair, 303
preventing disuse disabilities and, 191, 192
Prescription medicine, 59–60
Pressure sores. *See* Bedsores
Prognosis, 9–10
Psychological deterioration, 191
Public Health Department, 9
Pulling a patient, 83, 85
Pulse (pulse rate)
abnormal, 129–30
normal, 129
power and rhythm of, 130, 131
recording, 131
taking, 130
temperature and, 117–18
Pulse pressure, 137
Pushing a patient, 83–85

Quad canes, 36, *36*
Q-Tips, 58
Quilts, 44. *See also* Bedding

Radio, 102, 303
Rashes, reporting to doctor, 14
Reaching aids, 100–1, *100*
Reading aids, 100, *100*
Record players, 102, 303
Records, keeping detailed, 10–11, 16
Rectal/perineal area, 171
irrigations of, 173–76
Rectal temperature, 125–27, *127*
Registered nurses, 18–19
Relative and in-laws, visits from, 305
Relaxation, 180, 186–88
REM sleep, 181
Respiration
altitude and, 133
body temperature and, 133
rates of, 132–33
taking and recording, 134–35

temperature and, 117–18
types of, 132–34
Rest, 180, 184–85
Restlessness, reporting to doctor, 11–12
Retention enemas, 168–70
lubricating, 168–70
medicinal, 170
nutritional, 170
Ring cushions, 39, *39*
Rinse/shampoo tray, 27, *27*
Room cleaning, 301. *See also* House cleaning
making the bed and, 71
Room deodorant or freshener, 55
Room temperature, making the bed and, 71
Routine, 294–96
Rubbing, bedsores from excessive, 93
Rubbing alcohol, 56, 58

Safety strips for stall shower or bathtubs, *147*, 147–48
Saline/salt enema, 167
Sandbags for foot rotation protection, 111
Scales, 45
Schedules, 294–95
"Scotch" irrigation, 171
Scratches. *See* Cuts and scratches
Seat cushions (or pads), 38–39, *39*
Seats
bath, *148*, 148–49
toilet, 46
Sensitivity to irritants, 55
Sewage, 65
Shampoo, 58
dry, 27, 158, 159
Shampooing, 146, 157–59
Shampoo trays, 27, *27*
Shavers, electric, 45
Shaving, 146
Shaving equipment, 45
Sheepskin bed padding, *25*, 25–26, 94
Sheepskin heel cups, 104–7, *105*
Sheets, 27–28, 72. *See also* Bedding; Bottom sheet; Making the bed; Top sheet
changing, 28
draw. *See* Draw sheets
electric, 28
flat and fitted, 28, 74, 76
folding, 72
installing, 80
waterproof. *See* Waterproof sheets
Shower baths, 145, 147–52. *See also* Baths
bandages or casts and, 147
bath seats for, *148*, 148–49
for very debilitated persons, 150
drying patient after, 152
duration of, 150
giving, 150–52
guardrails and grabrails for, 149–50, *149*
pressure of water for, 150
safety strips and mats for, *147*, 147–48
temperature of water for, 150
Shower heads, portable, 154, *154*
Sickroom equipment, 20–55. *See also specific equipment*
sources of, 21
Sigh, 134
Sightless patients, feeding, 283–84
Sitz baths, 159–61, *160*
Sleep, 180–184
amount of, 181–82
NREM, 181
preparation for getting a patient to, 183–84
REM, 181
Sleep patterns, 182–83
Sleeping pills, 183
Sliding board, 45, *45*, 87
Slippers for toe protection, 108
Smiling, 319–20
Sneezing, transmission of disease by, 67
Soaking, feet, 103
Soap, 58, 142
Soap dish, 45
Soap enemas, 161–67, *165*
amount of, 162
equipment for, 162–64, *163*
giving, 164–66, *165*
high, 166
for infants and children, 162, 163, *163*, 166–67
proportions of soap and water for, 162
temperature of, 162
Sound, 4–5, 185
Speech, reporting to doctor slurred or difficulty in, 14
Sphygmomanometers, 45, 138–42, *139, 141*
aneroid, 138–40, *139*
electronic, *139*, 140
mercurial, 138–39, *139*
repair and testing of, 140
Sponge baths, 145, 154–55
Sponges, 142
Stair-climber walkers, 49–50, *50*
Stall shower. *See* Shower baths
Staphylococci, 63
Stereo system, 102
Stertorous breathing, 134
Stethoscope, 46, *139*
for taking blood pressure, 139–41
Stool, bath and shower, *148*, 149
Straws, drinking, 40
Streptococci, 63
Stridulous breathing, 134
Stroke patients
exercises for, 193–94
feeding, 282–83
Suffering in silence, 315–18
Sunshine for bedsores, 95
Surgical gloves, 41
Suspicions, patient's, 4

Swabs, cotton, 57, 58. *See also* Q-Tips
Swallowing, reporting to doctor difficulty in, 14
Swelling, reporting to doctor, 14
Systolic blood pressure, 136–37

Tables, bedside, 33, *33*
Talcum, 56
Tape players, 102, 303
Teeth, brushing, 57
Telephone, 96, 303
Television, 102, 303
Temperature. *See also* Body temperature
  of bath water, 145–46, 150, 160–61
  of room, 71
Thermometers, 46
  cleaning, 123
  electronic (automatic), 124–25
  markings on, 123
  mechanical (or glass), 122–23, *122*
  reading, 123
  shaking down, 123
  testing, 125
Thinness, bedsores and, 92
Thoracic breathing, 134
Tingling in the extremities, reporting to doctor, 14
Tips for canes and crutches, 36
Toe comfort board, 108
Toenails, care of, 112, *112*
Toes. *See also* Feet
  bedsore preventive devices, 108, *108*
  bedsores on, 94, 103–4
  exercises for, 112
Toilet
  assisting patient in, 303–4
  irrigating on a, 173–75
  portable. *See* Commode
  vaginal douches on a, 178–79
Toilet paper, 59
  for enemas, 164
Toilet safety frame, *46*, 47
Toilet seats, 46
Toothbrush, 47
  holders for, 98–99, *98*
Toothpaste and powder (dentifrice), 57, 59
Top sheet, 72. *See also* Sheets
  fitted, 76
  installing, 76–77, 80
Towels, 47, 142
  for enemas, 164
  for irrigations, 173
  transmission of disease and, 65, 69
  for vaginal douches, 178
Transfer board, 45, *45*
Transmission of disease, 66–70. *See also* Microorganisms
  airborne, 67
  by bite, 69
  by contaminated objects, 68
  by direct contact, 67–68
  fecal-and-oral, 69
Trapeze bars, *47*, 47–48, 101
  exercise with, 194–95
Tub baths, 145, 152
  bandages or casts and, 147
  for very debilitated persons, 153
  depth of water for, 153
  getting patient in and out of bathtub, 153
  giving, 154
Tub mat, safety, 147–48
Tumblers, 40

Ulcers, bed padding for prevention of, 23, 26
Unguents, 59
Unipod canes, 35, *35*
Urinals, *48*, 48–49, 303
Urinary tract infections, lack of exercise and, 190
Urination. *See also* Incontinence
  washing after, 142
Urine, measuring and recording, 290, 292–94
Utensils, washing, 65

Vacuum cleaning, 65
  mattresses, 42
  pillows, 44
Vaginal douche, 170, 176–80, *179*
  in a bathtub or bed, *179*, 179–80
  on a bidet, 179
  equipment for, 177–78
  flow of, 177
  giving, 178–79
  pressure for, 177
  solutions for, 177
  temperature of, 177
  on a toilet, 178–79
Vaseline, 59
Vectors, 64–65
Virulence of microorganisms, 63–64
Viruses, 62. *See also* Microorganisms
Visiting hours, 304
Visiting Nurse Service, 9, 18–21
Visiting with your patient, 296
Visitors, 304–7
  describing your patient's condition to, 306
  gifts from, 306
  length of visits, 306–7
  permission from patient for admitting, 305
  protecting patient against long-staying, 298, 304, 306
Vomit
  emesis basin for, 40–41, *41*
  reporting to doctor, 15

Walkanes, 36, *37*
Walkers, 49–50, *50*, 297
Washcloths, 50, 142
Washing. *See also* Baths
  face, 142–43
  feet, 103

feet, in bed, 156–57, *156*
hands, 65, 69, 142–43
nails, 143
to prevent spread of disease, 65, 68, 69
thermometers, 123
utensils, 65
Wastebag, 51, *51*
Wastebasket, 51, 304
Waste output, measuring and recording, 290, 292–94
Water, drinking, 37
in clear liquid diet, 220
Water beds or mattresses, 51, 94
Water pads (flotation pads), 51, 94
Water pitcher, 37
Water pressure for shower baths, 150
Waterproof sheets, 52, *52*
draw sheets and, 40
for enemas, 164
installing, 76, 80
for irrigations, 173
for vaginal douches, 178
Wedge pillows, bed, 23, 29, *29*
Wheelchairs, 52–55, *53, 54*
Eggcrate® padding for, 26
Wheel-mounted chair, *54*, 55
Wheeze, 134
Whispering, 5
Working full-time, 296
Worries, pain and, 196. *See also* Anxiety
Writing aids, 99, *99*
Written instructions, 10

Foods and Feeding Your Patient Index

Page numbers in italics refer to illustrations

Absorption, 197
Acid, 197
Alcoholic beverages, 202, 246
Alkali, 197
Amino acids, 197–98
Anabolism, 200
Animal fats, 199, 203
Apricot milk drink, 217
Aroma of food, 208–9

Banana milk drink, 218
Banana orange shake, 218
Basal metabolism, 198
Beverages. *See also specific beverages and diets*
alcoholic, 202, 246
between-meal, in general diet, 217–19
for low-cholesterol diet, 246
as sleeping aids, 183
Bland diet, 227
Breads, 202, 205. *See also specific diets*
in general diet, 213
for low-cholesterol diet, 246
in sodium-restricted diets, 263, 266
Breakfast, washing patient before, 142
Broth, in clear liquid diet, 220
Buttermilk-herb dressing, 252

Cakes. *See also specific diets*
for low-cholesterol diet, 246
Calcium, foods containing, 203
Calcium diets, 267
Calories, 198
Carbohydrates, 198. *See also* Cellulose; Starches; Sugars
foods that contain, 202–3
Carbonated beverages, in clear liquid diet, 220
Catabolism, 200, 201
Cellulose, 198–99
Cereals, 205. *See also other specific diets*
in full liquid diet, 221
in general diet, 213
in low-cholesterol diet, 246
in sodium-restricted diet, 263, 266
Children, feeding, 283, 284, 286
Cholesterol, 199, 245. *See also* Low-cholesterol diet
Clear liquid diet, 220–22

Coffee
in clear liquid diet, 220
as sleep aid, 183
Color of food, 207–8
Cookies. *See also specific diets*
for low-cholesterol diet, 246
Cooking. *See also* Meals, preparing and serving
meat, to reduce fat content, 249
vegetables, 210
Crumb crust for pie, 251

Dairy products, 199, 203–5
in general diet, 213
in low-cholesterol diet, 249
in sodium-restricted diets, 260–61, 265
Desserts. *See also* Cakes; Cookies; Pastries; *and other specific diets*
in low-cholesterol diet, 246
Dextrose. *See* Glucose
Diabetic diets, 268–78
menus for, 277–78
Diabetic food exchanges, 269–76
Diets, 205–80
balanced, 213
bland, 227
calcium, 267
choosing foods for, 206–12, 323
definition of, 199
diabetic, 268–78
general, 212–19
high-calorie, 231–33
high-protein, 238–42
liquid, 219–22
low-calorie, 233–38
low-cholesterol, 245–59
low-fat, 242–45
low-gluten, 267–68
low-residue, 228–30
low-sodium, 259–66
mechanically soft, 225–26
naturally soft or light, 222–25
phosphorous, 268
potassium, 268
tube-feeding, 278–80
ulcer, 227
Diet specialties in low-cholesterol diet, 247
Digestion, 199

Eating. *See* Diets; Foods; Meals; Nutrition
Eating aids, 96–99, *97, 98*
Elderly patients, feeding, 283
Eye appeal of foods, 207–8

Fat(s), 242. *See also* Low-fat diet; *and other specific diets*
foods with a high content of, 203
functions of, 199
in low-cholesterol diet, 247
monounsaturated, 200
polyunsaturated, 200
saturated, 200
sources of, 199–200
Fatty acids, 200
Feeding your patient, 280–86, 303, 322–25. *See also* Meals
handicapped patients, 280–84
intravenous, 200
sightless patients, 283–84
unwilling eaters, 284–86
Fish
in low-cholesterol diet, 247
in sodium-restricted diets, 261, 265
Flavorings. *See also* Seasonings
in low-cholesterol diet, 248
Food blender, 41, 226
Food coloring, artificial, 207
Food groups, basic, 204–5
in general diet, 213
Food intake, measuring and recording, 290–94
Foods. *See also* Diets; Feeding your patient; Meals; Nutrition
amount of, 324
attractive amounts of, 208
choosing, for diets, 206–12, 323
consistency of, 209–10
as disease-transmitting agents, 64
eye appeal of, 207–8
mouth appeal of, 209–11
nose appeal (aroma) of, 208–9
personal likes and dislikes of, 211–12
taste of, 210
temperature of, 210–12
trying new, 323–24
Foods, "maybe" allowed
in low-calorie diets, 235
in low-fat diets, 243
Foods, unlimited amounts or "free"
in diabetic diets, 275
in low-residue diets, 235
Foods, usually allowed
in high-calorie diets, 231
in low-calorie diets, 234, 235
in low-cholesterol diets, 246–55
in low-fat diets, 242
in low-residue diets, 228
in low-sodium diets, 260, 262–64, 265
in naturally soft or light diets, 223
Foods, usually avoided
in diabetic diets, 276
in low-calorie diets, 236
in low-residue diets, 229
in low-sodium diets, 261, 264, 265
in naturally soft or light diets, 224
Food substances, classes of, 202–5
Fruits, 205. *See also other specific diets*
in general diet, 213

in low-cholesterol diet, 248
in sodium-restricted diets, 262, 265
Full liquid diet, 221, 222

General diet, 212–19
Glucose, 200
Gluten, 267–68
Gravies, 249

Handicap eating aids, 96–99, *97, 98*
Handicapped patients, feeding, 280–86
Hemoglobin, 200
Herbs in low-cholesterol diet, 254
Herb sauce, 254
High-calorie diet, 231–33
High-protein diet, 238–42
Hormones, 199, 200
Hydrogenate, 199

Ingestion, 200
Inorganic, definition of, 200
Iodine, foods containing, 203
Iron, foods containing, 203

Jam in low-cholesterol diet, 248
Jelly in low-cholesterol diet, 248
Juice (juice drinks)
in clear liquid diet, 220
in low-cholesterol diet, 248

Kidney stones, lack of exercise and, 190
Kilocalorie, 198
Knives, for handicapped patients, 97, *97*

Light diet, 222–25
Liquid diets, 219–22
Low-calorie diets, 233–38
Low-cholesterol diet, 245–59
foods in, 246–55
recipes for, 250–54
sample 7-day menu for, 255–59
Low-fat diet, 242–45
Low-gluten diets, 267–68
Low-residue diet, 228–30
Low-sodium diets, 259–66

Margarine in low-cholesterol diet, 248
Mayonnaise, mock or imitation, 252
Meals, 303, 322–25
with the family, 302
getting ready for, 324–25
preparing and serving, 286–89, 324
washing before, 142
scheduling, 295
Meals-On-Wheels service, 296
Meat (meat group), 205. *See also other specific diets*
in general diet, 213
in low-cholesterol diet, 248–49
in sodium-restricted diets, 261, 265
Melon in low-cholesterol diet, 248
Menus. *See specific diets*
Metabolism, 200
basal, 198
Milk and milk products. *See* Dairy products
Minerals, 201. *See also specific minerals*
foods with a high content of, 203
trace, 202
Monounsaturated fats, 200

Naturally soft or light diet, 222–25
Niacin, foods containing, 204
Nutrient, definition of, 201
Nutrition, 197–206. *See also* Diets; Foods; Meals; *entries starting with* Food; *and specific topics*
definitions and descriptions of materials and actions involved in, 197–202
Nuts in low-cholesterol diet, 249

Odors of foods, 208–9
Oils
in low-cholesterol diet, 250
plant, 199, 203
Orange chiller, 218
Organic, definition of, 201
Overeating, 214
Oxygen, 201

Pancakes
in low-cholesterol diet, 250
wheat germ, 250
Pantothenic acid, foods containing, 204
Pastries in low-cholesterol diet, 251
Peach cooler, 218
Peanut butter in low-cholesterol diet, 251
Peristalsis, 201
Phosphorous diets, 268
Phosphorus, foods containing, 203
Pies
crumb crust for, 251
in low-cholesterol diet, 251
Pineapple-lemon shake, 219
Plant oils, 199, 203
Plate, inner-lip, *97*, 98
Polyunsaturated fats, 200, 203
Potassium, foods containing, 204
Potassium diets, 268
Poultry
in low-cholesterol diet, 251
in sodium-restricted diets, 261, 265
Protein, 201, 238. *See also* Amino acids; High-protein diet
complete, 203
foods with a high content of, 203
incomplete, 203

Relishes in low-cholesterol diet, 251
Roughage, 201

Salad dressings in low-cholesterol diet, 251–53
Salts, 201
Saturated fats, 200, 203
Sauces in low-cholesterol diet, 253–54
Scales, 45
Seasonings, 209, 210
  in low-cholesterol diet, 254
Shortening in low-cholesterol diet, 250
Sightless patients, feeding, 283–84
Snacks
  in low-cholesterol diet, 254
  as sleeping aids, 183
Sodium. *See also* Low-sodium diets
  foods containing, 204
Soft diet
  mechanically, 225–26
  naturally, 222–25
Sparer, 201–2
Spiced peach blossom, 219
Spoon holders, *97*, 98–99
Spoons
  for handicapped patients, 96–97, *97*
  measuring, 43
Spreads in low-cholesterol diet, 254
Starches, 202. *See also* Carbohydrates
Sugars, 202. *See also* Carbohydrates
Sweeteners in low-cholesterol diet, 254

Table service, 287–88
Tea in clear liquid diet, 220
Thickeners in low-cholesterol diet, 254
Trace minerals, 202
Tube-feeding diets, 278–80

Ulcer diet, 227
Urine, measuring and recording, 290, 292–94
Utensil hand clip, *97*, 98
Utensil holders, homemade, *98*, 98–99
Utensils for handicapped patients, 96–97, *97*

Vegetables, 205
  cooking and seasoning, 210
  in general diet, 213
  in low-cholesterol diet, 254–55
  in sodium-restricted diets, 262, 266
Vitamin A, foods containing, 204
Vitamin B_1 (thiamin), foods containing, 204
Vitamin B_2 (riboflavin), foods containing, 204
Vitamin B_6 (pyridoxine), foods containing, 204
Vitamin C, foods containing, 204, 205
Vitamin D, foods containing, 204
Vitamin E, foods containing, 204
Vitamin K, foods containing, 204
Vitamins
  fat-soluble, 202
  foods containing, 204, 205
  functions of, 202
  water-soluble, 202

Waffles in low-cholesterol diet, 250
Waste output, measuring and recording, 290, 292–94
Water, drinking, 202, 204, 304
  in clear liquid diet, 220
Wheat germ pancakes, 250

Yogurt dressing, 253